FOOD FOR THOUGHT

CHANGING HOW WE FEEL BY CHANGING HOW WE EAT

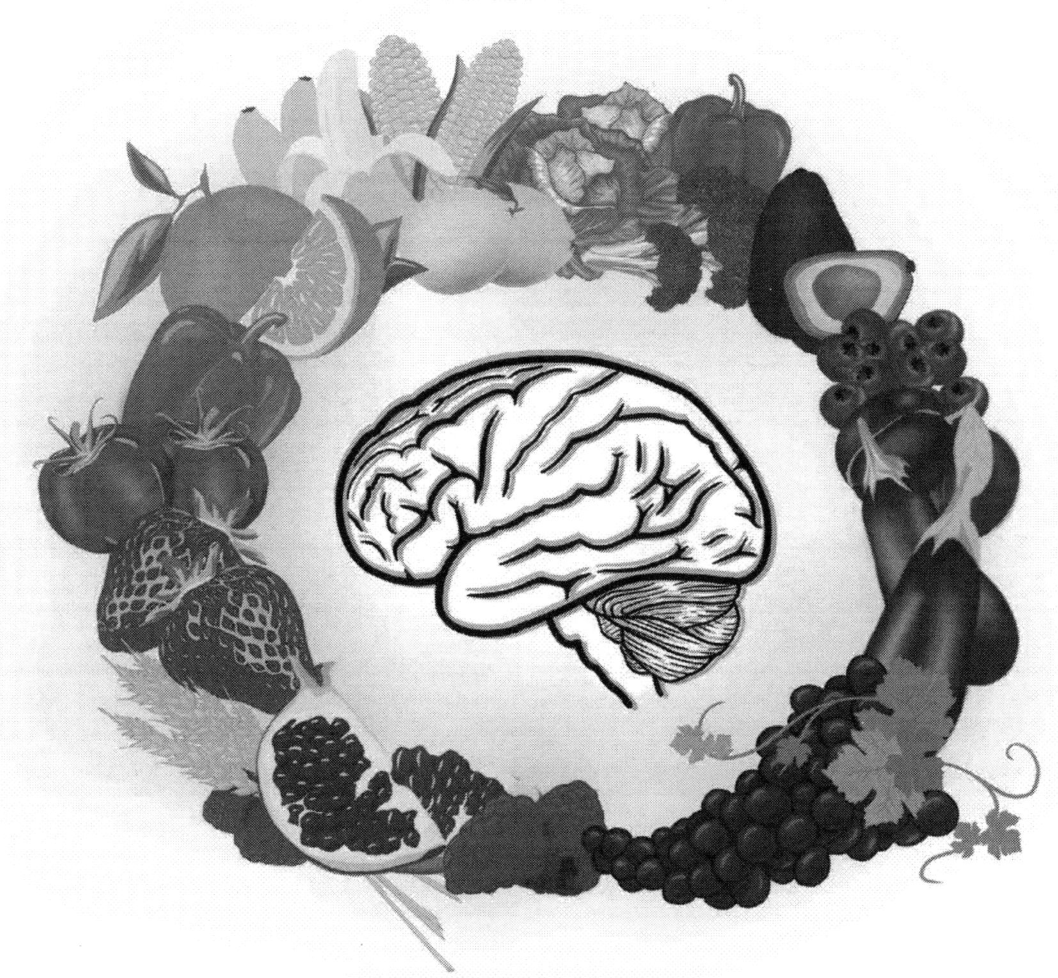

LISA E. GOEHLER, PhD.

Library of Congress Cataloging-in-Publication Data

Food for Thought: Changing How We Feel By Changing How We Eat, First Edition

ISBN: 978-0-9832465-7-2

Author: Lisa E. Goehler, Ph.D.
Editors: Jodie A. Trafton, Ph.D. and Joan M. Zimmerman, M.S.
Illustrator: Mara Gaykema

Copyright © 2023 by Institute for Disease Management, a division of Institute for Brain Potential (IBP).

Institute for Brain Potential (IBP) is a non-profit organization dedicated to presenting advances in the brain and behavioral sciences through publications, live conferences and online and recorded presentations. IBP is a 501 (c) 3 organization, tax identification number 77-0026830 was founded in 1984. Since its inception, IBP has taught over three million health professionals. IBP is the leading provider of accredited continuing education programs focusing on the brain and behavioral sciences.

Printed in the United States of America

Table of Contents

Earn up to 16 hours of continuing education by completing all or sections of Food for Thought: Changing How We Feel by Changing How We Eat (2023).

Lisa Goehler, Ph.D., (University of Virginia) is an acclaimed neuroscientist, educator, and inspired author. Food for Thought is unique in its coverage of stress, inflammation, nutrients, the gut-brain connection, and the way in which selected nutrients change how we feel and think.

The home study program can be taken in consecutive sections or in its entirety.   Key points are included at the end of each chapter and ingeniously simplifying cartoons can enable health professionals to develop a practical understanding for making health-related decisions.

Chapters 1-5: The Stress Connection: 3 CE Credits
- Describe how stress can undermine conscientious eating
- Learn how to reinterpret stressors as challenges
- Summarize how emotions can affect impulse control
- Identify pathways to manage emotional eating
- Discuss the body's language of eating and stress-related symptoms

Chapters 6-9: The Inflammation Connection: 3 CE Credits
- Discuss the interactions between shame, self-blame, inflammation, and weight gain
- Distinguish between healthy and harmful forms of inflammation
- State how inflammation can alter the way we think, feel, and eat
- Discuss how lifestyle can reduce age-related inflammation

Chapters 10-13: What is in Our Food: Sugar, Fats, and Antioxidants: 3 CE Credits
- List types of antioxidants and their common sources
- Explain how antioxidants can protect against oxidative stress
- Distinguish between harmful and healthful fats
- Identify sugars and white foods that increase inflammation and craving

Chapters 14-18: The Gut-Brain Connection: 4 CE Credits
- List several ways stress, inflammation, and the Western Diet can affect brain health
- Explain what is meant by the gut-barrier connection
- List ways that toxins, microbes, and stress can undermine gut health
- Discuss ways that probiotics can improve microbial balance
- Distinguish between harmful and healthful foods to improve the gut-brain connection

Chapters 19-21: Changing How We Feel and Think by Changing What We Eat: 3 CE Credits
- Name several psychological effects of inflammation
- Describe how sleep affects the immune system and eating habits
- Discuss practical guidelines for promoting gut-brain health
- Summarize key findings regarding how what we eat alters how we feel

Chapter 22 (not offered for CE credit) includes a neuroscience-informed set of diet practices and recipes. Learn more about this engaging text and home study program by emailing foodforthought@IBPceu.com

PROLOGUE: SCOPE OF THIS BOOK

To change how we feel by changing how we eat, it helps to understand what food means and how it affects the brain and body.

In this book, we will weave together the threads of stress, inflammation, gut health, and food to present an integrated in-depth picture of how choices that we make about food, and other aspects of lifestyle, affect our minds and bodies. The overall objective is to provide readers with enough evidence-based information to enable them to make and carry out informed choices about what they eat.

The goal of the text is to enable you to:

- Distinguish between health-enhancing and unhealthy foods
- Identify how stress encourages unhealthy food consumption and how to modify responses to stress
- Describe the links between food, psychological well-being, and the gut-brain axis
- Explain the importance of food choices in preventing and managing mood disorders and chronic medical conditions.
- Apply practical knowledge to optimize your diet and gut health, reduce stress and inflammation, and experience better well-being

Overall, the purpose of this book is to provide motivation and knowledge for anyone wishing to change their diet or for anyone wishing to help a client or loved one to improve their diet.

Chapter 1 introduces the complex interplay between the food we eat, our experience of the world, and health.

In chapters 2 through 4, we will begin by addressing stress. We will explore what stress is and when and how the brain responds to stress. This will allow us to understand how stress affects our food choices, and how stress can be effectively managed.

In chapter 5, we will learn about how we sense and respond to the internal state of our bodies. This sense is referred to as interoception and is central not only to sensing our internal environment, but also for shaping interactions between our diet and metabolism, the microbes that live in our gut, our immune system, and our brain and behavior.

In chapter 6, we explore the interplay between obesity and well-being, diet, inflammation, and social stress.

In chapters 7 through 9, we study inflammation. Because inflammation is the mechanistic link between diet and health, we will discuss what inflammation is, what it does to the body, and how different kinds of foods can either increase or decrease inflammation.

In chapters 10 and 11, we will learn about oxidation. We will learn how oxidation is innately tied to metabolism, and how it is both a crucial tool used to protect as well as a dangerous threat to our physiological well-being. Nature has developed elegant antioxidant systems to manage oxidation and protect cells from damage due to oxidation. We will explore these antioxidant systems and how diet may contribute to their availability and effectiveness.

In chapters 12 and 13, we will delve into fats and sugars. While fats and carbohydrates are crucial for nutrition, how they are consumed can have substantial impact on health and well-being. Here we learn about how differences in the form and processing of fats and sugars, both in the preparation of food and its metabolism, can influence health and behavior.

In chapter 14, we learn how dietary choices and stress can combine to produce metabolic disorders, including inflammation, diabetes, mood disorders, and even eventually dementia. We'll explore diet strategies to prevent the development and reverse the effects of metabolic disorders.

In chapters 15 through 18, we provide basic information about the gut and its microbes, as well as how to keep them healthy. The connections between the gut and the brain, via interoception, provide an important link between food, stress, mood, and decision-making.

In chapters 19 and 20, we explore how diet and inflammation interact with and influence emotional experience, particularly depression, anxiety, and pain. Next, we learn about interactions between sleep, diet, and metabolism, and ways of improving sleep.

Last, in chapter 21, we examine how food choices affect the health and function of our brains themselves. We learn how the high energy needs of the brain create special vulnerabilities, and consider findings on special diets designed to support brain health.

Throughout the book, these relationships will be discussed in the context of the emotional and cultural meanings of food. We will address the role of diet in specific medical conditions including obesity, metabolic diseases, gastrointestinal conditions, mental health, sleep, and chronic pain. We will discuss the relative merits of dietary strategies including exclusion diets, Mediterranean, and "keto" diets. In chapter 22, we provide easy-to-make recipes that include ingredients that have been shown to be associated with feeling well.

Why all the big words?

While this book does an occasional deep dive into complex biology, it is not necessary to understand or remember the details to learn the concepts and apply them to food choices. Understanding conceptual relationships between diet, physiology, behavior, and health will allow you to make and guide others towards better health behaviors, regardless of whether you can remember or even pronounce technical terms for actors in these relationships. Nevertheless, we have chosen to include technical language, even though it is not necessary to know or remember details about specific anatomy, brain circuits, and neurotransmitters. This technical language will enable those who want to explore underlying research more deeply to find and understand the academic literature in that area. Where understanding a complex process is key to understanding relationships between foods and health, we provide cartoons and/or analogies that we expect will enable understanding of the key concepts.

Because many specialty terms will be mentioned throughout the book, we have included a glossary in the back of the book. New terms will be defined at their first mention, and many will recur throughout chapters. We hope that the glossary will provide a quick refresher as needed.

Can changing your diet really change your life?

There are so many diet fads, drugs and supplements that claim to help lose weight, improve mood, and relieve pain. Unfortunately, any benefits tend to be temporary. Lifestyle changes require a commitment, but it can be easy to think that making such changes will not be worth it. But on the contrary, we have heard many stories from people we know or that we meet professionally who relate stories of how they suffered for years until they finally addressed their diet and their stress. Here is one story, in her own words:

"Since I was very young, I have been prone to strange chronic pain issues and inflammation. Always tested and prescribed, but never diagnosed with anything conclusively. Around age 18, I started to experience an escalation in my pain related symptoms. I was finding myself trapped in different scenarios where I could not physically get up from the floor because the pain was too intense. I was constantly in pain, barely sleeping, severely depressed, and too ill to continue my regular exercise routines. At this point I started to get extremely worried about my health. My blood panels and other tests came back mostly normal, and it was determined that I fit into the standard criteria for fibromyalgia. I felt a sense of relief to finally have answers, but I had no idea what that meant in terms of treatment.

After researching and talking to my mother about fibromyalgia, I was honestly a little bit skeptical that I could manage my symptoms simply with lifestyle and diet changes. Learning about inflammation and its primary causes, I realized that I had unknowingly been causing my flare ups by the choices I made on a daily basis. My stress levels were chronically high, my sleep habits were horrendous, and my eating habits were worse! Sugar, which happens to be the #1 trigger for fibro flare ups, was more than just a part of my usual diet. Lamenting over a pint of ice cream was my main method of coping with stress. I was astonished at how far away my diet was from what it needed to be. One thing I knew I had to do was forget my usual go-to meals. No more boxed pastas, no more processed meats, and most importantly, I needed to get my sweet-tooth under control. I started looking into what specific foods I could start using in meals that would help my symptoms, rather than exacerbate them. I focused on using colorful foods, fresh vegetables, wild rice and whole grains instead of white, and eating fresh fruit instead of sweet treats. Within two or three weeks I was already feeling more energetic and alert. I still had pain, but I wasn't finding myself on the floor wondering how long I would be there before the shooting pain jolting through my leg would cease.

After a year or so my stress levels were ever-growing, and because of this, I was starting to bail on my healthy habits and experiencing some of my old symptoms. I knew that red meat and sugar were two of the worst pro-inflammatory foods, but I ate them anyway. I started noticing a cycle of bad choices with food, feeling horrible, being stressed about it, and then in turn, making more bad choices with food. At this point I knew I had to start over. I needed to take my health back, otherwise I was going to wind up in a wheelchair or couch ridden before I was 30. I had to do something, so I took the plunge and went vegetarian. At first, I didn't know what to eat. I craved all the things I wasn't allowed to have and found it difficult to adjust to being vegetarian at social gatherings. It wasn't easy, but because it was such a major change, it helped me stick to the plan. I introduced various types of mushrooms, chickpeas, spinach, and kale into my diet; all anti-inflammatory sources of protein or iron. It didn't take long before the number of flare-ups I was experiencing started to dwindle, and my previously anemic blood work was improving. I could stand up through an entire double-shift at work, I could lift both my arms above my head, I could turn my head all the way to both sides, and I felt clear headed for the first time in years. In the years since I have managed to keep up my good habits, with fewer slip-ups. Today I am a much more active person, and even though I still experience the occasional flare up, they are far less debilitating. I have discovered so many delicious recipes that I don't even think about the stuff I used to crave.

Diet changes can have far-reaching health effects

I have heard many versions of this story, with diet changes having health benefits that go far beyond maintaining healthful weight and cardiovascular health. In this book, we will review science that helps to explain why and how diet changes can alter mood, cognition, pain, inflammation and immune response, cancer risk and health of all organ systems.

Although there are many challenges to making changes in the way we eat, it is absolutely worth doing. We will discuss the challenges and ways to deal with them in the following chapters, in hopes of enabling changes and fostering improved health and well-being.

CHAPTER 1: HOW CONSCIENTIOUS EATING CAN REDUCE STRESS AND INFLAMMATION

- INFORMATION OVERLOAD

- KNOWLEDGE IS POWER

- EATING IS EMOTIONAL

- THE LINK BETWEEN DIET, STRESS, AND DISEASE IS INFLAMMATION

- FOOD IS THE PROBLEM AND FOOD IS THE SOLUTION: CONSCIENTIOUS EATING

- THE GUT IS THE INTERFACE BETWEEN FOOD AND HEALTH

- BREAKING THE VICIOUS CYCLE

- KEY POINTS

"To do or not to do, that is the question:
Whether tis better in the body to suffer
The slings and arrows of exhaustion and fatigue,
Or to take action against a sea of listlessness
And by opposing act. To do—to get up.
No more sleep and to rest say: We end.
The somatic-ache and the thousand natural shocks of Getting out of Bed" *(Fully Sick, 2022)*

"Something was certainly wrong with this day! All animal nerves felt it. All human nerves felt it. All living things were irritable, restless, disturbed; sick without being sick; sad without being sad; annoyed without any apparent cause for annoyance!" *(Powys, 1932)*

How many people can relate to these feelings?

Fatigue, low mood, anxiety, and cognitive fuzziness are caused by many different factors, including social and societal adversity, as well as chronic illnesses that affect both the mind and body. The stress of these experiences can lead people to self-medicate by eating high energy, emotionally rewarding Western Diet foods. Unfortunately, such foods ultimately only worsen these symptoms.

Even though the links between diet and how we feel are well-documented, and good quality food is becoming more widely available, many people still choose highly processed, poor-quality foods, washed down with sugary drinks such as soda (Mialon 2017, National Center for Health Statistics 2018, Paula Neto 2017, Yu 2016, Morris 2016). These foods have been linked to depression and anxiety, as well as to the development of obesity, increased risk of diabetes, heart disease, chronic pain, and some forms of cancer. Indeed, worldwide, people eating a typical Western Diet too frequently suffer from preventable diseases, notably diabetes, obesity, and heart disease, that impair quality of life and overall health (Kim 2016, Paula Neto 2017, Willet 2019, Yu 2016). In the United States, between 67.8% (women) and 75% (men) of the population are overweight or obese. Since 2010, the percentage of "extreme obesity" has doubled in women to 8.7% (National Center for Health Statistics 2018). At the same time, the Western Diet's reliance on red meat and large-scale factory farming has led to widespread pollution of water and soil with animal waste and toxic pesticides and herbicides, with implications for human health and the health of the planet (Willet 2019).

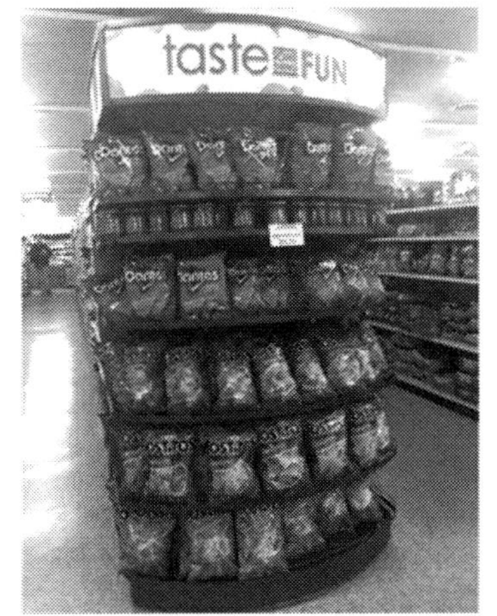

Why are such foods still so popular? To answer this question, we must address the many factors that contribute to eating behavior and food choice.

Information Overload

The internet allows anyone with access to a computer the ability to find a tremendous amount of information on nearly any kind of diet or health-related topic. Unfortunately, the quality of this information can be spotty, unreliable, or difficult to interpret. Sources range from easy-to-understand to only understandable by specialists, outdated to current, and inaccurate and intentionally misinforming scams to thoughtful and well-sourced papers (Mialon 2017, Azur 2017). Food and pharmaceutical companies use social media and other information outlets as marketing tools for products that may not be beneficial (Mialon 2017). These clever advertisements add to the confusion. Even among legitimate information sources, there are disagreements about recommendations on healthy diets. For instance, some sources treat saturated fats as undesirable, whereas other sources consider saturated fats to be healthy alternatives to unsaturated fats in certain circumstances. For anyone without a degree in food chemistry, it can be difficult to know which sources to believe.

Knowledge is Power

When people do not understand the mechanisms by which food influences health, they rely on habits when making food choices. Processed food has often been engineered to be highly valued by the reward-learning systems that regulate habits. Habit-driven choices tend to favor processed foods despite the longer-term harms they produce.

Most grocery stores have thousands of items to sell, including foods that are ready to eat. Many different fast-food restaurants tempt us with convenient and appetizing choices. Without information about the ways that such food compromises our bodies, these convenience foods can seem like a lifesaver to busy people who don't have the time or knowledge to cook good quality meals for themselves or their families.

On the other hand, understanding the basic ways in which diet supports the needs of the mind and body, and how what we eat affects the brain and immune system, can provide the motivation and confidence to make healthy choices about food.

Eating is Emotional

Food affects our lives in ways that go beyond simple nutrition. We may associate certain foods with comfort, such as chocolate desserts, chicken soup, or pasta with cheese. The types of food we find comforting can also be closely tied to the cultures that we grew up in (Tryon 2013, Viladrich 2016). Providing food for others is nurturing and eating meals with other people helps strengthen social bonds (Higgs 2016). Social bonds give us meaning in life and can help provide resilience against stress (Charuvastra 2008).

Indeed, probably the most insidious driver of poor eating behaviors is stress. If we are feeling stressed, we are more likely to choose sugary and fatty foods (Beebe 2013, Greer 2013). Some hormones released when we are stressed can increase appetite and encourage us to overeat (Chao 2017, Tryon 2013). Unfortunately, eating a poor diet when stressed exacerbates health problems, and paradoxically, leads to more stress.

How?

The Link Between Diet, Stress and Disease is Inflammation

Poorly regulated inflammation causes or contributes to chronic disease (Hernandez-Limas 2018, Ji 2016). Many studies are now showing that certain kind of foods can cause or increase inflammation by several different mechanisms (DiNicolantonio 2018, Paula-Nieto 2017). Poor-quality, processed food of low nutritional value increases inflammation (Paula-Nieto 2017). This increased inflammation exerts deleterious effects on body and mind and can drive chronic pain and mood disorders (Dantzer 2008, Franklin 2008, Iwata 2016). Pain and depression are stressful experiences, which increase inflammation, leading to a self-sustaining vicious cycle (Iwata 2016). How can we break this cycle?

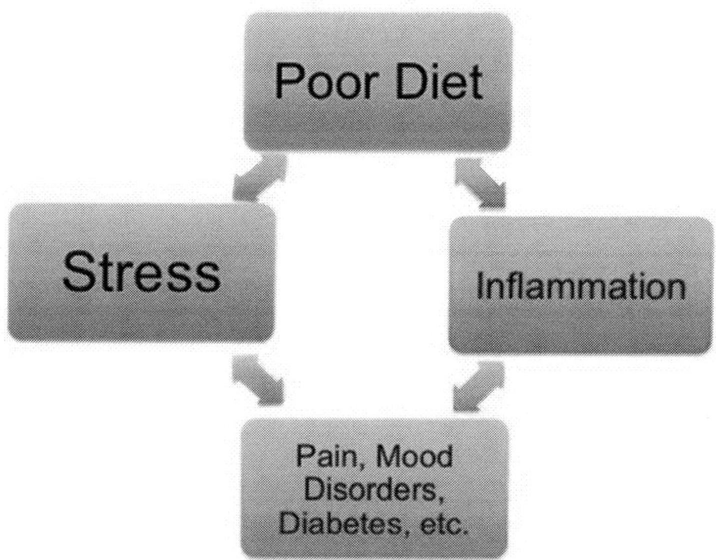

The Vicious cycle of Diet, Inflammation, and Stress

"Food is the Problem and Food is the Solution" (Finlay 2013): Conscientious Eating

How we feel, our well-being or *quality of life*, is a reflection of our current mood states, energy levels, and the kinds of challenges that we face. We face many types of challenges that may involve physical, mental, emotional, or health-related components. What and how we eat profoundly affects our quality of life, but accepting this idea and actually making dietary changes that will improve the way we feel can be much harder. The answer is that we really need to THINK about our diets and the way they affect our minds and bodies. This is where *conscientious eating* comes in.

Conscientious eating involves being purposefully aware of what we eat, how we eat it, and why we eat it. This means thinking about the quality of the nutrition in the foods that we eat, reading labels, and preparing food in ways that retain nutrients of the food. It means having a strategy guiding food choice that is informed by the source of the food (e.g., local farmers vs. large factory farms), the environmental and ethical impacts of things like the way food is grown/raised, the possible effects on our bodies, and transportation across continents or seas. It means knowing the specific ways that certain foods and cooking styles can increase or decrease inflammation. If we want to change the way we feel, we need to think about the way food affects our bodies.

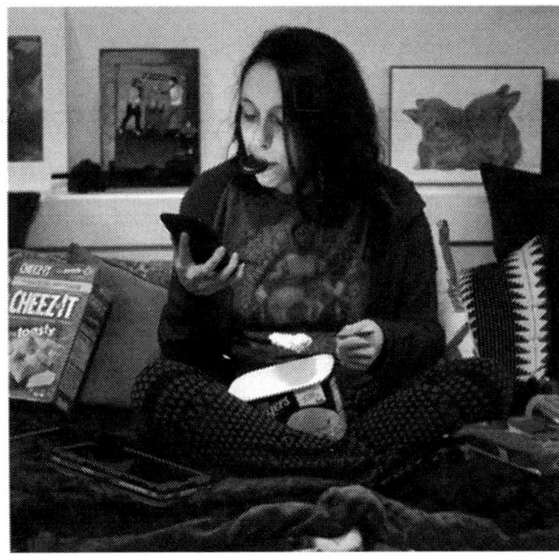

Do we eat convenience food alone while focusing on other things, or do we sit down with family or friends to eat home-cooked food made with fresh ingredients? The context in which we eat influences the kind of food choices we make. If we are mindlessly shoveling food down our throats, then we aren't paying attention to the quality of the food, and it is easier to fall into habits of eating junk food or processed food. These types of foods make stress, pain, and mood disorders worse. Thinking about why we are making certain food choices, especially when under stress, is critical to selecting those foods that can help decrease inflammation and reinforce a healthy mind and body. Conscientious eating can help us change the way we eat, and therefore change the way we feel.

The Gut is the Interface between Food and Health

The first place that food arrives after we eat it is the gut, where it is broken down and absorbed into the body. Because ingested food may also contain potentially dangerous things (e.g., toxins, pathogens, etc.,) the gut must decide what is nutritious and should be absorbed, and what is dangerous and should be attacked. For this reason, the immune system maintains a formidable presence in the gut. Indeed, the gut has been called the largest immune organ in the body. The gut plays a pivotal role in immune *homeostasis*, the maintenance of optimum immune functioning (Bingula 2017, Takiishi 2017).

The gut is also home to most of our commensal microbes: those bacteria, viruses, and fungi that not only peacefully co-exist with us, but also provide critical nutrients for cells of the gut. They also collaborate with our immune systems to prevent troublesome microbes from overgrowing and causing inflammation or other symptoms such as gas or bloating (Takiishi 2017).

What happens in the gut does not stay in the gut. Inflammation in the gut can cause malnutrition, as well as inflammation in other organs of the body (Takiishi 2017). In a process called immune programming, young immune cells become either pro-inflammatory or anti-inflammatory depending on interaction with microbes and other immune cells in the gut. Some of these cells can leave the gut and migrate into the blood or other tissues such as lung and release pro-inflammatory mediators that contribute to inflammation (Bingula 2017). In this way, the health of the gut can influence the health of other organs. So, if the gut is exposed to food containing things that it may consider dangerous, such as toxins or additives, the consequent gut inflammation and pro-inflammatory immune programming has serious implications for other parts of the body. Not only that, but the gut has a special link with the brain. Gut health can have marked effects on brain function and mental health (Dantzer 2008, Galland 2014). Thus, eating conscientiously, by choosing foods that keep the gut healthy, can help regulate inflammation in the rest of the body and help break the vicious cycle.

Is diet really the best part of the cycle to intervene?

Breaking the vicious cycle is challenging because the interactions of emotional and cognitive factors with signals from the body are complex and bi-directional. Signals from the gut can be hard to perceive and emotional factors can seem overwhelming.

In fact, making changes in what we eat can be the easiest first step. Once you make the decision to take back your health, you can begin the process of choosing foods that can help regulate inflammation and improve mood, pain, and cognition. What you will learn in this book will be specific, evidence-based information about how inflammation and stress interact with the brain, and the foods and diet patterns that have been shown to support a healthy mind and body.

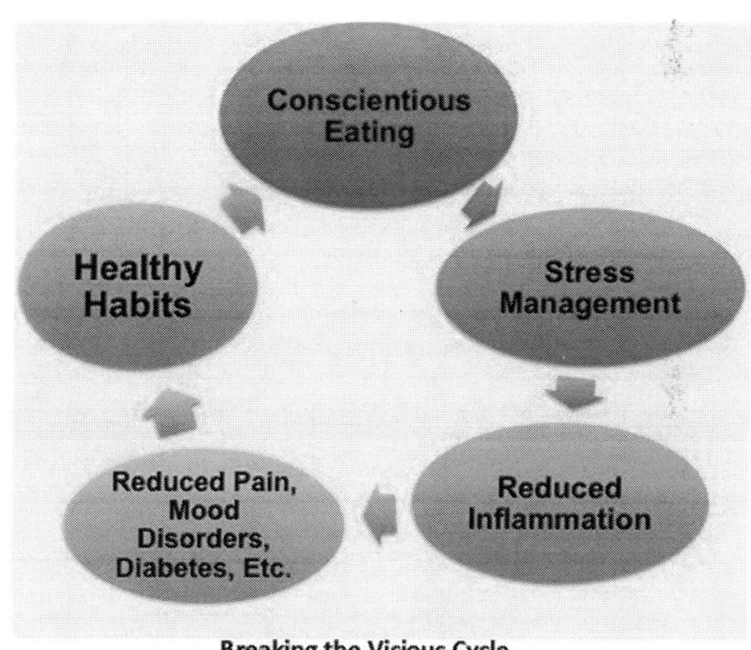

Breaking the Vicious Cycle

Key Points

- Emotion influences food choices.
- Information about diet in general media can be misleading and confusing.
- Stress can encourage poor diet choices that cause more stress.

- Poor diet can cause inflammation. Inflammation produces stress.
- Stress and inflammation drive development or worsening of a host of chronic health conditions, including chronic pain, mood disorders, diabetes, dementia, and metabolic disorders.
- The interplay between microbes living in the gut and immune system function in the gut has a huge impact on health throughout the body.
- Conscientious eating can break the vicious cycle of poor diet, stress, inflammation and disease, but it requires knowledge of the influence of diet choices on health.

References

Azer SA, Al Olayan TI, Al Gamadi MA, Al Sanea MA. Inflammatory bowel disease: an evaluation of health information on the internet. World Journal of Gastroenterology, 23:1676-1696, 2017.

Beebe DW, Simon S, Summer S, Hemmer S, Strotman D, Dolan LM. Dietary intake following experimentally restricted sleep in adolescents. Sleep, 36:827-834, 2013.

Bingula R, Filaire M, Radosevic-Robin N, Bey M, Berthon J-Y, Bernalier-Donadille A, Vasson M-P, Filaire E. Desired turbulence? Gut-lung axis, immunity and lung cancer. Journal of Oncology, 2017:5035371, 2017.

Chao AM, Jastreboff AM, White MA, Grilo CM, Sinha R. Stress, cortisol, and other appetite-related hormones: Prospective prediction of 6-months changes in food cravings and weight. Obesity, 25:713-720, 2017.

Charuvastra A, Cloitre M. Social bonds and Post-Traumatic Stress Disorder. Annual Review of Psychology, 59:301-328, 2008.

Dantzer R, O'Connor JC, Freund GG, Johnson RW, Kelley KK. From inflammation to sickness and depression: when the immune system subjugates the brain. Nature Neuroscience Reviews, 9:46-56, 2008.

DiNicolantonio JJ, Mehta V, Onkaramurthy N, O'Keefe JH. Fructose-induced inflammation and increased cortisol: A new mechanism for how sugar induced visceral adiposity. Progress in Cardiovascular Diseases, 61:3-9, 2018.

Finley, R. A Guerilla Gardner in South Central LA, TED.com Sept. 14, 2013.

Franklin TC, Xu C, Duman RS. Depression and sterile inflammation: Essential role of danger-associated molecular patterns. Brain Behavior and Immunity, 72:2-13, 2018.

Fully Sick. *To do or not to do*. Available at: https://allpoetry.com/Fully_Sick, accessed on September 25, 2022.

Galland L. The gut microbiome and the brain. Journal of Medicinal Food, 17:1261-1272, 2014.

Greer SM, Goldstein AN, Walker MP. The impact of sleep deprivation on food desire in the human brain. Nature Communications, 4:2259, 2013.

Hernandez-Limas E, Soto ME, Rosales C. Editorial: Integrative approaches to the molecular physiology of inflammation. Frontiers in Physiology, 9:1825, 2018.

Higgs S, Thomas J. Social influences on eating. Current Opinion in Behavioral Sciences, 9:1-6, 2016.

Iwata M, Ota KT, Li X-Y, Sakaue F, Li N, Duthell S, et al. Psychological stress activates the inflammasome via release of adenosine triphosphate and stimulation of the purinergic type 2X7 receptor. Biological Psychiatry, 80:12-22, 2016.

Ji R-R, Chamessian A, Y-Q Zhang. Pain regulation by non-neuronal cells and inflammation. Science, 354:572-577, 2016.

Kim Y, Keogh JB, Clifton PM. Differential effects of red meat/refined grain diet and dairy/chicken/nuts/whole grain diet on glucose, insulin and triglyceride in a randomized crossover study. Nutrients, 8:687, 2016.

Mialon M, Mialon J. Corporate political activity of the dairy industry in France: an analysis of publicly available information. Public Health Nutrition, 20:2432-2430, 2017.

Morris MC, Nutrition and risk of dementia: overview and methodological issues. Annals of the New York Academy of Science, 1367:31-37, 2016.

National Center for Health Statistics. Health, United States, 2017: With special feature on mortality. Hyattsville, MD. 2018.

Paula Neto HA, Ausina P, Gomez LS, Leandro JGB, Zancan P, Solao-Penna M. Effects of food additives on immune cells as contributors to body weight gain and immune-mediated metabolic dysregulation. Frontiers in Immunology, 8, article 1478, 2017.

Powys JP. *A Glastonbury Romance*. Simon & Schuster, 1932.

Takiishi T, Morales Fenero CI, Olsen Saraiva Camara N. Intestinal barrier and gut microbiota: Shaping our immune responses throughout life. Tissue Barriers, 5, e1373208, 2017.

Tryon MS, DeCant R, Laugero KD. Having your cake and eating it too: A habit of comfort food may link social stress exposure and acute stress-induced cortisol hyporesponsiveness. Physiology and Behavior, 114:32-37, 2013.

Viladrich A, Tagliaferro B. Picking fruit from our backyard trees: The meaning of nostalgia in shaping Latina's eating practices in the United States. Appetite, 97:101-110, 2016.

Willett W, Rockstrom J, Loken B, Springmann M, Lang T, Vermeulen S. Food in the Anthropocene: the EAT—Lancet Commission on healthy diets from sustainable food systems. The Lancet, 393:447-492, 2019.

Yu E, Rimm E, Rexrode K, Albert CM, Sun Q, Willett WC, Hu FB, Manson JE. Diet, Lifestyle, biomarkers, genetic factors, and risk of cardiovascular disease in the Nurses' Health Studies. American Journal of Public Health, 106:1616-1632, 2016.

- WHAT IS STRESS?

- HOMEOSTASIS, ALLOSTATIC LOAD, AND THE RELATIONSHIP OF STRESS TO CHALLENGE

- VIEWING STRESSORS AS CHALLENGES

- THE BRAIN "ORCHESTRATES" RESPONSES TO CHALLENGES

- THE PHYSIOLOGICAL CHALLENGE/STRESS RESPONSE

- FLIPPING THE SWITCH FROM THE CHALLENGE RESPONSE TO HOMEOSTASIS

- STRESS IS WHEN THE SWITCH FROM CHALLENGE TO RESOLUTION DOESN'T GET FLIPPED

- UNDERSTANDING CORTISOL: THE HORMONAL LINK BETWEEN STRESS, INFLAMMATION AND METABOLISM

- WHAT HAPPENS WHEN CORTISOL IS DYSREGULATED?

- EARLY LIFE HISTORY AFFECTS STRESS: ADVERSE CHILDHOOD EXPERIENCES (ACE) INCREASE INFLAMMATION, PROBLEMS MANAGING STRESS, AND RISK FOR OBESITY AND METABOLIC SYNDROME

- THE SPECIAL CHALLENGE OF SOCIAL RELATIONSHIPS AND SOCIAL STANDING

- THE PRICE OF LONELINESS

- KEY POINTS

Stress plays a pivotal role in the self-sustaining, vicious cycle of diet, inflammation, and stress, in which lifestyle and diet contribute to inflammation and chronic disease. Not only does stress influence decisions about what we eat, but stress alone can induce inflammation. Therefore, any attempt to regain health and to establish healthy lifestyle habits and diet must address stress. To do so it is necessary to understand just what stress is and is not, the types of situations that are likely to become stressful, and what kind of treatments and coping responses are most likely to enable us to manage stress.

What is Stress?

As an experience, stress is a noxious feeling that can be accompanied by physical or emotional pain and negative emotions such as anger, frustration, anxiety, or depression. The term "stress" was borrowed by pre-eminent stress researcher Hans Selye from the field of structural engineering, where it had been defined as "the applied force or system of forces that tends to deform a body" (NDT Education Resource Center, 2001-2014). Such deformation can cause a structure to fail (Parsons 2017). Thus, "stress" conveys the idea that certain circumstances can cause damage, or the risk of damage, to the mind or body. According to Selye (1950) "Anything that causes stress endangers life, unless it is met by adequate adaptive responses".

Over the years, however, researchers and practitioners have expanded the idea of stress, such that now many people even endorse the idea that there is such a thing as "good stress" (Lu 2021, Szabo 2017). But how can something that could cause a structure or a body to fail ever be good? The answer lies in the way that we conceptualize stress.

Situations that lead to the feeling of "good stress" are ones in which some kind of challenge is met. Meeting a challenge leads to feelings of reward and satisfaction. Because life is full of challenges, this reward can motivate us to make the effort to meet them. But if we fail to meet challenges, the opposite emotion is experienced—the feeling of stress.

Homeostasis, Allostatic Load, and the Relationship of Stress to Challenge

For our bodies to function well and stay healthy, many processes need to be regulated. The term *homeostasis* refers to the mechanisms by which the body maintains optimum physiological conditions. Homeostasis involves sensory systems that detect changes from a normal state, such as a drop in blood sugar, and primarily neurological systems that determine and activate responses that can bring the body back to its optimal state. These responses are terminated by negative feedback mechanisms that detect when the response has been successful, rather like a thermostat shutting off a heater when the desired temperature is achieved.

Allostasis is a term that extends the idea of homeostasis to describe how the body responds to physical or psychological threats, as opposed to normal perturbations. It denotes the response of the body to stressors as it attempts to maintain its optimal state. *Allostatic load* refers to the price that the brain and body pay as a consequence of dealing with threats (McEwen, 1998, McEwen 2020). If the challenge of the threat is effectively and efficiently met, the load is low. If the threat cannot be effectively or consistently addressed, this higher allostatic load leads to symptoms associated with stress response, including inflammation and mood disorders (McEwen, 2020). Higher allostatic load is particularly common when stressors are uncontrollable or unpredictable and persistent. These uncontrollable chronic stressors present unresolved, repetitive challenges beyond what our response systems are designed to anticipate and manage.

Viewing Stressors as Challenges

The idea that there is a separate regulatory mechanism specific for threats seems intuitively attractive, but it can be misleading. This is because the same systems and responses that manage everyday homeostatic disturbances are used to address threats or stress. There are no specific hormones or neurotransmitters that are only involved in signaling threats or the stress response. For example, although adrenal hormones are critically involved in signaling stress, they are also involved in responding to challenges and to positive states. The difference between homeostasis and allostasis is one of degree, such that small challenges result in small responses, whereas large challenges (threats) induce bigger responses. So, what we have, rather than a stress response system, is a *challenge response system*. This difference has important implications for how we can effectively manage challenges to prevent damage due to stress. The concept of challenge implies the ability to cope with the situation, and successfully meet the challenge. Challenge suggests the possibility of solving the problem presented. In contrast, stress implies a negative experience that is more likely to encourage an avoidant, passive, or protective response. Stress suggests an external, uncontrollable force that must be avoided or absorbed. Whereas avoidant, passive, or protective responses may provide immediate safety, they do not address the challenge, and do not ensure that a solution will be enacted. Instead that stress can go on to produce deleterious effects on physical and mental health.

Nonetheless, the concept of allostatic load is a cogent way of thinking about why it is so important to manage challenges. A high allostatic load is associated with an unregulated or maladaptive response to challenges that can compromise motivation to engage in a healthy lifestyle, and impair homeostasis and healing. In this way, the idea of a load conveys the emotional meaning of the consequences of stress, such as the heavy emotional weight of worries.

The Brain "Orchestrates" Responses to Challenge

Because challenges large and small are a constant part of living, managing them requires adjustments in the functioning of every tissue of the body. During large challenges, resources from tissues that are not directly involved in managing the challenge may be redirected to those that are central to the response. For example, under a threat that requires flight, blood flow is redirected from reproductive and gastrointestinal tract tissues that aren't crucial for the flight response, to the cardiovascular and brain tissues that enable successful escape. These adjustments must be tightly and rapidly coordinated by the nervous system, in concert with the endocrine and immune systems (McEwen 2020).

The sophisticated way that the nervous system organizes our behavior and physiology in the context of challenges has been described as a "neurosymphony" (Joels 2009). It involves carefully orchestrated and complex interactions between many different players (e.g., neurons). This analogy can be taken further to illuminate some general features of how the brain works. Our thoughts, emotions, and cognitions are generated by the combined activity of neurons and other cells in many brain regions. The neurons in the different brain areas function like musicians in the orchestra, where the individual activity of each set of musicians working in synchrony creates the music. What the music sounds like depends on which musicians are playing at any time, how intensely they are playing, and how well they are listening and communicating with each other. Similarly, our moods, thoughts, and emotions, as well as unconscious activities of the brain, depend on groups of neurons working well together. The activity pattern of the neurons, or the "music" of the brain, determines our experience of life. Our thoughts and experiences are an emergent property of neuronal activity across the brain and nervous system.

In an orchestra, certain instruments may be featured more prominently than others, depending on the type of music being played. The same is true in the brain, depending on the type of behavior, mood, or challenge that needs to be addressed. In an orchestra, if someone is missing, or not playing well, the music is affected. Similarly, deficiencies in one part of the brain can disrupt the delicate balance needed for proper functioning of the whole brain. Orchestras can adapt to the loss of a particular instrument by arranging the music such that a similar instrument can play the part (e.g., substitute tenor sax for bassoon). Musicians can learn new music through innovation or imitation, plus training and practice, just as brains can learn new information, and train in new patterns of functioning. This learning occurs through a process called *plasticity*, where brain circuits are modified in response to patterns of activity. Thinking about brain activity as a neurosymphony provides an elegant way to conceptualize the complexity of functional systems that can be difficult even for scientists to get their heads around.

So what happens in the brain/orchestra when there is a challenge? This will depend on the type of challenge, which is determined by sensory information coming in from the body. Sensory information associated with a possible threat can be diverse, such as the sound of footsteps behind you when walking down a deserted street, the smell of natural gas in the house, or a visual image of a venomous snake. This sensory information alerts a constellation of brain regions that assess the threat to determine if it is truly dangerous. This is likely experienced as anxiety or fear. If the situation seems actually dangerous, behavioral responses are engaged. This is often called the "fight or flight response," and may involve hiding, running away, or engaging the threat. At the same time, cognitive systems continue to evaluate the threat while continuing to produce feelings of alertness, anxiety, and fear.

How does the brain manage this information? Recent neuroimaging studies in humans have identified networks of brain regions that are functionally connected and play together during specific challenges, such as cognitive, emotional, or physiological challenges. Four overlapping functional networks have been identified as particularly relevant to managing challenges and provide insight into how they work together. Activity in these networks is altered by stress. First, a network often referred to as the Salience Network (SN) scans incoming information and decides which data warrant attention and which can be ignored (Redkay 2018). The SN determines the importance of the potential threat and helps to prioritize responses in relation to other activities. Simultaneously, Executive Control Networks (ECNs) integrate information about challenges and rewards to select and modulate behavioral and emotional responses (Hobkirk 2019, Chahal 2021). These ECNs help choose responses to address the challenge. A third network contributes appropriate emotional responses and determines the relevance of the incoming information or challenge to the self (Raichle 2015). This network of brain regions is often active even when a person is not directly focused on completing a task. Because most brain imaging studies focus on task-related brain activity, this network has been called the Default Mode Network (DMN), referencing the network activity patterns that the brain defaults to when not task-focused. Together the SN, ECN, and DMN assess and plan key responses to a challenge, including the magnitude of the response, and appropriate behavioral and emotional responses. Importantly, together they help identify and recognize when the challenge has been met.

The body must be ready to support behavioral responses, and a network of brain regions called the Central Autonomic Network (CAN) collectively interacts with the other networks to identify, and then carry out, appropriate physiological responses (LaMotte 2021). This includes activation of neuroendocrine and nervous system changes that provide energy and increased blood supply, etc. needed to manage the threat.

Some threats arise internally, such as infection, inflammation, or damage, but the physiological response to internal and external threats is basically the same. Internal threats are detected by a sensory modality called *viscerosensation* or *interosensation*. This sensory system constantly monitors the internal conditions of the body, providing crucial information about internal state to the CAN. Through communication with the SN, ECN, and DMN plus information from interosensory systems, the CAN works to control homeostasis and enact responses to larger challenges.

Breaking the response process into these interacting networks helps to explain how the brain parses problem-solving in response to a challenge, tailoring attention (SN), thought and behavioral plans (ECN), emotional response (DMN), and physiological response (CAN) to try to address the potential threat. As depicted below, each of these networks includes brain regions with specific functions in this challenge

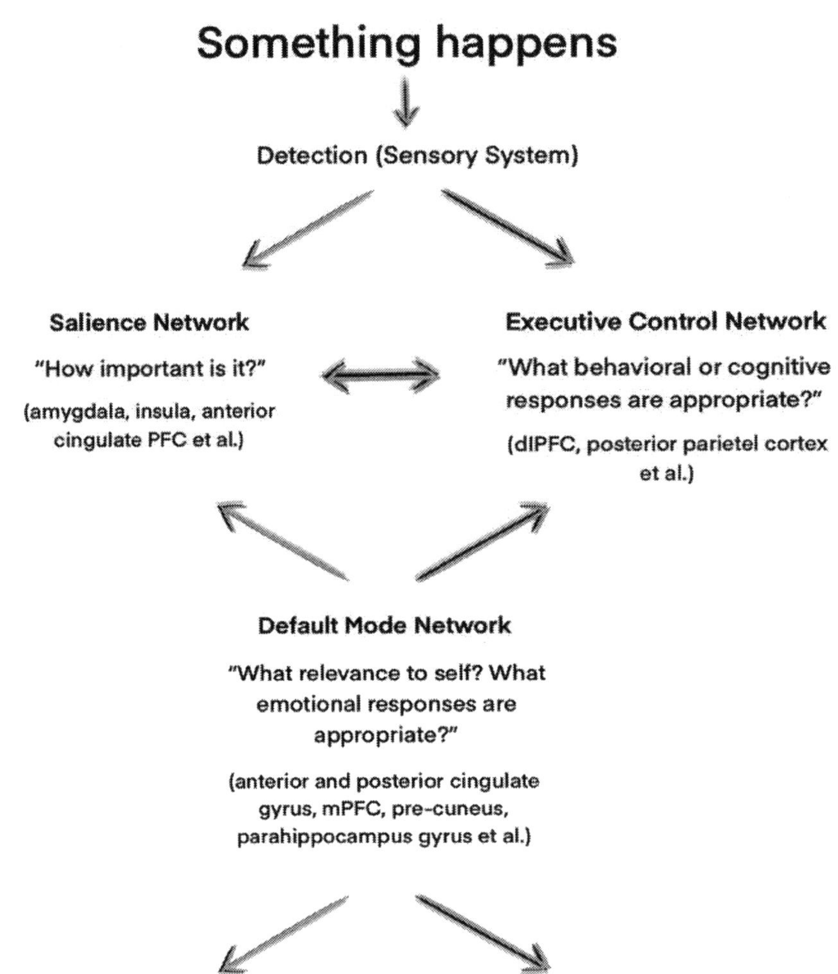

response system. We will introduce some of these regions in more detail later in the book, but provide their names here for reference.

The Physiological Challenge/Stress Response

A part of the CAN called the hypothalamus plays a pivotal role in the integrating emotional experiences with physiological responses to challenge (Lamotte 2021). The hypothalamus is located at the bottom of the brain and receives signals from the body via interosensory systems or *interoception* (Chapter 5), and from the SN, DMN, and ECN. The hypothalamus then initiates neuroendocrine adjustments via the hypothalamo-pituitary adrenal (HPA) axis, and peripheral nervous system responses via the autonomic nervous system (ANS). The ANS is part of the peripheral nervous system and innervates all our internal tissues, blood vessels and skin.

Neuroendocrine responses: Hypothalamo-Pituitary-Adrenal (HPA) axis:

One of the two ways the hypothalamus acts to help manage challenges is by inducing the release of the hormone cortisol from the adrenals. It does this indirectly by first releasing a substance called corticotropin- releasing hormone "CRH" into blood vessels that supply the pituitary gland, located right below the hypothalamus. CRH signals the pituitary to release a hormone called adrenocorticotropic hormone (ACTH). ACTH then travels in the general circulation to the adrenal gland, where it signals the adrenals to release the hormone cortisol. Cortisol levels then increase in the blood, helping the body to prepare for managing the challenge or threat. This process takes several minutes, and we are not usually consciously aware of it. Cortisol is able to enter the brain and when it does, it attaches to receptors that actively signal the hypothalamus to stop releasing CRH onto the pituitary gland, in a classic negative feedback mechanism that turns off the response (McEwen 2020).

As we will learn later, cortisol is not only central to the response to challenges, but also to regulation of eating patterns, use of sugar by the body, and stress-related eating. Cortisol's intertwined role in responding to challenges and regulating food consumption and energy use make challenge response, food, and eating behaviors inseparably linked.

Autonomic Nervous System (ANS):

At the same time it regulates cortisol levels, the hypothalamus activates other brain regions that are part of the CAN, including the spinal cord to activate the sympathetic nervous system (SNS), which is one branch of the autonomic nervous system (ANS). The SNS provides the very rapid signaling that is necessary for the fight-or-flight responses to threats. It also mobilizes the immune system to help it prepare for any tissue damage or infection that may occur due to the threat (Dhabhar 2018).

The SNS response feels nearly immediate. It is responsible for the rapid increase in heart rate and blood pressure, dilation of pupils, and the sweating we experience when we feel we are in danger. The SNS response also increases blood sugar, again tying together challenge response to the body's use of food. This rapid response is mediated by the release of the neurotransmitter norepinephrine (NE) into the heart, blood vessels, and glands. The SNS also signals the adrenal gland to release other hormones, including epinephrine and endogenous opiates.

Flipping the Switch from the Challenge Response to Homeostasis

When the challenge or threat has been resolved, the sympathetic nervous system steps back and the other part of the ANS, the parasympathetic nervous system (PNS), takes over. The PNS brings the body back to its previous resting state. The major nerve of the PNS, the vagus nerve, slows down heart rate and reduces blood pressure. The primary neurotransmitter of the PNS, acetylcholine, also has anti-inflammatory actions that serve to down-regulate immune functions such as inflammation. This shift to parasympathetic activity is akin to flipping a switch from the active challenge response to a recuperative or resolution phase that restores homeostasis.

Stress is when the Switch from Challenge to Resolution Doesn't get Flipped

Under some circumstances, the challenge response does not transition into a resolution phase. The switch does not get flipped. This is usually because the challenge has not been met. Unresolved stress leads to persistent activation of the HPA axis and the SNS, with blood pressure, blood sugar, and levels of circulating cortisol remaining elevated, along with the persistence of the noxious feeling of emotional stress. Persistent SNS and HPA activation also induces or increases inflammation in the body, and even in the brain, where it is called *neuroinflammation* (DiSabato 2016). Consequently, it is the unresolved stress, rather than the challenge itself, that is associated with the increased risk of metabolic, cardiovascular, and neurological diseases that result from chronic SNS and HPA activation.

One of the most important ways that stress affects brain function is by impairing neuronal plasticity (Sweatt 2016). As explained in the previous analogy comparing the brain to an orchestra, plasticity is the general term for the many mechanisms via which brain activity changes in response to experience. Plasticity is also the basis for learning and is essential for effective adaptation to challenges and changing conditions. Plasticity may involve changes or adaptations in synapses between neurons, or changes in patterns of activity in the circuits that control behavior and cognition. Any impairment in plasticity can be expected to have negative consequences for coping with challenges, thereby increasing stress and contributing to the vicious cycle of stress, inflammation, and disease. In short, effective plasticity is critical for emotional well-being and fostering health behaviors.

An inability to manage challenges is associated with imbalances in the functional connectivity of the networks that control emotions and determine cognitive and behavioral responses. Parts of the DMN (e.g., medial prefrontal cortex, interacting with the insula and amygdala) that govern negative emotions including fear, anxiety, and depression, become uncoupled from the ECN and other prefrontal cortex areas. This makes it harder to regulate these negative emotions, likely contributing to the persistence of stress. Using the symphony analogy, here the orchestra conductor has lost control, and the sections that contribute angry, frustrated, or depressing music are playing too loud, and so repetitiously that nothing else can be heard.

Part of the brain's challenge response systems, including those that use the neuromodulator dopamine, involve regulating motivation, reward, and arousal (Baik 2020, Farr 2016, Koob 2016). The lack of resolution prevents the experience of reward associated with meeting challenges. When the inability to resolve challenges becomes chronic, this reward deficiency can lead to compensatory reward-seeking behaviors, such as overeating or craving for palatable foods (Sinha 2018). Together these contribute to the association of stress with mood disorders and addiction (Koob 2016, Ruisoto 2019).

Understanding Cortisol: The Hormonal Link Between Stress, Inflammation and Metabolism

Many of the deleterious effects of unresolved challenges and a high allostatic load are consequences of dysregulation of the HPA axis, which lead to persistently increased levels of cortisol. To understand the consequences of HPA dysregulation, it is necessary to appreciate the many functions of cortisol in the body.

Cortisol's main role is to facilitate the body's adaptation to physical or psychological challenges (McEwen, 2020). Thus, cortisol is highly *pleiotropic*, meaning that it has many different kinds of actions in all tissues of the body. It has powerful effects on metabolism to ensure that there is sufficient fuel, specifically blood glucose, available to manage a challenge. Cortisol also promotes fat deposition, and helps prime some immune responses to help manage infections. It also regulates these responses, as it has powerful anti-inflammatory actions. Indeed cortisol, or drug analogs of cortisol, are often used to treat disorders associated with poorly controlled immune response, such as autoimmune diseases, or suppression of immune rejection of implanted organs. Cortisol also influences cell function in the brain, whereby it can boost cognition and memory to help ensure that appropriate behavioral coping measures are taken (Joels, 2018, McEwen 2020).

One of cortisol's principal roles in physiology is to regulate circadian rhythms. Homeostasis requires that the many different functions and systems of the body work together in a coordinated way. Under normal circumstances, physiological systems are entrained or linked to the time of day. A part of the brain called the suprachiasmatic nucleus (SCN) is responsible for monitoring light levels and thereby inferring time of day. Most tissues also contain so-called "clock genes" that regulate their function according to daily cycles, but these clock genes do not have direct access to information about light levels or time of day. Thus, the SCN must convey its information about time of day to the rest of the body. It does this in part by influencing cortisol release (Koch 2016). The SCN converts information about light and time of day into fluctuations in cortisol levels in the blood. This cortisol signal is distributed along with blood to all tissues in the body, providing cells with information about time of day. In the cell, cortisol regulates transcription and expression of clock genes, thus patterning clock gene activity in alignment with the light and time of day information. In this system, cortisol acts as a messenger, bringing orders from the SCN regarding planned daily cycles to cells where clock genes can enact cyclic patterns of cell function (Mavroudis 2012, Spencer 2018, Wiley 2016). Thus the cortisol rhythms and the regulation of clock genes in other body tissues can be thought of as an important "day job" of cortisol, in addition to its well-characterized role in responding to challenges (Spencer 2018, Wiley 2016).

Cortisol levels are higher during the daytime, probably to support our daily activities, and very low at night (Liiyanarachchi 2017). Levels begin to rise in the hours before waking, and there is a little peak right before awakening, possibly to support arousal to get us up and going. The highest peak occurs around 9 AM, after which it declines, then peaks again around noon, then declines again through the afternoon, peaking once more at about 6 PM before declining again until the next morning. This cortisol rhythm correlates with mealtimes and may be related to cortisol's important role in regulating metabolism (Rasz 2015, Greulich 2016). The peaks may also contribute to daily appetite-related rhythms of maintaining nutrient availability during the day.

Cortisol is an enigmatic hormone, however, in that it can have very different and even opposite actions depending on the context in which it is induced. For instance, cortisol can either increase or decrease immune functions such as inflammation or antibody responses (Xavier 2016). When challenges are not prolonged or high in intensity, cortisol facilitates brain functions such as memory (McEwen 2020). But if cortisol levels are high, such as when experiencing a trauma, or are prolonged, cortisol can profoundly impair cognition and memory (McEwen 2020).

Part of the apparent inconsistencies in its effects may stem from the fact that cortisol has two different modes of action, depending on timing and on whether or not a challenge has successfully been met. Cortisol has rapid effects on cells that occur within minutes of being released into the blood. These support immediate responses to challenges (Joels 2018). At the same time, cortisol has genomic effects, initiating changes in the expression of many genes. The changes in gene expression are thought to facilitate longer-term adaptions to chronic situations (Joels 2018).

What Happens when Cortisol is Dysregulated?

Because cortisol has many different functions, and because many of these functions rely on factors such as time of day, ongoing behaviors (such as eating), and the circadian rhythms driving cortisol release, must be tightly regulated. Dysregulated cortisol is associated particularly with psychiatric disorders (Joseph 2018). Because of cortisol's close relationship with the immune system, dysregulation contributes to chronic inflammation (Joseph 2018). Elevated levels of cortisol at awakening have been associated with development of insulin resistance, potentially linking cortisol dysregulation to diabetes risk (Joseph 2018). Thus, perturbations in cortisol release can have widespread implications for every tissue of the body.

Cortisol dysregulation is manifested by changes in the rhythm and volume of daily cortisol release, including elevated levels on awakening, "blunted" or flatter peaks during the day, and overall higher levels of daily release. Chronic stress seems to be one of the main contributors to dysregulated cortisol, although lifestyle habits, such as disrupted circadian rhythms due to shift work or irregular sleeping habits, may also contribute (Koch 2017). Similarly, diet patterns that involve eating late at night can expected to dysregulate cortisol, given that cortisol levels need to be low at night and a meal will induce a cortisol response (Gu 2020, Koch 2017). The dietary regime known as time-restricted eating, which involves limiting food consumption to 8-10 hours during the day can help control eating behavior, possibly by helping to normalize cortisol rhythms (Ravussin 2019).

Early Life History Affects Stress: Adverse Childhood Experiences (ACE) Increase Inflammation, Problems Managing Stress, and Risk for Obesity and Metabolic Syndrome

Stressful experiences in childhood, such as parental separation, neglect, beatings, and sexual abuse are called Adverse Childhood Experiences (ACE). People who have had ACE grow up to have higher levels of inflammation and poorly regulated endocrine systems, especially the cortisol system (Brown 2009, Iob 2021, Luo 2005, Wiley 2016). This results largely from epigenetic changes that influence how genes are activated or expressed. Over the course of development, some genes only need to be active temporarily, and so when their jobs are done, they are epigenetically silenced, while the gene itself remains unaltered. These epigenetic mechanisms can also affect other genes, in ways that either turn them off, or make them active when they shouldn't be active.

Epigenetic changes can also occur as a response to the environment, including under- or over-nutrition. These epigenetic changes are a major mechanism by which "nurture" influences "nature." People with ACE are at much higher risk than others for mood disorders and addiction, as well as disorders involving inflammation and pain, including irritable bowel syndrome, fibromyalgia, and preterm birth (Iob 2021, Brown 2009, Luo 2005). Abuse, especially sexual abuse, is associated with obesity and metabolic syndrome in adulthood (Pandey 2018; Rosenbaum 2015, Wildes 2008). The shame associated with abuse, especially sexual abuse, complicates efforts to address the role of ACE in obesity or eating disorders. Abused children are usually warned to never tell anyone and are manipulated into feeling responsible for the abuse, often leading them to carry the weight of the shame and guilt into adulthood. Some hypothesize that the physical weight is a manifestation of that burden, which can serve as a physical barrier against the world when there is no protection from psychological pain (Ross 2009). It is therefore important for practitioners to address the possible contribution of abuse with people who have persistent problems with weight.

The Special Challenge of Social Relationships and Social Standing

Probably the most challenging of challenges are those involving social situations, including those associated with the workplace, our families, or our friends. Humans are social animals, and our close relationships can have profound effects on our behavior, health, and ability to confront challenges. Importantly, social experiences have a reliable influence on levels of inflammation, which may explain the outsized impact of social stress as compared to other stressors on health. The chronicity of many social stresses, such as relationship stress, can drive dysregulation of cortisol and the SNS.

The link between social function and inflammation is well-documented. Social stress activates the SNS, which drives immune system activation, contributing to inflammation (Laurent 2013). Specifically, the SNS neurotransmitter norepinephrine (NE) directly activates immune cells to incite inflammation. Even relatively mild levels of relationship stress, such as marital discord, can lead to elevated levels of markers of inflammation in the blood, especially among women (Kiecolt-Glaser 2010, Rohlender 2014).

Our standing in society, frequently referred to as socio-economic status (SES), also influences levels of stress and health outcomes. People with low SES suffer from higher levels of many kinds of stress, including social stress, and experience higher rates of chronic disease and psychiatric symptoms (Luo

2005). More unequal societies have higher rates of physical and mental disorders (Rohleder 2014). Some of this effect may be accounted for by disparities in access to health care, but other contributions are more direct. Chronic social stress can lead to epigenetic changes that enhance inflammation and dysregulated stress responses (McRory 2019). Poor diets are also associated with lower SES, with an over-reliance on cheap, highly processed, highly refined carbohydrate foods (Darmon 2008). In this way, low SES can induce both psychological and physical stress.

The Price of Loneliness

Loneliness is an important risk factor for inflammation and both mental and neuropsychiatric and medical disorders (Eisenberger 2017). People who report feeling lonely have higher levels of inflammation, and experiments designed to temporarily induce feelings of loneliness show that just a brief experience of feeling excluded can increase measures of inflammation (Rohleder 2014). It is important to note that loneliness is distinct from personality features such as introversion, where people genuinely desire less social interaction as compared with others. Rather, loneliness refers to the negative emotion people experience when they, for example, would like to have more friends but for reasons beyond their control, they feel emotionally isolated. Persons with mental illness, stigma, physical isolation, and disability may be particularly vulnerable to loneliness.

Loneliness is particularly common in the elderly. As we age it can be harder to make friends, and the transient nature of many jobs may lead many to not settle down long enough anywhere to make and retain strong friendships. By the time we are retired, we may not have developed or maintained close friendships that can survive changing life circumstances. For older people there is also the loss, through death, of friends and family. This loss can be compounded with a loss of mobility that makes it hard to get out and make new friends. Not surprisingly, then, aging is associated with increased inflammation and mood disorders (Bektas 2018, Meyer 2020). In addition, many older people become caregivers to relatives, often spouses, who develop serious diseases. The demands of caregiving are considerable, and can involve physical challenges, including sleep loss, as well as psychological challenges related to the loss of a life partner. These issues are particularly relevant for caregivers of people with dementia (Gilhooly 2016, Rohleder 2014). The constant demands of monitoring and caring for someone who is losing mental, but not necessarily physical, capacity can be both emotionally and physically draining. The resulting isolation can lead to loneliness. It is therefore not surprising that caregivers sometimes pass away before the partner with dementia.

Key Points

- To stay healthy, we must be conscious about the challenges we face, and how we manage them.
- What we usually think of as "stress" can be more accurately thought of as challenges that are not met.
- Our challenge response systems exert body-wide influences that are designed to support coping with threats or challenges. The challenge response is "turned off" by the parasympathetic nervous system, especially by vagus nerve activity that returns the body back to its resting condition.

- Conceptualizing possible stressors, or stressful situations, as challenges encourages a positive, problem-solving approach that is more likely to lead to meeting the challenge, and thus preventing the stress.
- Adverse Childhood Experiences result in increased inflammation, and increased risk for obesity and metabolic syndrome, highlighting a link between stress and weight problems.
- Social stressors, including socio-economic stress and loneliness, have outsized effects on inflammation and brain health.

References

Baik J-H. Stress and the dopaminergic reward system. Experimental and Molecular Medicine, 52:1878-1890, 2020.

Bektas A, Schurman SH, Sen R, Ferrucci L. Aging, inflammation and the environment. Experimental Gerontology, 105:10-18, 2018.

Brown DW, Anda RF, Tiemeier H, Felitti VJ, Edwards, VJ, Croft JB, Giles WH. Adverse childhood experiences and the risk of premature mortality. American Journal of Preventative Medicine, 37:389-396, 2009.

Chahal R, Kirshenbaum JS, Miller JG, Ho TC, Gotlib IH. Higher executive control network coherence buffers against puberty-related increased in internalizing symptoms during the COVID-19 pandemic. Biological Psychiatry: Cognitive Neuroscience and Neuroimaging, 6:79-88, 2021.

Dhabhar FS. The short-term stress response- Mother Nature's mechanisms for enhancing protection and performance under conditions of threat, challenge, and opportunity. Frontiers in Neuroendocrinology, 49:175-192, 2018.

Di Sabato D, Quan N, Godbout JP. Neuroinflammation: The devil is in the details. Journal of Neurochemistry, 139:136-153, 2016.

Darmon N, Drewnowski A. Does social class predict diet quality? American Journal of Clinical Nutrition, 87:1107-1117, 2008.

Eisenberger NI, Moieni M, Inagaki TK, Muscatell KA, Irwin MR. In sickness and in health: the co-regulation of inflammation and social behavior. Neuropsychopharmacology, 42:242-253, 2017.

Farr OM, Li C-SR, Mantzoros CS. Central nervous system regulation of eating: Insights from human brain imaging. Metabolism, 65:699-713, 2016.

Gilhooly KJ, Gilhooly MLM, Sullivan MP, McIntyre A, Wilson L, Harding E, Woodbridge R, Crutch S. A meta-analysis of stress, coping and interventions in dementia and dementia caregiving. BMC Geriatrics, 16:106, 2016.

Greulich F, Hemmer MC, Rollins DA, Rogatsky I, Uhlenhaut NH. There goes the neighborhood: Assembly of transcriptional complexes during the regulation of metabolism and inflammation by the glucocorticoid receptor. Steroids, 114:7-15, 2016.

Gu C, Brereton N, Schweitzer A, Cotter M, Duan D, Borsheim E, Wolfe RW, Pham LV, Polotsky VY, Jun JC. Metabolic effects of a late dinner in healthy volunteers- a randomized crossover clinical trial. Journal of Clinical Endocrinology and Metabolism, 105:2789-2802, 2020.

Hobkirk AL, Bell RP, Utevsky AV, Huettel S, Meade CS. Reward and executive control network resting-state functional connectivity is associated with impulsivity during reward-based decision making for cocaine users. Drug and Alcohol Dependence, 194:32-39, 2019.

Iob E, Baldwin JR, Plomin R, Steptoe A. Adverse childhood experiences, daytime salivary cortisol, and depressive symptoms in early adulthood: a longitudinal genetically informed twin study. Translational Psychiatry, 11:420, 2021.

Joels M, Baram TZ. The neurosymphony of stress. Nature Reviews Neuroscience, 10:459-466, 2009.

Joels M. Corticosteroids and the brain. Journal of Endocrinology, 238:R121-R130, 2018.

Joseph JJ, Golden SH. Cortisol dysregulation: the bidirectional link between stress, depression, and type 2 diabetes. Annals of the New York Academy of Sciences, 1391:2034, 2018.

Kiecolt-Glaser J, Gouin J-P, Hantsoo L. Close relationships, inflammation, and health. Neuroscience and Biobehavioral Reviews, 35:33-38, 2010.

Koch CE, Leinweber B, Drengberg BC, Blaum C, Oster H. Interaction between circadian rhythms and stress. Neurobiology of Stress, 6:57-67, 2017.

Koob GF, Volkow ND. Neurobiology of addiction: a neurocircuitry analysis. Lancet Psychiatry, 3:760-773, 2016.

Lamotte G, Shouman K, Benarroch EE. Stress and central autonomic network. Autonomic Neuroscience: Basic and Clinical, 235:102870, 2021.

Laurent H, Powers SI, Granger DA. Refining the multisystem view of the stress response: Coordination among cortisol alpha-amylase, and subjective stress in response to relationship conflict. Physiology and Behavior, 119:52-60, 2013.

Liyanarachchi K, Ross R, Debono M. Human studies on the hypothalamo-pituitary-adrenal axis. Best Practice & Research Clinical Endocrinology & Metabolism, 31:459-473, 2017.

Lu S, Wei F, Li G. The evolution of the concept of stress and the framework of the stress system. Cell Stress, 5:76-85, 2021.

Luo Y, Waite LJ. The impact of childhood and adult SES on physical, mental and cognitive well-being later in life. Journal of Gerontology B, Psychological Sciences and Social Sciences, 60:S93-S101, 2005.

Mavroudis PD, Scheff JD, Calvano SE, Lowry SF, Andreoulakis, IP. Entrainment of peripheral clock genes by cortisol. Physiological Genomics, 44,11: 607-21, 2012.

McEwen BS. Protective and damaging effects of stress mediators. Seminars in Medicine at the Beth Israel Deaconess Medical Center. New England Journal of Medicine 338:171-179, 1998.

McEwen BS, Akil H. Revisiting the stress concept: Implications for affective disorders. Journal of Neuroscience, 40:12-21, 2020.

McCrory C, Fiorito G, Ni Cheallaigh C, Polidoro S, Karisola P, Alenius K, Layte R, Seeman T, Vineis P, Kenny RA. How does socio-economic position (SEP) get biologically embedded? A comparison of allostatic load and the epigenetic clock. Psychoneuroendocrinology, 104:64-73, 2019.

Meyer JH, Cervenka S, Kim M-J, Kreisl WC, Henter ID, Innis RB. Neuroinflammation in psychiatric disorders: PET imaging and new targets. Lancet Psychiatry, 7:1064-1074, 2020.

NDT Education Resource Center, 2001-2014, The Collaboration for NDT Education, Iowa State University, www.nde-ed.org

Pandey N, Ashfaq SM, Dauterive EX, MacCarthy AA, Copeland LA. Military sexual trauma and obesity among women veterans. Journal of Women's Health, 27(3): 305-310, 2018.

Parsons J, Cena V. "Engineering Stress: Definition & Equation." *Study.com*, 27 November 2017, available at study.com/academy/lesson/engineering-stress-definition-equation.html, 2017.

Raichle M. The brain's default mode network. Annual Review of Neuroscience, 38:433-447, 2015.

Rasz B, Duskova M, Vondra K, Sramkova M, Hill M, Starka L. Daily profiles of steroid hormones and their metabolites related to food intake. Physiological Research, 64:S219-S225, 2015.

Ravussen E, Beyl RA, Poggiogalle E, Hsie DS, Peterson CM. Early time-restricted feeding reduces appetite and fat oxidation but does not affect energy expenditure in humans.Obesity, 27:1244-1254, 2019

Redkay E, Warnell KR. A social-interactive neuroscience approach to understanding the developing brain. Advances in Child Development and Behavior, 54:1-43, 2018.

Rohlender N. Stimulation of systemic low-grade inflammation by psychosocial; stress. Psychosomatic Medicine, 76:181-189, 2014.

Rosenbaum S, Stubbs B, Ward PB, Steel Z, Lederman O, Vancamfort D. The prevalence and risk of metabolic syndrome and its components in people with posttraumatic stress syndrome: a systematic review. Metabolism, 64:926-933, 2015.

Ross CA. Psychodynamics of Eating Disorder Behavior in Sexual Abuse Survivors. American Journal Of Psychotherapy, 63:211-226, 2009.

Ruisoto P, Contador I. The role of stress in drug addiction. An integrative review. Physiology and Behavior, 202:62-68, 2019.

Selye H. Stress and the general adaption syndrome. British Medical Journal, 1(4667):1384-1392, 1950.

Sinha R. Role of addiction and stress neurobiology on food intake and obesity. Biological Psychology, 131:5-13, 2018.

Spencer RL, Chun LE, Hartsock MJ, Woodruff ER. Glucocorticoid hormones are both a major circadian signal and major stress signal: How this shared relationship signal contributes to a dynamic relationship between the circadian and stress systems. Frontiers in Neuroendocrinology 49:52-71, 2018

Sweatt JD. Neural plasticity and behavior- sixty years of conceptual advances. Journal of Neurochemistry, 139:179-199, 2016.

Szabo S, Yoshida M, Filakovsky J, Juhasz G. "Stress is 80 years old: From Hans Selye original paper in 1936 to recent advances in GI ulceration. Current Advances in Pharmaceutical Design, 23:4029-4041, 2017.

Wildes JE, Kalarchian MA, Marcus M, Levine MD, Courcoulais AP. Childhood maltreatment and psychiatric morbidity in bariatric surgery candidates. Obesity Surgery, 18:306-313, 2008.

Wiley JW, Higgins GA, Athey BD. Stress and glucocorticoid receptor transcriptional programming in time and space: Implications for the brain-gut axis. Neurogastroenterology and Motility, 28:12-25, 2016.

Xavier AM, Anunciato AKO, Rosensock TR, Glezer I. Gene expression control by glucocorticoid receptors during innate immune responses. Frontiers in Endocrinology, 7:31, 2016

CHAPTER 3: UNDERSTANDING EMOTIONAL EATING

- WHY DO WE HAVE TO EAT?

- HOMEOSTATIC SIGNALS CAN INFLUENCE WHEN WE EAT AND WHEN WE STOP: "GUT FACTORS"

- MOTIVATION, REWARD, AND FOOD: HEDONIC EATING

- EMOTIONAL EATING CONTRIBUTES TO OBESITY AND INFLAMMATION

- STRATEGIES TO MANAGE STRESS-INDUCED EATING

- KEY POINTS

Stress can influence eating in many ways. The emotions that come with not being able to meet a challenge are unpleasant, even painful. That feeling of being unrewarded can drive us to crave foods that we associate with pleasure (Berthoud 2017). Stress and sleep deprivation can cause us to choose unhealthy foods like donuts, deep-fried Twinkies, or ice cream, even if we normally prefer more healthy foods (Zellner 2006). And if we know these sugary, high-fat foods aren't good for us, we will sometimes feel even worse from self-stigma and regret. Stress can be overwhelming, making it harder to find the energy to shop for and cook nutritious food, leading to reliance on prepared, highly processed food. It can be easy to give up on trying to eat well. The low mood that can accompany chronic stress can make a healthy diet seem unattainable or unimportant. To learn how to make healthy food choices when stressed, we must first be mindful of the many different factors driving appetite.

Why Do We Have to Eat?

The cells in our bodies must have constant fuel. Additionally, our bodies need "raw materials" to replace old or damaged molecules, membranes, etc. We are literally "not who we were ten years ago," as the molecules that make up our tissues are replaced or renewed over time.

We must obtain metabolic substances and raw material from outside the body. To do this, we need to detect when foods are available, and be motivated to go get them. We then need to eat the food and break it down into smaller molecules, such as glucose, fructose, amino acids, and lipids, and absorb it into our bodies. The absorbed molecules are then made available to cells, most commonly through blood circulation, and any extra energy is stored internally as sugar in the liver, or fats in adipose tissue, in case it becomes hard to find food.

This whole process involves communication between the brain, responsible for the motivation and behavior needed to acquire food, and the body, which knows how much fuel we have in our blood, how much fat is stored, and how much food we have in the gut (Berthoud 2017). Thus, appetite is regulated by factors relevant to both body ("gut factors") and mind ("head factors").

Homeostatic Signals Can Influence When We Eat and When We Stop: "Gut Factors"

When food is ingested, it enters the mouth, or the beginning of the gut. In the mouth, the tongue has receptors that sample the food and report to the brain at least five basic tastes: sweet, sour, bitter, salt, and umami, which is the taste of glutamate or protein. The aroma of the food also activates olfactory receptors in the nose, which together with taste gives food its "flavor." The principal jobs of these sensory receptors are to determine whether what is in the mouth is actually food and initiate either swallowing or spitting it out. Sweet, salty, and umami tastes seem to be innately preferred, likely because they signal nutrition, whereas sour and bitter tastes can signal poisonous or unripe items. Preferences for sour and bitter tastes need to be learned. Sweet tastes, especially, also induce a cephalic phase of digestion, which involves release of insulin and digestive enzymes from the pancreas (Woods 2016). This serves to prepare the gut for the food that, after being chewed in the mouth, must be broken down for absorption into the body. In this way, sensory receptors in the mouth influence both ingestive behavior and digestion.

Once food arrives in the stomach, chemosensory cells that line the stomach release a hormone called ghrelin. Ghrelin travels in the blood to the brain, where it crosses the blood-brain barrier to interact with cells in the hypothalamus and brainstem to increase appetite (Berthoud 2017, Horner 2020). In general, circulating levels of ghrelin are higher when we are hungry, and it acts to increase motivation for food (Jacubwisz 2012, Kroemer 2012). When food is broken down sufficiently so that it can be absorbed into the body, it is sent into the small intestine.

The lining of the small intestine also has chemosensory cells, most of which are sensitive to nutrients, especially fats of different kinds (Maljaars 2007). These cells release peptides, such as cholecystokinin (CCK), peptide YY (PYY), glucagon-like peptide (GLP), and serotonin, to control digestion and modify eating behavior (Berthoud 2017). Many gut peptides bind to the vagus nerve that is associated with the parasympathetic nervous system, and that connects internal organs with the brain. This pathway is part of interoception (Chapter 5), a sensory pathway that influences activity in the Central Autonomic Network (CAN) and other brain networks that respond to challenges. These gut peptides can signal the brain via a neural route, and/or they travel in the blood, like ghrelin does, to influence behavior directly (Berthoud 2017). Intestinal peptides generally induce satiety or reduce the amount of food eaten (Maljaars 2007).

Another hormone that influences appetite, called leptin, is not produced in the gut, but rather by fat cells. Leptin can signal the vagus nerve and also act directly in the brain, where its role is to let the brain know that fat cells are full. As such, leptin levels are lower in lean people and higher in those who are overweight. Leptin acts to reduce appetite and motivation for rewards (Di Spiezio 2018). Unfortunately, obesity can be associated with leptin resistance, wherein the brain does not respond to high leptin levels (Berthoud 2017, Woods 2016). Leptin resistance can make it hard for obese people to regulate their appetites.

The pancreas secretes the hormone insulin, which prompts cells to absorb glucose and amino acids. Insulin also plays a role in regulating appetite (Woods 2016). Most insulin is released when food is absorbed into the body, especially after a carbohydrate-rich meal. Insulin acts in the brain to reduce the attractiveness of food (Kroemer 2012, Tiedeman 2018) and contributes to the experience of satiety by decreasing motivation to eat.

There are other signals from the body that contribute to controlling appetite, but the theme is the same. Signals generated early in a meal, such as ghrelin, or when metabolic fuels are low, act to increase appetite and motivation for food. Signals that are generated during or shortly after a meal, or hormones like leptin that are associated with more than adequate fuel storage, are associated with reductions in motivation for food. Interestingly, most of the endocrine cells that produce satiety hormones such as CCK and GLP1 are activated by fats and proteins in the meal (Paton 2020, Modvig 2021, Steiner 2016). This may be why foods containing fats and proteins tend to be more satiating than low-fat, sugary foods that do not stimulate these gut peptides.

Motivation, Reward and Food: Hedonic Eating

"Head factors" involve aspects of food that are mediated by the brain, such as palatability or "tastiness," learned preferences or aversions, emotional rewards, cultural norms, and habits. These factors can drive hedonic eating, or eating for pleasure rather than for nutrition (Coccurello 2018).

Decisions to seek out food, and to actually eat it, follow from interactions of a motivational brain network with the Executive Control Network (ECN) and the Salience Network (SN) described in Chapter 2. These brain networks receive signals from gut factors indicating need or lack of need for food. In this way the brain integrates "needs" with "wants" (Woods 2016). Notably, the brain networks that regulate appetite are the same networks that control our responses to challenges in general, and that are dysfunctional in the context of stress (Sinha 2014).

The motivation network consists of the mesolimbic dopamine pathway, which originates in the ventral tegmental area of the midbrain and drives subcortical areas such as the striatum to activate reward or relief-seeking behaviors (Koob 2010, Woods 2016). Activation of this pathway can be associated with the emotional experience of craving, discussed in more detail later in this chapter (Koob 2010). This system is influenced by other areas related to emotion, such as the amygdala. Hedonics, the pleasurableness of the taste or smell of the food, are signaled by nucleus accumbens neurons and some cortical areas, as well as by gut factors such as ghrelin, which seems to increase the hedonic or pleasurable value of food (Schellekens 2013).

Executive/decision-making functions are carried out by the ECN of brain regions located mostly in the frontal and parietal lobes. The frontal lobe integrates information about sensory features of food with information about emotional state and cognitive beliefs, intentions, and expectations. The frontal lobe thus combines information about the look, taste, smell, texture, and even sound associated with food or eating, with cognitive and emotional information such as learned associations of food with pleasure or pain, knowledge of food value and healthfulness, and also the goals of eating, like increasing or decreasing consumption of specific foods or amounts (Gluck 2017, Rolls 2005, Spetter 2020). The network then directs behavior based on the relative salience of the various factors related to need for food, habit, drive for pleasure, social and emotional factors, and quality of food. Salience is a term referring to the importance or relevance of a given factor, and how noticeable it is. The SN determines this quality of salience and interacts with autonomic and neuroendocrine systems, such as the HPA axis, to coordinate the brain's response to biologically relevant stimuli such as food.

In humans, head factors and hedonic eating seem to play dominant roles in when, what, and how much we eat (Berthoud 2017, Cocurello 2018, Farr 2016). Thus, understanding how emotions drive eating can develop healthy eating strategies.

Emotional Eating Contributes to Obesity and Inflammation

Our first experience of being nurtured, and having our needs met, is when we are nursed by our mothers when we are newborns. It is therefore not surprising that we have a tendency to turn to food when we are stressed. When my youngest daughter was a newborn, she had to have her hearing tested, and the procedure completely freaked her out. She was returned to me hysterical, desperately seeking my breast. Only by nursing was she able to calm herself down. This early experience of associating food with security likely contributes to the powerful, and sometimes unconscious, association between food and relief from stress.

Sometimes the connection is quite conscious, as this excerpt from a New York Times article illustrates:

"Oh, hello, nice to see you, have a seat — let's stress-eat some chips together. Let's turn ourselves, briefly, into dusty-fingered junk-food receptacles. This will force us to stop looking, for a few minutes, at the bramble of tabs we've had open on our internet browsers for all these awful months: the articles we've been too frazzled to read about; the TV shows we've been meaning to watch; the useless products we keep almost impulse-buying; the sports highlights and classic films that we digest in 12-second bursts every four days; that little cartoon diagram of how to best lay out your fruit orchards in Animal Crossing. Eating these chips will rescue us, above all, from the very worst things on our screens, the cursed news of the outside world — escalating numbers, civic decay, gangs of elderly men behaving like children. That is the great virtue of chips: They are here for us to eat them. So that is what we will do. I will put the first chip, now, into my mouth. I will set it delicately on my tongue like a communion wafer. Instantly, the flavor snaps against my taste buds — that earthy, cheesy tang — flashing like a firecracker, lighting up the whole wet cave of my mouth and radiating out, further, to fill my whole head, my whole being. These chemicals are transcendent, Proustian, as powerful as any drug: They trigger nodes of memory that stretch back years, decades, back to old Super Bowls and family reunions, back to the outside world that I am trying to forget. Another chip. Another chip" (Anderson 2021).

Clearly, food and eating serve functions beyond the homeostatic regulation of energy availability for our cells. Food and beverages facilitate social interaction, and because food is always available in Western societies, we can plan meals around other activities. Being able to schedule meals means we do not have to rely on homeostatic signals from the body to decide when we will eat a meal. Indeed, regular mealtimes entrain the metabolic systems, including cortisol rhythms, such that we become conditioned to become hungry at specific times of day. If we always eat lunch at noon, for example, we will tend to feel hungry just before then. If we have adopted a habit of snacking in the mid-afternoon, we will likely become hungry around that time even if we ate a decent lunch.

Emotional eating refers to consuming palatable, highly-rewarding foods, usually fats and sweets, or salty things, for the purpose of improving mood rather than driven by physiological need or schedule (Bourdier 2018, van Strien 2018). Because food is necessary for survival, motivation to eat is hard-wired into the neurocircuitry of our brains (Berthoud 2017). Eating behavior is highly rewarding, ensuring that we will reliably eat. The pleasurable experiences of eating, however, involve the same brain mechanisms as do other motivated behaviors, including sex, social interaction, and unfortunately use of substances that can cause addiction, such as cocaine, amphetamine, and heroin (Sinha 2018, Singh 2014). One critical feature of reward is that it improves mood, and indeed, emotional eating is associated with depressive symptoms, a state commonly linked to a lack of experience of reward (Singh 2014, Kontinen 2019, Felger 2016). Chronic stress can also increase the likelihood of eating palatable foods when acutely stressed (Singh 2014, Tryon 2013a, Tryon 2013b). Negative emotions such as stress and depression can be momentarily improved by eating foods, such as fats and sweets, that strongly drive brain reward mechanisms.

Although stress-induced eating can immediately ameliorate negative emotions, it comes with unfortunate long-term consequences (Tomiyama 2019). Emotional eating contributes to overweight and obesity (Bourdier 2018). Depression and obesity are linked most strongly via emotional eating (Ouakinin 2018). Dieting to manage weight gain can make this worse due to feelings of self-deprivation, and of having to ignore signals from the body that are necessary for both homeostasis and mood regulation (Simmons 2017). Excessive weight disturbs the body's energy balance, contributing to inflammation in a variety of ways (Chapter 14). The typical foods consumed during emotional eating are sugary, starchy, refined carbohydrates and fried fatty foods (Chao 2017, Sinha 2018) that can induce inflammation (Chapters 10-13). This increased inflammation can in turn increase low mood, especially depression, creating a feed-forward cycle that can drive further emotional eating. In this way, coping with stress by eating rewarding but unhealthful food induces a downward spiral of worsening mood, increasing inflammation, and dysregulated body weight control.

Food Craving

Once we discover that certain foods can improve negative emotions, the brain learns to associate that food with rewards, beyond the purpose of eating (Lender 2020). The brain's reward learning circuits can then initiate drives for the rewarding food whenever there is stress or low mood. This happens in part via activation of the mesolimbic dopamine system, leading to the experience of craving (Morales 2020, Singh 2014). Craving is an intrusive desire for those food items such as ice cream, donuts, and other sweet or fatty comfort foods that normally activate brain reward pathways. This food craving produced by similar brain circuits and mechanisms as craving for drugs of abuse. Craving is a driver of emotional eating, and because it is a learned habit, craving can be very hard to manage. A particular challenge is that food craving links stress with consumption of high-energy foods. (Chao 2018). Interestingly, cravings tend to differ by gender. Men tend to crave fats, whereas women tend to crave sweets. As people learn to alleviate feelings of stress and negative emotions with rewarding food, resulting food cravings can contribute to inflammation, which can further drive feelings of stress and negative emotions.

Strategies to Manage Stress-Induced Eating

Stress Management and Resilience

Emotional eating is strongly linked to stress (Singh 2014). Stress seems to increase levels of ghrelin, which increases the rewarding value of food (Schellekens 2013). This disrupts the normal regulation of eating and dysregulates the balance between hedonic and executive brain circuits. As emotions and stress-related signals become more salient, the executive network becomes less engaged with behavioral control mechanisms (Sinha 2018). This can lead to unfortunate food choices (e.g. junk food) and overeating.

The experience of stress is a psychological phenomenon, deriving from challenges that are difficult, or even impossible to meet. Therefore, the only way to effectively address stress is by active psychological and behavioral approaches. Whereas it is critical to develop a healthy relationship with food, such that food is not being used as a drug to improve mood, it is also imperative to actively address the issues that are driving the stress experience.

Positive attitudes and feelings of self-efficacy, or possessing the confidence to meet specific challenges, are strongly associated with resilience to stress (Penacoba 2021). Self-efficacy and positive emotions can support changes in eating behaviors (Teizeira 2015). The opposite state, characterized by negative emotions and low self-efficacy, are particularly related to emotional eating and becoming overweight (Kontinnen 2010). Low self-efficacy for engaging in healthy behaviors, such as exercise or limiting unhealthy food choices, are especially relevant. This implies that positive self-talk, or getting "psyched up" to meet the challenges of health behavior change can help promote resilience. Because loneliness and social exclusion can drive emotional eating and preference for palatable comfort foods, having supportive friends and relationships can help buffer the effects of difficult challenges (Giel 2021).

Regulation of Emotions

One of the biggest challenges for all of us is managing negative emotions. It is sometimes hard to avoid despairing when challenges aren't met, and stressful states persist. The basic problem with emotional eating is that it provides only short-term relief from symptoms of low mood and does not confront the issues that drive the low mood (Klatzkin 2019, van Strien 2019). The immediate relief may limit efforts to explore causes of the low mood, analyze them, and make decisions about what behaviors or attitudes would be most helpful for managing the challenge. In this way, emotional eating is a passive coping response. To develop a healthy relationship with food, we must be able to actively regulate negative emotions. Regulating emotions is critical to stress resilience, which we will discuss in more detail later.

An easy and effective technique for managing emotions is called mindfulness (Schuman-Olivier 2020). Mindfulness is a technique of approaching ourselves and the world in an objective, observing, and accepting way. For example: "Oh, I notice I'm feeling depressed right now, and that's okay. What just happened that might have triggered this feeling?" Stepping back a bit reduces the intensity of the emotion, and allows a cognitive assessment of it. Accepting the experience helps reduce catastrophizing and a cycle of self-recrimination. In the case of anxiety, acceptance helps prevent one from being "anxious about being anxious". Mindfulness-based stress reduction techniques, including acceptance strategies, have been shown to help with a wide variety of stress-related problems, and also show promise in helping people to change their eating behaviors (Schuman-Olivier 2020, Warren 2017).

Key Points

- Signals from the body, or "gut factors", can influence our motivation for food and how much we eat.
- "Head factors" involve not just our conscious decisions about what we will eat, but also emotional aspects, such as hedonics, or how pleasurable we expect the food to be. Higher-level "head factors" integrate information regarding cognitive, emotional, and "gut factors."
- Because a major objective of the challenge response is to provide sufficient metabolic fuel for managing challenges, stress from unmet challenges increases drive for high-energy comfort foods.
- Emotional eating may seem to improve mood and make us feel better in the short-term, but habits of eating, or overeating, sugary and/or fatty foods contribute to inflammation and feeling worse in the longer term.
- Emotion regulation is key to managing tendencies toward stress-induced eating.
- Food preferences can be learned, as can preferences for comfort foods.

References

Anderson, S. I Recommend Eating Chips. New York Times, January 13, 2021.

Berthoud H-R, Munzberg H, Morrison CD. Blaming the brain for obesity. Gastroenterology, 152:1728-1738, 2017.

Bourdier L, Orri M, Carre A, Gearhardt AN, Romo L, Dantzer C, Berthoz S. Are emotionally driven and addictive-like eating behaviors the missing links between psychological distress and greater body weight? Appetite, 120:536-546, 2018.

Chao AM, Jasteboff AM, White MA, Grilo CM, Sinha R. Stress, cortisol, and other appetite-related hormones: Prospective prediction of 6-month changes in food cravings and weight. Obesity 25:713-720, 2017.

Coccurello R, Maccarrone M. Hedonic eating and the "delicious circle": From lipid-derived mediators to brain dopamine and back. Frontiers in Neuroscience, 12: article 271, 2018.

Di Spiezio A, Sandin ES, Dore R, Muller-Fielits H, Storck SE, Bernau M, Mier W, Oster H, Johren O, Pietrzik CU, Lehnert H, Schwaninger. The LepR-mediated leptin transport across brain barriers controls food reward. Molecular Metabolism, 8:13-22, 2018.

Farr OM, Li C-s R, Mantzoros CS. Central nervous system regulation of eating: insights from human brain imaging. Metabolism, 65:699-713, 2016.

Felger JC, Li Z, Haroon E, Woolwine BJ, Jung MY, Hu X, Miller AH. Inflammation is associated with decreased functional connectivity within corticostriatal reward circuitry in depression. Molecular Psychiatry, 21:1358-1365, 2016.

Giel KE, Schurr M, Zipfel S, Junne F Schag K. Eating behavior and symptom trajectories in patients with a history of binge eating disorder during COVID-19 pandemic. European Eating Disorders Review, 29:657-662, 2021.

Gluck ME, Viswanath V, Stinson EJ. Obesity, appetite, and the prefrontal cortex. Current Obesity Reports, 6:380-388, 2017.

Horner K, Hopkins M, Finlayson G, Gibbons C, Brennan L. Biomarkers of appetite: is there a role for metabolomics? Nutrition Research Reviews, 33:271-286, 2020.

Jakubwicz D, Froy O, Wainstein J, Boaz M. Meal timing and composition influence ghrelin levels, appetite scores and weight loss maintenance in overweight and obese adults. Steroids, 77:323-331, 2012.

Klatzkin RR, Dasani R, Warren M, Cattaneo C, Nadel T, Nikodem C, Kissileff HR. Negative affect is associated with increased stress-eating for women with high perceived stress. Physiology and Behavior, 210:112630, 2019.

Konttinen H, Silventoinen, Sarlio-Lahteenkorva S, Mannisto S, Haukkala A. Emotional eating and physical activity self-efficacy as pathways in the association of depressive symptoms and adiposity indicators. American Journal of Clinical Nutrition, 92:1031-1039, 2010.

Konttinen H, van Strien T, Mannisto S, Jousilahti P, Kaukkala A. Depression, emotional eating and long-term weight changes: a population-based prospective study. International Journal of Behavioral Nutrition and Physical Activity, 16:28, 2019.

Koob GF, Volkow ND. Neurocircuitry of addiction. Psychopharmacology, 35:217-238, 2010.

Kroemer NB, Krebs L, Kobieel A, Grimm O, Vollstadt-Klein S, Pilhatsch, M, Bidlingmaier M, Zimmermann U, Smolka MN. Fasting levels of ghrelin covary with the brain response to food pictures. Addiction Biology, 18:855-862, 2012.

Lender A, Miedl SF, Wilhelm FH, Miller J, Blechert J. Love at first taste: Activation in reward-related brain regions during single-trial naturalistic appetitive conditioning in humans. Physiology and Behavior, 224:113014, 2020.

Maljaars J, Peters HPF, Masclee AM. Review article: the gastrointestinal tract: neuroendocrine regulation of satiety and food intake. Alimentary Pharmacology and Therapeutics, 26:241-250, 2007.

Modvig IM, Kuhre RE, Jepsen SL, Xu SFS, Engelstoft MS, Egerod KL, Schwartz TW, Orskov C, Rosenkilde MM, Holst JJ. Amino acids differ in their capacity to stimulate GLP-1 release from the perfused rat intestine and stimulate secretion by different sensing mechanisms. American Journal of Physiology Endocrinology and Metabolism, 320:E874-E885, 2021.

Morales I, Berridge KC. "Liking" and "wanting" in eating and food reward: Brain mechanisms and clinical implications. Physiology and Behavior, 227:113152, 2020.

Ouakinin SRS, Barreira DP, Gois CJ. Depression and obesity: integrating the role of stress, neuroendocrine dysfunction and inflammatory pathways. Frontiers in Endocrinology, 9:431, 2018.

Paton CM, Son Y, Vaughan RA, Cooper JA. Free fatty acid-induced Peptide YY expression is dependent on TG synthesis rate and Xbp1 splicing. International Journal of Molecular Sciences, 21:3368, 2020.

Penocoba C, Catala P, Velasco L, Carmon-Monge FJ, Garcia-Hedrera FJ, Gil-Almagro F. Resilience and anxiety among intensive care unit professionals during the Covid-19 pandemic. Nursing in Critical Care, 2021:1-8, 2021.

Rolls ET. Taste, olfactory and food texture processing in the brain, and the control of food intake. Physiology and Behavior, 85:45-56, 2005.

Schellekens H, Dinan TG, Cryan JF. Taking two to tango: a role for ghrelin receptor heterodimerization in stress and reward. Frontiers in Neuroscience, 7:148, 2013.

Schuman-Olivier Z, Trombka M, Lovas DA, Brewer JA, Vago, Gawande R, Dunne JP, Lazar SW, Loucks EB, Fulwiler C. Mindfulness and behavior change. Harvard Review of Psychiatry, 28:371-394, 2020.

Simmons WK, DeVille DC. Interoceptive contributions to healthy eating and obesity. Current Opinion in Psychology, 17:106-112, 2017.

Singh M. Mood, food, and obesity. Frontiers in Psychology, 5:925, 2014.

Sinha R. Role of addition and stress neurobiology on food intake and obesity. Biological Psychology, 131:5-13, 2018.

Spetter MS, Higgs S, Dolmans D, Thomas JM, Reniers RLEP, Rotshtein P, Rutters F. Neural correlates of top-down guidance of attention to food: an fMRI study. Physiology and Behavior, 225:113085, 2020.

Steiner RE, Beglinger C, Langhans W. Intestinal GLP-1 and satiation: from man to rodents and back. International Journal of Obesity, 40:198-205, 2016.

Teixeira PJ, Carraca EV, Marques MM, Rutter H, Oppert JM, De Bourdeauhuij I, Lakerveld J, Brug J. Successful behavior change in obesity interventions in adults: a systematic review of self-regulatory mediators. BMC Medicine, 13:84, 2015.

Tiedemann LJ, Schmid SM, Hettel J, Giesen K, Franke P, Buchel C, Brassen S. Central insulin modulates food valuation via mesolimbic pathways. Nature Communications, 8: 16052, 2018.

Tomiyama AJ. Stress and Obesity. Annual Review of Psychology, 70:703-718, 2019.

Tryon MS, DeCant R, Laugero KD. Having your cake and eating it too: A habit of comfort food may link chronic social stress exposure and acute stress-induced cortisol hyporesponsiveness. Physiology & Behavior, 114:32-37, 2013b.

Tryon MS, Carter CS, DeCant R, Laugero KD. Chronic stress exposure may affect the brain's response to high calorie food cues and predispose to obesogenic eating habits. Physiology & Behavior, 120:233-242, 2013a.

van Strien T. Causes of emotional eating and matched treatment of obesity. Current Diabetes Reports 18:35, 2018.

van Strien T, Ginson EL, Banos R, Ceboll A, Winkens LHH. Is comfort food actually comforting for emotional eaters? A (moderated) mediation analysis. Physiology and Behavior, 211:112671, 2019.

Warren JM, Smith N, Ashwell M. A structured literature review on the role of mindfulness, mindful eating and intuitive eating in changing eating behaviors: effectiveness and associated potential mechanisms. Nutrition Research Reviews, 30:272-283, 2017.

Woods SC, Begg DP. Regulation of the motivation to eat. Current Topics in Behavioral Neuroscience, 27:15-35, 2016.

Zellner DA, Loaiza S, Gonzalez Z, Pita J, Morales J, Pecora B, Wolf A. Food selection changes under stress. Physiology and Behavior, 87:789-793, 2006.

- WHAT DO WE MEAN BY RESILIENCE?
- RESILIENT PEOPLE COPE ACTIVELY WITH CHALLENGES
- RESILIENT PEOPLE KEEP POSITIVE, OPTIMISTIC ATTITUDES
- EMOTION REGULATION: HOW WE THINK ABOUT CHALLENGES DETERMINES HOW WELL WE MANAGE THEM
- MINDFUL AWARENESS CAN IMPROVE EMOTION REGULATION
- RESILIENT PEOPLE WORK TO KEEP SITUATIONS AND EVENTS IN PERSPECTIVE
- RESILIENT PEOPLE FIND MEANING IN LIFE
- RESILIENT PEOPLE MAINTAIN CONNECTIONS WITH OTHER PEOPLE
- KEY POINTS

Because food and eating behaviors are markedly influenced by stress, if we want to change the way we eat, we must address the ways in which we approach challenges. Challenges, both great and small, are integral parts of life. Meeting a challenge provides a sense of mastery, boosting self-confidence, and providing an opportunity to grow emotionally. The rather cliché saying, "that which doesn't kill you makes you stronger," is often used as a joke, but it is true. Unmet challenges to well-being become stress, which contributes to chronic disorders both in the body and in the mind, as well as the feeling of not being well. If we want to change the way we feel, we must learn to accept the challenge.

Studies of stress and coping have identified a feature termed resilience that is associated with successful coping. Understanding what it is that makes people resilient, and knowing how to incorporate resilience into our lives, can enable us to manage challenges and stressors and to make good choices about the foods we eat.

What Do We Mean by Resilience?

Resilience is a term that describes the ability to confront challenges, and even endure horrific situations, and emerge psychologically healthy. It involves successful physiological and psychological adaption to challenges, and even stressors. The study of resilience was inspired by survivors of the Nazi Holocaust (Frankl 1959). Many people left the camps broken and unable to heal from the privation, and the loss of family and friends they endured. But others were able to move on, and live happy, productive, and even long, lives.

What makes someone resilient?

Resilient People Cope Actively with Challenges

Often, when we are faced with challenges we think we may not be able to meet, the impulse is to shut down, and try to reduce the experience of stress by being passive. Unfortunately, a passive coping response nearly guarantees that the challenge will not be met. In contrast, if the potentially stressful situation is viewed as a challenge, a natural response it to think about how to meet the challenge. For example, suppose you need to make dinner, but you don't have ingredients or a way to get to the store. A passive coping response might be to feel frustrated and think "I'm just going to have to go hungry!" It will be hard to not feel depressed. In contrast, an active coping response might be "Well, this is a challenge. I wonder if my neighbor has the ingredients I need or will let me borrow their car." Or "How close does the bus go to the store?" Or "What do I have here that I can make into a decent dinner?" The difference in these two types of responses is that the first, passive, response assumes failure and thereby guarantees stress, whereas the second, challenge-oriented response involves problem-solving and encourages a sense of control over the challenge.

This active coping is critical to avoid the transition from challenge to stress. Even when stress is unavoidable, such as workplace or family stress, an active coping, problem-solving style can help find ways to mitigate the effects of stress. For instance, someone with an active coping style may be more willing to seek out social support, exercise, or mind-body modalities such as yoga, meditation, or psychotherapy that are established to help mitigate the effects of stress on the mind and body. In contrast, a passive style of coping response can lead to social isolation and stress-induced eating.

Active coping itself can be a challenge, however, in the context of chronic stress or disease. As we will see, inflammation associated with illness and chronic stress can induce a behavior pattern that, in encouraging protective recuperative behavior, tends to encourage passive coping with challenges. Nonetheless, there are other aspects of coping strategies and approaches to life that have been shown to boost psychological resilience and reduce inflammation.

Resilient People Keep Positive, Optimistic Attitudes

Many studies have shown that negative, pessimistic attitudes are associated with increased levels of inflammation, and thus increased risk for chronic diseases, including cardiovascular disease, Alzheimer's disease, and mood disorders (Friedman 2019). The good news is that the opposite is true: people with positive attitudes and an optimistic outlook have lower risks for chronic diseases, do better when they do have a chronic disease, and have greater longevity than people with pessimistic, cynical, and other negative attitudes (Friedman 2019).

A tendency towards either positive or negative attitudes has been considered to part of psychological temperament, which seems to be strongly influenced by heredity (Zwir 2020). This idea, unfortunately, has led to the assumption by many that if you have a negative-tending temperament, you are just stuck with it. This assumption reinforces passive coping behaviors.

As it happens, even those of us who think of ourselves as Negative Nellies can learn to be more optimistic and positive. Grandma's advice to "Count your blessings" has been supported by studies showing that when people pay attention to the good things in their lives, they feel better and are healthier (Harshberger 2005). Because positive attitudes and active coping styles are associated with better mental and physical health, and overall quality of life, it is worthwhile to optimize the way we respond to challenges (Friedman 2019, Kubansky 2018). Attitudes and behaviors are really just habits, things that our brains have doing so long it can feel impossible to change. But the brain is an activity-dependent place, such that the more you do something, the easier it is to do it. The learning that comes with practicing active coping is associated with strengthened connections in neural networks that mediate thoughts and behaviors. In fact, the genes that are associated with temperament are strongly linked to learning pathways (Zwir 2020). Thus, the brain can learn to adopt new thinking patterns and attitudes, but this does take practice. In neurosymphony terms, the orchestra needs more rehearsal time for pieces that are unfamiliar. But the orchestra can learn to play new music, and it would be rather dull if it just played the same thing over and over.

I can personally attest to the fact that attitudes and coping styles can change. My childhood and adolescence were marked by low mood, pessimism, and negative emotions such as jealousy. I wished that I could be happier and more outgoing, like my popular classmates, but felt I was just stuck. At one point in high school, though, I decided to try to make a change. I had a friend whose face would light up with big grin, and would say "Hi!", whenever she would see me or any other friends. It made me feel better every time I saw her. I decided to see if I could do that too. So, I practiced in the mirror, smiling and saying "Hi!" at the same time. When I deployed my new greeting to people, the results were amazing. People looked a little surprised, and then gave me a big grin back. It made me feel more connected, and happy that I brightened someone's day a little. This success encouraged me to tackle other issues about my attitudes, using informal versions of what are now tried and true techniques for cognitive and behavior change: cognitive re-appraisal, thought-stopping, and mindfulness.

Emotion Regulation: How We Think About Challenges Determines How Well We Manage Them

One of the hardest but most important factors in maintaining active coping and positive attitudes is being able to regulate emotions in the face of a challenge, especially one that is difficult or where a safe outcome may not be controllable. Emotion regulation involves actively addressing negative emotions (Schafer 2017). In addition to being important for supporting active coping, effective regulation of emotion is critical to making good decisions, especially about food. Indeed, both emotion regulation and healthful eating behaviors are more difficult in the face of difficult or uncontrollable challenges or highly noxious stress.

One of the best techniques for regulating emotions is called cognitive re-appraisal (Schafer 2017). Cognitive re-appraisal involves changing the way that a situation is viewed in a way that makes it less distressing. An example of re-appraisal would be to re-conceptualize a stressful event as simply a challenge to be met. This re-appraisal can then reduce anticipatory negative emotions that induce a passive, protective response. Active, problem-solving approaches are more likely to be effective at managing the challenge, and thus preventing stress.

Distraction refers to active efforts to reduce negative emotions (Hunt 2017, Schafer 2017), and can involve attention shifting or thought-stopping. With these strategies, attention is shifted from the thoughts that drive the negative emotion towards thoughts that are more positive. For example, according to a research participant considered resilient to stress, "when something upsetting happens, I try to stop thinking about it and instead I think about something that is positive or interesting" (Hunt 2017). I, also, have found that thought-stopping and immediately substituting a negative with a more positive thought is very effective for training my brain to respond in more adaptive, less negative ways. Indeed, distraction as a coping strategy has been linked to stress resilience and effective emotion regulation in research studies (Hunt 2017).

Mindfulness Awareness Can Improve Emotion Regulation

Being able to regulate emotions first requires being aware of them. This requires awareness of both signals from the body, called interoception, and the conscious experiences of an emotion. Negative emotions, however, are often uncomfortable or painful. Some may impulsively avoid thinking about negative emotions, a form of passive withdrawal. Because negative emotions are typically experienced in the context of challenges, they do need to be confronted, rather than avoided (Schafer 2017).

One effective technique for increasing awareness of emotions that is conducive to addressing and understanding them is called mindful awareness, or mindfulness. Mindfulness is an ancient mind-body practice that focuses on feeling consciously present in the moment, as opposed to being distracted with the past, or preoccupied with the future. One notices what is happening, right now in both the external world (including sights, sounds, events, and other people) and the internal world of the body and mind. External focus may include attending to sights, sounds, smells, sensations, expressions on other people's faces, and other details of the environment. Internal focus may include awareness of breath, emotional response, and/or thoughts and interpretation. Importantly, these experiences are observed in a non-judgmental way. When practicing mindfulness, these experiences are observed and absorbed without a drive to react automatically to the experience. The practice of mindfulness can be used to manage stress in a program called mindfulness-based stress reduction, and in psychotherapeutic applications such as mindfulness-based cognitive therapy. Studies have shown these techniques are helpful for regulating emotions and reducing stress-related symptoms, including anxiety and depression (Keng 2017, Schuman-Olivier 2020). Use of mindfulness-based stress reduction techniques has been associated with reduced inflammation as well. Mindfulness-based training has also been shown to buffer the cortisol responses to stressors, further supporting the idea that learning to modulate emotional responses can mitigate the effects of stress in meaningful ways (Lindsay 2018).

Mindful awareness involves learning to be consciously aware of physical, emotional, and cognitive responses to challenging situations, by noticing them in a calm and non-judgmental way. For instance, one might notice that "I feel angry right now." A key feature of mindful awareness concerns acceptance (Lindsey 2018). Acceptance is a non-judgmental attitude towards emotions being perceived. So, after noticing that I am angry, rather than becoming more immersed in the emotion, suppressing it, or thinking "I shouldn't be angry," with mindful awareness the next thought might be "I wonder why? What just happened that made me feel this way?" In this way, the practice takes some of the emotion out of the emotion. One observes and evaluates the experience rather than getting wrapped up in the response patterns that the emotion or experience triggers. By doing this, it becomes easier to determine whether the emotional response was appropriate, or if there are steps to be taken to avoid or mitigate situations that cause the negative emotions.

Part of mindfulness involves becoming aware of sensations from the body. In this way, mindfulness can support interoception— the sensory system that reports on the condition of the body (Craig 2002, Price 2018). Interoception pathways provide information about pain and inflammation, as well as hunger and satiety. This system will be discussed shortly, but to preview, interoceptive awareness is a measure of the conscious perception of the body, including such things as heart rate. Low interceptive awareness is associated with psychological disturbances, including eating disorders and depression, probably due to the important role of feedback from the body for the perception of emotion (Chapter 5) (Badoud 2017, Eggart 2019). Certainly, being aware of and monitoring signals from the gut, including satiety factors, can help tremendously to rebalance drives for food, and reduce the over-reliance on hedonic eating that is common in Western society and the hallmark of emotional eating. Mindful awareness of emotional states and physiological status (hunger versus satiety) can help interpret bodily signals, such as distinguishing between the sensation of hunger and indigestion, which can seem similar without conscious attention.

The other principal aspect of mindful awareness is a relaxation of the body, and a conscious focus on breathing. This facilitates the adoption of the calm attitude that is necessary to face the experience of difficult, negative emotions, and replace them with more positive ones. Intentional breathing can dial down anxiety, possibly via interoceptive effects on the amygdala. The amygdala is a major player in responses to challenges and stress, and some of its activity contributes to the expression of negative emotions, including fear and anxiety (Gilpin 2015). In addition, mindfulness and interoceptive meditation activate the vagus nerve. Vagus nerve activation can both improve interoceptive awareness and down-regulate inflammation (Zila 2017). In this way, mindful awareness can facilitate the development of emotional resilience: the ability to maintain positive emotions and recover quickly from negative emotional experiences.

Resilient People Work to Keep Situations and Events in Perspective

One reason that regulation of negative emotions is so important is that the perception or fear of stress can induce anxiety and encourage a cognitive/emotional response called catastrophizing. Catastrophizing involves over-focusing on the negative aspects of a situation and extrapolating the worst outcome. When catastrophizing, one may over-interpret the severity of a stressor and respond excessively with amplified physical, emotional, cognitive, and behavioral responses. Not surprisingly, catastrophizing is generally associated with passive coping styles and can lead to chronic negative emotional states. Catastrophizing worsens inflammatory conditions and is the most robust predictor of higher levels of suffering and poor quality of life in chronic pain conditions such as fibromyalgia (Braun 2020, Ellingson 2018). Thus, cognitive appraisal that involves keeping situations in perspective is imperative in managing stress and inflammation. Mindful awareness with acceptance, which focuses on relaxation and positive emotions, can also be helpful.

Resilient People Find Meaning in Life

Many studies investigating resilience have found that people who report having meaning in their lives are more resilient to stress from challenges, such as trauma or chronic illness (Frankl 1959, Ostafin 2020). Although researchers can rarely define meaning in life, one can infer the definition from descriptions of factors associated with meaning, such as spirituality, and activities such as hobbies and volunteering in the community (Ettun 2014). It seems that meaning, for most individuals, is conferred by a feeling that one or one's activities are important, even if only to another person or to a god. Finding meaning in life often involves a connectedness to other people, and a philosophy of life that helps make sense of the relative importance of life events, attitudes, and behaviors.

Finding meaning seems to be especially helpful in situations where the main challenges are not controllable, such as caregiving, terminal disease, or grieving. Indeed, in these cases the challenge become focused on coping. Meaning-focused coping involves a set of strategies that specifically focus on enhancing meaning in life (Folkman 2008). In this manner of coping, one strategy might involve reorganizing priorities to address whatever is most personally important in life.

One positive emotion that is associated with meaning and seems to contribute importantly to resilience is gratitude (Kreitzer 2019, McGuire 2021). Dispositional gratitude is the tendency to be aware of positive outcomes, blessings, or good deeds and to feel grateful. Dispositional gratitude is protective against stress-related disorders such as depression, anxiety, PTSD, suicidality, and substance use disorder (McGuire 2021). People who may not already habitually feel grateful can learn to incorporate a practice of gratitude into their lives. One easy method is the Three Gratitudes exercise. This involves taking time before bedtime to identify three good things that happened during the day and writing them down. The good things can be small, like a tasty meal. While writing them down, think about why the good thing happened and why you feel good about it. Each week, look back over the things written down and notice how you feel about them and if there are any themes. A large study of people facing serious health challenges found that this simple intervention helped reduce their experiences of stress, and the effects were greater with more time spent with the practice (Kreitzer 2019).

Resilient People Maintain Connections with Other People

Social integration, the extent to which we feel connected to other people and society, is associated with better physiological functioning across the lifespan (Cunliffe 2016, Yang 2016). Social relationships can modulate inflammation (Ditzen 2014, Kiecolt-Glaser2010). Relationship deficits are stressors, and loneliness and social exclusion are associated with increased inflammation, and its consequences, including depression, cardiovascular disease, and pain. (KiecoltGlaser 2010, Nersesian 2018).

Socio-economic stress (SES) is similarly deleterious. Unequal societies have higher rates of physical and mental disorders, and neglect or deprivation can lead to epigenetic changes that enhance inflammation and dysregulated stress responses (Williams 2019, Friedman 2019). On the other hand, programs for at-risk youth, parenting training, and other programs that support parents, buffer SES stress on children. Social ties can also help connected communities buffer individuals from society-wide stress (Ditzen 2014). This may be due to the perception that in connected communities there is social support, which has been found to be protective against the deleterious effects of stress (Neergheen 2019). The perception that help is available when needed can reduce the impact of challenges in a community.

What can we do to strengthen or maintain social connectivity? This is a challenge in our current society in which many people move around a lot and/or away from social support from family and established friendships. This challenge is magnified for older people who have retired from working and lose the social interactions they may have had with their jobs. Aging can be associated with loss of mobility, further exacerbating loneliness.

Nonetheless, there are ways of helping establish social bonds. Social media can help connect people who share the same interests, and because it is online, mobility is not an issue. Online connections can be made with people in different geographical areas. For those of us who can get out, joining clubs related to interests, hobbies, or sports can introduce us to people who have the same interests. Many local senior centers offer different types of activities and opportunities to make new friends. For people of faith, joining a congregation can help connect people who share habits and dogma that may supply meaning. Volunteering time and expertise to a charity or other group can both enlarge social circles and help add purpose and meaning to life. In recent years, community musical groups have formed all over the country, offering opportunities to dance, sing or play instruments in choirs, band, or orchestras. Active efforts to establish engaged social networks and connections can improve resilience.

Key Points

- Resilience refers to the ability to confront challenges, even trauma, and be able to heal, move on, and live a happy productive life.
- Resilient people have positive, solution-focused attitudes, and they keep events and situations in perspective. They don't catastrophize. They maintain healthy relationships with other people and have work or other activities that provide meaning to their lives.
- Active coping with challenges can prevent or mitigate the effects of stress.
- Being able to regulate emotions is key to resilience. Mindful awareness practices can help with recognizing emotions as they occur and strengthen mind-body connections that support emotion regulation.
- Many lifestyle choices can help promote resilience. Healthy diet and exercise can help reduce or prevent inflammation.

References

Badoud D, Tsakiris M. From the body's viscera to the body's image: Is there a link between interoception and body image concerns? Neuroscience and Biobehavioral Reviews, 77:237-246, 2017.

Braun A, Evdokimov D, Frank J, Pauli P, Uceyler N, Sommer C. Clustering of fibromyalgia patients: A combination of psychosocial and somatic factors leads to resilient coping in a subgroup of fibromyalgia patients. PLOS One,15: e0243806, 2020.

Craig AD. How do you feel? Interoception: the sense of the physiological condition of the body. Nature Reviews Neuroscience, 3:655-666, 2002.

Cunliffe VT. The epigenetic impacts of social stress: how does social adversity become biologically imbedded? Epigenomics, 8:1653-1669, 2016.

Ditzen B, Heinrichs M. Psychobiology of social support: The social dimension of stress buffering. Restorative Neurology and Neuroscience, 32:149-162, 2014.

Eggart M, Lange A, Binser MJ, Queri S, Muller-Oerlinghausen B. Major depressive disorder is associated with impaired interoceptive accuracy: A systematic review. Brain Sciences, 9:131, 2019.

Ellingson LD, Stegner AJ, Schwabacher IJ, Lindheimer JB, Cook DB. Catastrophizing interferes with cognitive modulation of pain in women with fibromyalgia. Pain Medicine, 19:2408-2422, 2018.

Ettun R, Schultz M, Bar-Sela G. Transforming pain into beauty: On art, healing, and care for the spirit. Evidence-Based Complementary and Alternative Medicine. 2014:789852, 2014.

Frankl V. Man's search for meaning. Beacon Press, 1959/1992.

Friedman E, Shorey C. Inflammation in multimorbidity and disability: An integrative review. Health Psychology, 38:791-801, 2019.

Folkman S. The case for positive emotions in the stress process. Anxiety, Stress and Coping. 21:3-14, 2008.

Gilpin NW, Herman MA, Roberto M. The central amygdala as an integrative hub for anxiety and alcohol use disorders. Biological Psychiatry 77:859-869, 2015.

Hershberger PJ. Prescribing Happiness: Positive psychology and family medicine. Family Medicine 37:630-637, 2005.

Hunt C, Cooper SE, Hartnell MP, Lissek S. Distraction/Suppression and Distress Endurance diminish the extent to which generalized conditioned fear is associated with maladaptive behavioral avoidance. Behavior Research and Therapy. 96:90-105, 2017.

Keng S-L, Tan ELY, Eisenlohr-Moul, Smoski, MJ. Effects of mindfulness, reappraisal, and suppression on sad mood and cognitive resources. Behavior Research and Therapy, 91:33-42, 2017.

Kiecolt-Glaser JK, Close relationships, inflammation, and health. Neuroscience and Biobehavioral Reviews, 35:33-38, 2010.

Kreitzer MJ, Telke S, Hanson L, Leininger B, Evans R. Outcomes of a gratitude practice in an online community of caring. The Journal of Alternative and Complementary Medicine. 25:385-391, 2019.

Kubansky LD, Huffman JC, Boehm JK, Hernandez R, Kim ES, Koga HK, Feig EH, Lyoyd-JonesDM, Seligman MEP, Labarthe DR. Positive psychological well-being and cardiovascular disease. Journal of the American College of Cardiology, 72:1382-1396, 2018.

Lindsay EK, Young S, Smyth JM, Brown KW, Creswell JD. Acceptance lowers stress reactivity: Dismantling mindfulness training in a randomized controlled trial. Psychoneuroendocriniology, 87:63-73, 2018.

McGuire AP, Fogle BM, Trai J, Southwick SM, Pietrzak RH. Dispositional gratitude and mental health in the U.S. veteran population: Results from the National Health and Resilience Veterans Study. Journal of Psychiatry Research. 135:279-288, 2021.

Neergheen VL, Topel M, Van Dyke ME, Sullivan S, Pemu PE, Gibbonds GH, Vaccarino V, Quyyumi AA, Lewis TT. Neighborhood social cohesion is associated with lower levels of interleukin-6 in African American women. Brain, Behavior, and Immunity, 76:28-36, 2019.

Neresesian PV, Han H-R, Yenokyan G, Blumenthal RS, Nolan MT, Hladek MD, Szanton SL. Loneliness in middle age and biomarkers of systemic inflammation: Findings from Midlife in the United States. Social Science Medicine,209:174-181, 2018.

Ostafin BD, Proulx T. Meaning in life and resilience to stressors. Anxiety, Stress, and Coping, 33:603-622, 2020.

Price CJ, Hooven C. Interceptive awareness skills for emotion regulation: Theory and approach to Mindful Awareness in Body-Oriented Therapy (MABT). Frontiers in Psychology, 9:798, 2018.

Schafer JO, Nauman E, Holnes EA, Tuschne-Caffier B, Samson AC. Emotion regulation strategies in depressive and anxiety symptoms in youth: A meta-analytic review. Journal of Youth and Adolescence, 46:261-276, 2017.

Schuman-Olivier Z, Trombka M, Lovas DA, Brewer JA, Vago, Gawande R, Dunne JP, Lazar SW, Loucks EB, Fulwiler C. Mindfulness and behavior change. Harvard Review of Psychiatry, 28:371-394, 2020.

Williams DR, Lawrence JA, Davis BA, Vu C. Understanding how discrimination affects health. Health Services Research, 54:1374-1388, 2019.

Yang YC, Boen C, Gerkin K, Li T, Schorpp K, Harris KM. Social relationships and physiological determinants of longevity across the human life span. Proceedings of the New York Academy of Sciences, 113:578-583, 2016.

Zila I, Mokra D, Kopincova J, Kolomaznik M, Javorka M, Calkovska A. Vagal-immune interactions involved in cholinergic anti-inflammatory pathway. Physiological Research, 66:S139-S145, 2017.

Zwir I, Arnedo J, Del-Val C, Pulkko-Raback L, Konte B, Yang SS et al. Uncovering the complex genetics of human temperament. Molecular Psychiatry, 25:2275-2294, 2020.

CHAPTER 5: INTEROCEPTION: FOOD, EMOTIONS AND THE BODY'S INNER LANGUAGE

- INTEROCEPTION: THE "MATERIAL ME"

- INTEROCEPTION: TURNING UP OR DOWN THE VOLUME OF THE "NEUROSYMPHONY" OF THE BRAIN

- INTEROCEPTION AND EMOTION

- EMOTIONAL MEANINGS OF FOOD

- INTEROCEPTION AND THE "SELF"

- "BEING VERSUS DOING": THE DEFAULT MODE NETWORK AND THE "SELF-BOX"

- INTEROCEPTION, STRESS, AND INFLAMMATION: MIND-BODY LINK

- KEY POINTS

Eating is more than simply acquiring nutrients. What happens in our bodies, and especially our guts, influences our minds, both consciously and unconsciously. Interoception, the sense of the conditions in our bodies, including pain, inflammation, hunger, and satiety, provides this information to our brain. Many of the words and phrases we use to describe our emotions are derived from our experiences of eating. For instance, to express disgust, we might say something like "This makes me want to vomit!" Indeed, the word "disgust" literally means "bad taste." To express the feeling of something enjoyable, we might say that it was "yummy." And we often mention "gut feelings" when making decisions or evaluating situations. These are just a few examples of the ways in which information from the body influences the way that our mind interprets our experiences. Understanding the scope and mechanisms of these mind-body interactions is critical for our ability to make conscientious decisions about what we eat, and thereby take control of how we feel.

Interoception: The "Material Me"

"As humans, we perceive feelings from our bodies that relate our state of well-being, our energy and stress levels, our mood and disposition. How do we have these feelings? What neural processes do they represent? Recent functional anatomical work has detailed an afferent neural system in primates and in humans that represents all aspects of the physiological condition of the physical body. This system constitutes a representation of 'the material me', and might provide a foundation for subjective feelings, emotion and self-awareness." A.D "Bud" Craig, 2002 (Craig 2002)

In the years since Bud Craig published this delineation of the concept of interoception, it has become clear that the sensory system that monitors the internal milieu plays fundamental roles in maintaining the health of the body and in managing the body's response to both physiological and psychological challenges. It is also clear that this system profoundly influences functions associated with the mind, notably cognition, memory, and emotion.

The connections between mind and body are carried out principally by nerves of the autonomic nervous system (ANS), in which the vagus nerve seems to play a particularly important role. Originally, interoception was classified as only concerning visceral organs, such as the heart, lung, and gastrointestinal tract. However, it is clear that nervous system pathways that carry the signals about potentially damaging, nociceptive, conditions that typically evoke the experience of pain from the entire body are organized more like visceral pathways, rather than the exteroceptive pathways that carry sensory information from the environment to the body, such as touch, vision and hearing. Nociceptive nerves and viscerosensory nerves are sensitive to inflammation, and they influence mood and behavior. Thus, they are considered together to form the sensory modality of interoception.

Interoceptive information enters the nervous system via a direct-to-cortex primary sensory pathway via the spinal cord and brainstem. Signals from this pathway propagate through the thalamus to terminate in the insula, which constitutes the primary interoceptive cortex (Craig 2002, Quadt 2018). This pathway seems to contribute to conscious awareness of internal bodily sensations, including the experience of pain, breath, and heartbeat (Pace-Schott 2019). After interoceptive information enters the brainstem, it also branches off into several indirect pathways. These pathways target brain regions controlling responses to physiological perturbations and external challenges. These pathways influence arousal systems that use the neuromodulators serotonin, norepinephrine, and acetylcholine, as well as the hypothalamus, which regulates metabolism and influences cardiovascular functions (Gaykema 2011). Interoceptive information also drives activity in brain structures associated with the limbic midline/medial networks associated with emotions and memory, including the amygdala, hippocampus, medial temporal lobe, cingulate cortex, and medial prefrontal cortex (Pace-Schott 2019, Quadt 2019). In this way, interoceptive information is distributed throughout the brain and influences nearly every aspect of experience.

Compared to other sensory modalities, interoceptive signals such as pain, hunger, or thirst are hard to ignore. In addition to its role as the primary cortical region that specifically processes interoceptive information, the insula is a key node in the Salience Network. Thus, interoceptive information is wired to be preferentially treated as important. The prefrontal cortex also is strongly influenced by interoceptive information, and it plays a critical role in coordinating functions of different regions and networks, functioning rather like an orchestra conductor. The frontal lobes decide what we pay attention to, and in what behaviors we do or don't engage. Interoception particularly influences orbito- and medial prefrontal cortex (OMPFC) regions that are critical for motivation, decision-making, and emotion (Rich 2018, Seabrook 2020). Interestingly, much of OMPFC activity is concerned with eating behavior and all aspects of the quality of food (taste, smell, appearance, desirability, etc.), underlining how important food is for both physical and psychological motivation. With such a strong influence on the insula and frontal cortex, it is not surprising that food plays such an outsized role in our psychological and social functions.

Finally, although interoceptive information is usually transmitted via the peripheral nervous system, endocrine signals also interact with interoceptive nerves and/or brain regions, such as the hypothalamus and hippocampus, that integrate interoceptive information. One example is leptin, which is produced by adipose tissue and released into the circulation to reach the brain, where it informs the hypothalamus regarding body fat content (adiposity). Another example is the gut hormone ghrelin, which enhances appetite. In this way, hormone and other endocrine signals can influence signaling through these interoceptive pathways and their many targets.

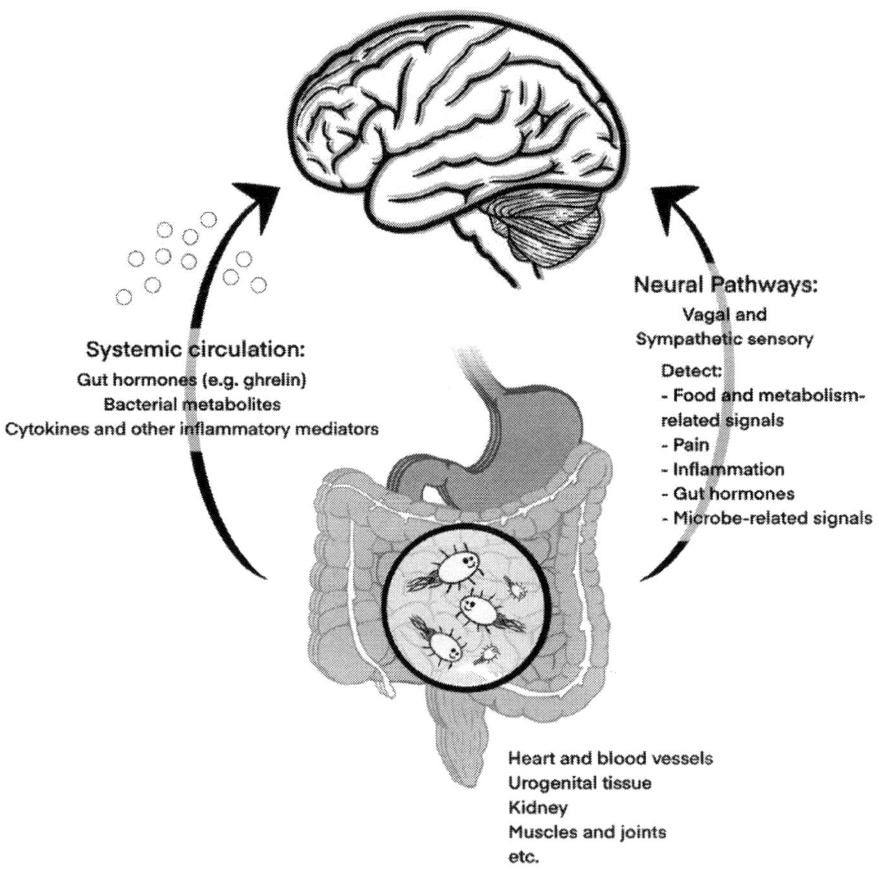

Figure Legend: Information about the state of our gut and other organs is sent to the brain both directly through neurons and indirectly via chemical signals in the blood stream.

Interoception: Turning Up or Down the Volume of the "Neurosymphony" of the Brain

From the foregoing, it is clear that interoception contributes to the regulation of emotions and behavior. However, unlike the other classic sensory systems of vision, taste, smell, light touch, and hearing, much of interoception is unconscious. So how does interoception exert its influences? Using the orchestra analogy, one may consider these interoceptive signals about the condition of the body as either turning up or turning down the volume of the ongoing "neurosymphony." Interoceptive signals are making the brain-music that is associated with positive or negative emotions, motivation, and thoughts either louder or softer. For instance, hunger or the early phases of a meal release the gut hormone ghrelin, which acts on brain pathways such as the mesolimbic dopamine pathways, whose activity gives rise to increased motivation to eat and think about food (Kroemer 2012). In this way, we are made aware of our hunger, as this interoceptive signal amplifies the volume of neural music associated with eating and overwhelms the sounds of other ongoing activities.

In contrast, many interoceptive signals associated with inflammation seem to turn down the volume on activity associated with memory and cognition, and motivation for rewards. This lowered volume can make it difficult to get it together to do anything. This lowered motivation, and poor memory and cognition are some of the core features of sickness behavior. Sickness behavior follows in part from bottom-up interoceptive pathways inhibiting the activity of the brain's arousal systems (Gaykema 2011, Felger 2017, Felger 2016). The brainstem arousal systems, which act to coordinate activity throughout the brain, function rather like the percussion section in an orchestra in that they set the tempo or pace of brain activities (Venkatraman 2017). At the same time, sickness behavior turns the volume up on activity associated with negative emotions through pathways involving the amygdala, insula, anterior cingulate cortex, medial prefrontal cortex, and others. This can lead to the experience of suffering or depression. When these experiences get loud, they can drown out any other activity, becoming the dominant experience.

Interoception and Emotion

Much of the information relayed by interoceptive channels is used to regulate physiology and behaviors, such as eating and escape from threats, that support homeostasis (Simmons 2017). These signals regulate physiology to maintain optimum conditions in the body. But interoception is also important for what we can think of as emotional homeostasis as well. Indeed, both the regulation of emotions and impaired interoception are characteristic of many psychological disturbances, including mood disorders, autism, schizophrenia, and eating disorders (Donofrey 2016, Khalsa 2018, Sliz 2012).

Why should emotions be so tied up with homeostasis? Homeostasis requires not only physiological adjustments, but behavioral responses as well (Strigo 2016). We need to be motivated to look for food and finding food must be rewarding so that we will keep doing it. To avoid damage, we need to avoid predators and other dangerous situations, and the emotions of fear and pain provide the motivation for escape.

Whereas it is intuitive to think that our emotions are generated and perceived by the brain, in fact perception of emotion occurs as a kind of brain-body-brain loop (James 1884, Bechara 2000, Pace-Schott 2019). When the brain perceives a situation that should be associated with emotion, it activates the ANS to produce bodily sensations associated with that emotion such as "butterflies" in the stomach,, tingling skin, tears, or a lump in the throat. These bodily sensations in turn are conveyed to the brain via interoception, where they are interpreted as emotion. When interoceptive pathways are deficient, or the interoceptive information is not properly used by the brain, we are not able to perceive our emotions adequately or infer the emotions of others (Quigley 2021, Hubner 2021). This can lead to difficulty in regulating our emotions, and in maintaining positive relationships with other people. Perhaps surprisingly, impaired interoception also leads to poor decision-making (Bechara 2000). This is probably because emotion is the most important factor driving decisions and choices (Bechara 2000). Emotions have substantial consequences for behavior and social relationships, and effective emotion regulation is central to making good decisions about eating and diet.

Emotional Meanings of Food

Unlike most other animals, we humans do not need to spend our entire lives acquiring necessary nutrients and can spend our time in other activities. Even so, many of those other activities involve food. Food is more than just necessary nutrients. Indeed, our earliest experience of safety, learning that our needs will be met, and the contentment of satiety is when we nurse as newborns, establishing a deeply rooted connection between food and positive emotions.

Eating, and the kind of foods we eat, forms a basis for many of our social interactions. What we commonly eat is an expression of who we are in our communities (Johnston 2012). Many religious faiths have strict rules about what food can, and cannot be eaten, and how that food should be prepared. Food is prominent in many religious and non-religious holidays as well. We use food as an expression of how much we care about other people. We give chocolate as a gift, prepare meals for the grieving, treat friends to lunch or dinner or a home-cooked meal. Many social occasions focus on food as a way to attract people, such as wine and cheese parties, food festivals, or pizza-fueled meetings. In this way food serves as the social glue that binds our human communities.

Commonalties between dietary preference and political views suggest that choice of food is an extension of our personalities (Pfeiler 2018). Preferences for food can make us consciously, or unconsciously, identify with groups of people who have the same preferences, and can be associated with prejudiced attitudes towards people who eat a different diet (Earle 2017). In this way, our choice of diet can be extension of our identity. Unfortunately, an identification with a certain type of diet with personality and self can be a daunting barrier to developing conscientious eating habits if that diet is not a healthy one.

Interoception and the "Self"

It has been noted that a "coherent relationship with self" is critical to emotion regulation, and emotion regulation is critical to making good decisions about food (Price 2018, Swan 2018). As pointed out previously, many studies now indicate that interoceptive cues are critical to emotion regulation and our sense of self (Quigley 2021). This is important because a strong sense of self predicts healthy psychological functioning and resilience to stress (Koban 2021).

However, trying to understand what exactly the "self" is can be challenging, both empirically in studies and conceptually (Frewen 2020, Wozniak 2018). Neuroimaging studies consider the "self" as slippery, because the activation patterns that you observe in the brain depend on what self-related task you are studying (Frewen 2020). Social psychologists have argued that the self does not really exist, because personality inventories can vary depending on when people are tested. Some strains of Buddhism posit the same thought. Nonetheless, most people feel like they do have a self. But what exactly is a self? Certainly, it is a feeling that we are separate from other people, but it also seems to involve qualitative things like our memories and opinions, and even diagnoses ("I am a depressive person"). This kind of conceptualization can become a barrier to psychological growth because it can make learning different ways to manage challenges seem inauthentic or impossible. Similarly, healing from traumatic or stressful experiences, negative attitudes, or loneliness can be challenging to address when these experiences are believed to contribute to or define one's self.

My favorite conceptualization of the self was put forth by a student in a Developmental Psychology class I once taught. She argued that the self is not our memories, opinions, and emotions, but rather the self is like a box that holds all those things. The "self-box" constructs the boundaries between us, the outside world, and other people. It holds all the opinions, preferences, memories, habits. and other experiences that we associate with our own originality. These contents of the self-box can change, but there is a continuity of identity and self-awareness such that we always feel like we are the same person, even if our values and opinions are different than they were 20 years ago. In this way, we can make choices about what we want in our self-box and realize that everything in there is a choice. For example, if one is a person who relies on food to treat emotional hurts ("I am an emotional eater"), one can reconceptualize this to: "Eating is one of the tools I keep in my self-box that I use to manage stress." They can then decide to either keep it or throw it out and replace it with another kind of tool for managing stress. In this way, thinking of ourselves as more than just the collection of our habits and emotions can make it more possible to change both our attitudes and diets.

"Being versus Doing": The Default Mode Network and the "Self-Box"

Whereas the concept of self-box can be useful for thinking about the self and its relationship to behavior and decision-making, is there a basis in neurological reality for it? In fact, the Default Mode Network (DMN) seems to contribute importantly to features of the self. The DMN is a collection of brain regions that are most active when we are resting or daydreaming, rather than when we are engaging in specific tasks or behaviors (Reikle 2015). It is active when we are "being" rather than "doing". The DMN defines the physical and cognitive boundaries, as well as the perception of the emotional self and coordinates many of the functions that could be attributed to a self-box (Koban 2021).

What we know about the neurological basis of the self derives from neuroimaging studies of activation, or increased blood flow, in specific brain regions of people, who are imaged while at rest, or while being asked to think about some aspect of themselves. Resting state connectivity studies assess the extent to which such activated brain regions function as a network. Changes in resting state connectivity may reflect how well the regions are working together. Using the orchestra analogy, activation implies that a specific region is contributing actively to the music, whereas connectivity indicates how well sections are playing together. If the network exhibits low connectivity, the music will not sound coherent or coordinated. If connectivity is too high, it may be that the network is over-focused on itself and ignoring other players. For a clinical example, major depressive disorder is often associated with reduced activity in medial prefrontal regions that form part of the anterior DMN, while overall connectivity of the network is increased (Reikle 2015). The increased connectivity is thought to underlie a preoccupation with self and negative emotions, and this increased connectivity may contribute to the resistance of the depressed brain to engage in other activities that could alleviate the depression. In contrast, in Alzheimer's disease, which is characterized by memory loss and a disorganized sense of self, resting state connectivity of the DMN is reduced (Chabran 2020). In this way, maintaining an optimal connectivity in the DMN seems critical for maintaining a sense of self that can be flexible enough to respond to challenges.

The DMN is organized generally into two sub-networks: the posterior DMN and the anterior DMN. Core regions of the posterior DMN include the posterior cingulate cortex, precuneus, medial temporal lobe, hippocampus, and temporal-parietal junction. Together they seem to coordinate perceptions of our physical boundaries, autobiographical memories, self-referential cognition, and social cognition (Yeshurun 2021). In contrast, the anterior DMN includes the medial prefrontal, anterior cingulate, and orbitofrontal cortices, which seem to construct our emotional selves, attach value to rewards, and make decisions (Zhang 2019). Together, the components of the DMN construct an awareness of ourselves as continuous, separate, individual beings capable of interacting with the non-self-world. Reduced connectivity between components of the DMN is associated with lack of self-awareness and reduced sensitivity to interoceptive cues from the body, as well as reduced sensitivity to rewarding effects of drugs (Zhang 2019). Conceptually, this lack of connectivity could result in a weak or leaky self-box, with a reduced awareness of personal boundaries or feelings of satiety, and a feeling of emptiness. Notably, reduced connectivity within components of the DMN has been reported in substance use disorders, autism, depression, and borderline personality disorder, all conditions with disturbances in social functioning and self (Zhang 2019, Nair, 2020, Soares 2017, Quattrini 2019).

Importantly, interoception is a key driver of activity in both the posterior and anterior DMN. The insula, considered to be the primary interoceptive cortex and thus the major direct target of signals from bodily tissues, has been demonstrated by neuroanatomical and functional neuroimaging studies to be closely linked to both nodes of the DMN. Electrical stimulation of the vagus can improve DMN connectivity implying that interoceptive information influence the ability of DMN to function well (Liu 2020). These findings provide a mechanistic rationale for mind-body modalities or interventions that engage interoceptive pathways in the treatment of emotional conditions that are associated with impaired functioning of self. An example of such a mind-body modality is vagus nerve stimulation for treatment of depression.

Mind-body modalities such as mindfulness, meditation, massage, and yoga operate through interoceptive pathways, and have been used for millennia to address mood and other psychological conditions. A key component of many of these techniques involve control of breath, one of the interoceptive sensations that is easy to consciously perceive (Weng 2021). Breath control engages the parasympathetic nervous system while modulating sympathetic function, which seems to balance the relationship between the two branches of the autonomic nervous system (Weng 2021). Notably, stress-related disorders including PTSD, depression, and anxiety are often associated with imbalance in autonomic function, typically overactivity in the sympathetic nervous system. Thus, modalities that involve breath control, such as mindfulness, yoga, and exercise have shown great promise in ameliorating mood problems and stress (Price 2018, Weng 2021).

Interoception, Stress and Inflammation: A Mind-Body Link

The influence of interoception goes beyond mental health and emotion. The ventromedial prefrontal cortex, a key component of the anterior DMN and target of interoceptive pathways, is sometimes called the visceromotor cortex. While the ventromedial prefrontal cortex (PFC) receives information from much of the rest of the frontal lobe, its output is principally to the brain regions that control bodily functions via the autonomic and neuroendocrine systems (e.g., amygdala, hypothalamus, brainstem). Key targets include the HPA axis and the immune system. Using these connections, the ventromedial PFC, and thus the DMN/self-box, directs the brain's control over bodily functions. This forms a bi-directional link between mind and body and is crucial for regulating inflammation (Koban 2021, Lopez 2018).

This arrangement implies that that what is going on in the body, such as inflammation and/or pain, can impact mental states via interoception. In turn, interoception can either positively or negatively impact inflammation, pain, and even social behavior (Eisenberger 2017). For instance, negative emotions can drive inflammation and set up a loop that increases suffering, negative emotion, pain, and so on. On the other hand, positive attitudes, active coping styles, a supportive social network, and meaningful activities and hobbies are all associated with less chronic disease, and better prognosis for disease. A strong self and optimally connected DMN support a resilient lifestyle and contribute to a longer, happier life (Koban 2021). In this way, interoceptive pathways provide the mechanistic link between what is happening in our minds and what is happening in our bodies.

Key Points

- Interoception is the sense of the condition of our bodies. This sense contributes not only to helping the brain control physiological processes that maintain health and homeostasis, but also influences our motivation, feeling of reward, and emotion.
- Interoception also contributes to our sense of self. A healthy sense of self enables good decision-making, resilience in stressful situations, healthy social relationships, and maintenance of positive attitudes.
- Interoception is a key indicator of how we feel.
- What we eat is an expression of who we are in our society, and influences our emotions, motivation, and social interactions. What we eat also affects conditions in our bodies. Interoception provides the information from the body through which food can influence the mind.

References

Bechara A, Damasio H, Damasio AR. Emotion, decision making and the orbitofrontal cortex. Cerebral Cortex, 10:295-307, 2000.

Chabran E, Noblet V, Louriero de Sousa P, Demuynck C, Philippi N, Mutter C, Anthony P, Martin-Hunyani C, Cretin B, Blanc F. Changes in gray matter volume and functional connectivity in dementia with Lewy bodies compared to Alzheimer's disease and normal aging: implications for fluctuations. Alzheimer's Research and Therapy, 12:6, 2020.

Craig AD. How do you feel? Interoception: the sense of the physiological condition of the body. Nature Reviews Neuroscience, 3:655-666, 2002.

Donofry SD, Roecklein KA, Wildes JE, Miller MA, Erickson KI. Alterations in emotion generation and regulation neurocircuitry in depression and eating disorders: A comparative review of structural and functional neuroimaging studies. Neuroscience and Biobehavioral Reviews, 68:911-927, 2016.

Earle M, Hodson G. What's your beef with vegetarians? Predicting anti-vegetarian prejudice from pro-beef attitudes across cultures. Personality and Individual Differences, 119:52-55, 2017.

Eisenberger NI, Moieni M, Inagaki TK, Muscatelli KA, Irwin MR. In sickness and in health: The co-regulation of inflammation and social behavior. Neuropsychopharmacology, 42:242-253, 2017.

Felger JC, Li Z, Haroon E, Woolwine BJ, Young MY, Hu X, Miller AH. Inflammation is associated with decreased functional connectivity within corticostriatal reward circuitry in depression. Molecular Psychiatry, 21:1358-1365, 2016.

Felger JC, Treadway MT. Inflammation effects on motivation and motor activity: role of dopamine. Neuropsychopharmacology Reviews, 42:216-241, 2017.

Frewen P, Schroeter ML, Riva G, Cipresso P, Fairfield B, Padula C, Kemp AH, Palaniyappan L, et al. Neuroimaging the consciousness of self: Review, and conceptual-methodological framework. Neuroscience and Biobehavioral Reviews, 112:164-212, 2020.

Gaykema RP, Goehler LE. Ascending caudal medullary catecholamine pathways drive sickness-induced deficits in exploratory behavior: brain substrates for fatigue? Brain, Behavior and Immunity, 25:43-460, 2011.

Hubner AM, Trempler I, Gietmann C, Schobotz RI. Interoceptive sensibility predicts the ability to infer others' emotional states. PLoS ONE, 16:e0258089, 2021.

James W. What is an emotion? Mind, 9:188-205, 1884.

Johnston L, Longhurst R. Embodied geographies of food, belonging and hope in multicultural Hamilton, Aotearoa New Zealand. Geoforum, 43:325-331, 2012.

Khalsa SS, Adolphs R, Cameron OG, Critchley HD, Davenport PW, Feinstein JS, Feusner JD, et al. Interoception and mental health, a roadmap. Biological Psychiatry: Cognitive Neuroscience and neuroimaging, 3:501-513, 2018.

Kroemer NB, Krebs L, Grimm O, Pilhatsch M, Bidlingmaier M, Zimmerman US, Smolka MN. Fasting levels of ghrelin covary with the brain response to food pictures. Addiction Biology, 18:855:862, 2012.

Koban J, Gianaros PJ, Kober H, Wager TD. The self in context: brain systems linking mental and physical health. Nature Reviews Neuroscience, 22:309-322, 2021.

Liu C-H, Yang M-H, Zhang G-Z, Wang X-X. Li B, Li M, Woelfer M, Walter M, Wang L. Neural networks and the anti-inflammatory effect of vagus nerve stimulation in depression. Journal of Neuroinflammation, 17:54, 2020.

Lopez RB, Denny BT, Fagundes CP. Neural mechanisms of emotion regulation and their role in endocrine and immune functioning: A review with implications for treatment of affective disorders. Neuroscience and Biobehavioral Reviews, 95:508-514, 2018.

Nair A, Jolliffe M, Lograsso YSS, Bearden CE. A review of Default Mode Connectivity and its association with social cognition in adolescents with Autism Spectrum Disorder and Early-Onset Psychosis. Frontiers in Psychiatry, 11:614, 2020.

Pace-Schott EF, Amole MC, Aue T, Balconi M, Bylsma LM, Critchley H, Demaree HA, Friedman BH et al. Physiological feelings. Neuroscience and Biobehavioral Reviews, 103:267-304, 2019.

Pfeiler TM, Egloff B. Examining the "Veggie" personality: Results from a representative German sample. Appetite, 120:246-255, 2018.

Price CJ, Hooven C. Interoceptive awareness skills for emotion regulation: Theory and approach of mindful awareness in body-oriented therapy (MABT). Frontiers in Psychology, 9:798, 2018.

Quattrini G, Pini L, Pievani M, Magni LR, Lanfredi M, Ferrari C et al. Abnormalities in functional connectivity in borderline personality disorder: Correlations with metacognition and emotion dysregulation. Psychiatry Research Neuroimaging, 283:188-124, 2019.

Quadt L, Critchley HI, Garfinkel SN. The neurobiology of interoception in health and disease. Annals of the New York Academy of Sciences, 1428:112-128, 2018.

Quigley KS, Kaonoski S, Grill WM, Feldman Barret L, Tsakiris M. Functions of interoception: From energy regulation to the experience of the self. Trends in Neuroscience, 44:29-38, 2021.

Raichle ME, The brain's default mode network. Annual Review of Neuroscience, 38:433-447, 2015.

Rich EL, Stoll FM, Rudebek PH. Linking dynamic patterns of activity in orbitofrontal cortex with decision making. Current Opinions in Neurobiology. 49:24-32, 2018.

Seabrook LT, Borgland SL. The orbitofrontal cortex, food intake and obesity. Journal of Psychiatry and Neuroscience, 45:304-312, 2020.

Simmons WK, DeVille DC. Interoceptive Contributions to Healthy Eating and Obesity. Current Opinion in Psychology, 17:106-112, 2017.

Soares JM, Marques P, Magalhaes R, Santos NC, Sousa N. The association between stress and mood across the adult lifespan on default mode network. Brain Structure and Function, 222:101-112, 2017.

Sliz D, Hayley S. Major Depressive Disorder and alterations in insular cortical activity: a review of current functional magnetic imaging research. Frontiers in Human Neuroscience, 6:323, 2012.

Strigo IA, Craig AD. Interoception, homeostatic emotions and sympathovagal balance. Philosophical Transactions of the Royal Society B 371:20160010, 2016.

Swan E, Bouwman L, Aarts N, Rosen L, Hiddink GJ, Koelen M. Food stories: Unraveling the mechanisms underlying healthful eating. Appetite, 120:456-463, 2018.

Venkatraman A, Edlow BL, Immordino-Yang MH. The brainstem in emotion: A review. Frontiers In Neuroanatomy, 11:15, 2017.

Weng HY, Feldman JL, Leggio LL, Napadow V, Park J, Price CJ. Interventions and manipulations of interoception. Trends in Neurosciences, 44:52-62, 2021.

Wozniak M. "I" and "Me": The self in the context of consciousness. Frontiers in Psychology, 9:1656, 2018.

Yeshurun Y, Nguyen M, Hasson U. The default mode network: where the idiosyncratic self meets the shared social world. Nature Reviews Neuroscience, 22:181-192, 2021.

Zhang R, Volkow ND. Brain default-mode network dysfunction in addiction. Neuroimage, 200:313-331, 2019.

- THE BRAIN IN PERSONS WITH OBESITY

- WHY ARE PSYCHOSOCIAL STRESSORS SUCH A RISK FOR OBESITY?

- ABUSE AS QUINTESSENTIAL "SOCIAL SELF" STRESSOR

- BEING POOR PREDISPOSES TO OVERWEIGHT AND OBESITY

- THE SPECIAL CHALLENGE OF MINORITY STATUS

- SHAME AND FAT STIGMA

- STRESS, VISCERAL FAT, AND INFLAMMATION SET UP THE VICIOUS CYCLE

- HOW DOES INFLAMMATORY FAT CONTRIBUTE TO HOW WE FEEL?

- BODY WEIGHT IS "DEFENDED"

- IMPROVING INTEROCEPTIVE AWARENESS AND STRESS EFFECTS ON EATING: MINDFUL AND INTUITIVE EATING

- FURTHER ISSUES THAT STILL NEED TO BE ADDRESSED

- KEY POINTS

At the intersection of stress, Western diet, and inflammation, we find obesity. Obesity is usually defined as having a body mass index (BMI) value of 30 kg/m^2 or higher. Sixty percent of Americans are overweight, defined as having BMI of 25 kg/m^2 or higher, or obese. Worldwide, 650 million people are obese, and rates appear to be increasing (Chung 2019). Obesity is directly associated with much higher risk of a variety of other dangerous chronic disease conditions, including diabetes, metabolic syndrome, Alzheimer's disease, mood disorders, osteoarthritis, and chronic pain (Wang 2017).

Why are so many people overweight or obese? At the most basic level, overweight/obesity occurs because too many calories are taken in. The body stores the extra calories as fat in adipose tissue, leading to an excess in body fat mass (Schwartz 2017). This is a very important survival strategy because throughout human history, sources of food have been unreliable due to famine, drought, or insect infestation. When food access is unreliable, it is highly adaptive to store energy when food is plentiful to protect against starvation when it is not.

Access to food became much easier for most humans in the second half of the twentieth century. Food production became industrialized, leading to easy availability of cheap food. Food science developed methods of processing food to make it more rewarding, shifting decision-making about what and how much to eat to favor cravings over nutritional need. Advertising has further optimized methods of triggering food cravings and driving consumption, encouraging people to eat for reasons far afield from nutritional hunger. More career opportunities for women, and economic changes that often require both parents to be employed, have made it difficult for many families to prepare healthy meals and control family food access. This has led to the proliferation of fast food, which while palatable and convenient, is usually high-energy and calorie-rich, but not necessarily nutritious. This shift to processed, fast-food comprises what is called the Western diet.

Calorie expenditure depends on metabolic rate, diet, and activity levels, with genetic and epigenetic, lifestyle, cultural, economic, and stress-related factors moderating these relationships (Reddon 2018). Gut microbe populations additionally contribute to how food is absorbed, and thus alter risk for obesity (Martinez 2017, Reddon 2018). While there is currently intense focus on lifestyle factors, including amount of exercise, or quality and quantity of food choices, studies report that 40-75% of variability in body weight is due to genetic factors (Reddon 2018). A key question is: How do these genetic factors influence the development and maintenance of obesity?

Research is still needed to fully answer this question. To date, only a few genes have been linked to obesity, accounting for a relatively small contribution to variability in body weight. Nonetheless, characterizing the function of these obesity-related genes has emphasized the complex nature of weight regulation and the close relationships among eating behaviors, stress, and inflammation. Many genes considered to contribute to obesity are involved in the regulation of metabolism and eating behavior (Goodazi 2018). These effects involve the hypothalamus, a brain region deeply involved in regulation of not only appetite, but also adrenal cortisol release. Notably, some genes linked to obesity are involved in the regulation of cortisol receptors and inflammation (van der Valk 2018, Zhu 2020, Hotamisligil 2017). This is potentially important because cortisol receptors regulate both metabolism and brain responses to challenges. Obesity has been associated with disrupted regulation of cortisol receptors (van der Valk 2018). Disrupted cortisol receptor regulation is common in mood and behavior disorders and is a key feature of developmental programming following Adverse Childhood Experiences (ACE). This suggests that part of the genetic contribution to obesity may be related to epigenetic effects associated with stress or inflammation. Taken together, these findings support the idea that some genetic components of obesity are related to regulation of inflammation and metabolism in the context of stress.

Interestingly, some genes linked to obesity are also associated with tendencies toward particular lifestyle choices, such as how active we are, preferences for high-energy foods (such as fats and sweets), how fast we eat, and our tendencies to overeat in response to stress (Reddon 2018). Thus, the factors that influence lifestyle choices may be more complex than previously assumed, and the relationships between genetic predisposition, environment, and behavior are closely intertwined.

The Brain in Persons with Obesity

Neuroimaging studies of people with obesity provide insight into factors that drive overeating and illustrate the complexity of responses to food. To review, interoceptive information related to metabolic status is relayed to brain regions, including the amygdala, insula, and part of the prefrontal cortex, all of which contribute to the Salience Network (SN). The SN determines the relative importance of information to ongoing behaviors. Interoceptive information also contributes to the activity of reward pathways that control motivation, and to Default Mode Network (DMN) areas such as medial prefrontal cortex, which integrate emotional and self-referential responses to food. Finally, the Executive Control Network (ECN) integrates all this with decision-making related to what and whether to eat.

In the context of obesity, neuroimaging studies verify that activity in the ECN is weaker in the context of palatable food (Donofrey 2020, Gluck 2017). This reduced activity impairs the ability to make sensible decisions, especially in the face of choices that while harmful overall or in the longer term, also provide immediate reward (Donofrey 2020, Farr 2016). Additionally, people with obesity have been reported to have SN function, particularly activity in the insula, that seems over-focused on hunger signals (Borowitz 2020, Ding 2020). Simultaneously, medial pre-frontal cortical regions that are central to the DMN and which regulate emotions and impulsivity, are less able to modulate the influence of reward, leading to increased motivation to consume the high-energy sweets and fats typical of the Western diet (Donofry 2020).

Thus, overeating occurs due to a dysregulation of the interoceptive, bottom-up signals related to hunger and satiety in the context of impaired top-down, or executive, decision-making regarding what and how much to eat (Seabrook 2020, Schwartz 2017, Simmons 2017, Ding 2020). In neurosymphony terms, it seems that the volume is turned up on interoceptive drive related to hunger, food-related cues, and reward pathways, while the volume is turned down on cognitive functions related to decision-making. Although the observations are not surprising, they suggest important targets or strategies for addressing regulation of appetite to address overeating and weight control. For instance, awareness of the imbalance in the salience of interoceptive cues related to hunger and satiety (such that hunger is perceived as more important) may help control the emotional drive to eat. In other words, if one can recognize that the intensity of hunger feelings may not accurately reflect the need for food, one may enable to gain cognitive control over emotional eating. These findings underline the importance of regulating emotions for managing appetite.

The pattern of brain responses to food in obese people exhibit similarities to brain activity during stress, suggesting that chronic stress may play a role in the development of obesity. Resting-state connectivity in the DMN has been reported to be increased in both chronic stress and obesity, which may reflect preoccupation with stress, emotions, and sense of self (Soares 2017). Whereas not all obese people report feeling stressed, studies have indicated that in general, obese children and adults report more symptoms of stress than lean people (Tomiyama 2019). However, most neuroimaging studies that assess eating behavior in obese people do not assess stress, so the contribution of stress to differences in eating behavior and overeating are still hypothetical. Nonetheless, given the overlap between brain networks that contribute to challenge responses and those that mediate goal-directed behaviors, such as eating and reward, it is hard to imagine that stress is not a critical factor in the overeating that leads to obesity.

Although many people engage in stress-eating from time to time, this can become a problem for people who experience chronic stress, as the unmet challenges continue to drive appetite and impair regulation of drives and emotion (Cotter 2018). Not all challenges/stressors, however, are equally associated with appetite and weight. Rather, the kinds of challenges that increase cortisol are most closely linked to obesity and metabolic disorders, at least in part due to the pivotal role of cortisol in regulating metabolism, and during challenges in particular. What kind of stressors are linked to cortisol?

Why are Psychosocial Stressors such a Risk for Obesity?

While acute challenges activate both the sympathetic nervous system and HPA axis, evidence exists of some specificity in stress response. This specificity is informed by emotional states, such that the HPA axis, with cortisol as its principal endpoint, is most reactive to social stresses (Dickerson 2004). In particular, social stresses that impact the *social self*, such as threats to social esteem, status, acceptance, and shame, produce greater increases in cortisol (Dickerson 2004). Compared to other challenges/stressors, social and evaluative stress most effectively recruits, and then dysregulates, the HPA axis (Dickerson 2004, Tomiyama 2014). Thus, because cortisol is a principal link between challenge, stress, and metabolism, threats to the social self can carry outsize risks for obesity.

Chronic psychosocial stress is associated with disrupted regulation of HPA axis function. Indeed, Trier Social Stress Test studies, comparing responses between obese and normal-weight people to a social evaluative task, show that obese individuals have blunted cortisol responses, particularly among obese people who report social stress or stigma (Heraus 2018). This could be indicative of a long-term adaptation to chronic stress (Jung 2020). Endocrine disruption is a major factor in the development of the serious health consequences of obesity, such as type 2 diabetes and metabolic syndrome. In addition, implications of dysregulated cortisol also include increases in inflammation, which is a principal pathophysiological feature of metabolic diseases. Whereas negative emotions in general modulate responses to stress, shame seems particularly linked to inflammation (Dickerson 2004).

What is the link between threats to the social self, cortisol, and inflammation? A principal neurological link operates most likely through the medial prefrontal cortex (PFC). In particular, the ventromedial PFC (vmPFC), which is part of the DMN, serves as a controlling neuroendocrine and autonomic nervous system link that contributes to social behavior, mood control, and motivational drive, all of which are important components of an individual's personality (Reichle 2015). The output of the vmPFC provides drive on the HPA axis, thus informing the HPA axis of the state of the self and emotional functioning. The dorsomedial PFC (dmPFC), adjacent to the vmPFC and functionally coupled to it, processes self-referential mental activity. The medial prefrontal cortex constitutes a major node in the DMN, one that becomes impaired in the context of chronic stress and obesity. In this way, a "damaged self-box" may be less able to regulate emotional response to food, and based on neuroimaging studies, be vulnerable to increased drive from reward systems that can compensate for negative emotions. Within the context of a dysregulated HPA axis, this could predispose one to eat for comfort, leading to increased fat storage and development of obesity.

Abuse as a Quintessential "Social Self" Stressor

The relationships between stress, the "social self," and weight are seen clearly in the context of physical, emotional, or sexual abuse, in both children and adults. These types of stressors fundamentally threaten or damage a person's feeling of self-worth and may be accompanied by feelings of guilt for "deserving" the abuse (Ross 2009). At the same time, problems with eating, food, and weight are very common among survivors of abuse (Davies 2016, Bartlett 2018). Moreover, the severity of the problems correlates with the severity of abuse (Hemingsson 2014, Alhalal 2018).

Whereas experience of any kind of abuse raises the risks for obesity and disordered eating, sex abuse, especially incest is associated with both shame and increased inflammation (Smith 2010, Bertone-Johnson 2012). Although most research has focused on children and adolescents, unwanted sexual experiences in adulthood are also associated with eating disorders and elevated weight. Both male and female military service members are at risk for sex abuse, and higher rates of obesity and disordered eating occur among service members who experienced sex abuse compared to those who did not (Morris 2013, Pandey 2018). These effects seem to be independent from combat stress or PTSD, which are also associated with obesity.

Relationships with intimate partners are particularly emotionally salient. Physical and/or psychological and emotional abuse is linked to increases BMI and obesity (Davies 2016). For example, the experience of intimate partner violence by young women predicted weight gain over five years, implying that these experiences may have significant implications for weight over a lifetime, with associated risks for negative health-related consequences. Intimate partner violence is particularly problematic for people who also have Adverse Childhood Experiences (ACE). These experiences already increase risk for obesity and metabolic disorders, and further abuse during adulthood leads to markedly higher BMI, as well as depression and PTSD (Alhalal 2018).

The mechanistic connections among abuse, food and weight are complex, multilayered, and poorly understood. However, they clearly involve intertwined psychological, neurological, endocrine, and metabolic components. High-energy, palatable comfort foods might soothe or compensate for the loss of nurturing experiences in those affected by childhood physical and emotional abuse. For sex abuse survivors, weight gain is theorized to serve as a protective buffer between self and the outside world, by making the body "unattractive" (Ross 2009).

Abuse survivors with disordered eating or weight problems often report feeling spiritually empty, with an "empty hole" in their abdomen or chest (Ross 2009). This location implies an interoceptive hole, and that overeating, or eating comfort food, may be an attempt to fill the perceived emptiness.

Sensations of food in the gut provide interoceptive drive on reward pathways and the anterior DMN, which may temporarily alleviate negative emotions and "fill the hole." This idea is supported by findings showing that vagus nerve stimulation tempers anterior DMN responses to trauma-related images in people who had previously experienced trauma, but who do not have PTSD (Wittbrodt 2020). The vagus nerve is the principal interoceptive nerve linked to the gut and is activated by food. This finding that vagal stimulation can correct brain activity related to trauma response, potentially links food consumption to improved neurologic response to emotion.

For abuse survivors, feelings of emptiness are often accompanied by disordered or negative sense of self. Survivors may report that "I don't know myself anymore" or "I feel like an object not a person" (Lanius 2020). This damaged sense of self likely contributes to disordered eating and the mood disorders that commonly accompany history of abuse. Abnormal functioning of the anterior DMN is common in ACE, trauma, and Major Depressive Disorder (Smith 2010). Importantly, stimulation of the vagus nerve seems to increase anterior DMN connectivity in people with depression, thereby reducing depression symptom severity (Fang 2016). These findings support the idea that stress-eating may serve as a way for survivors to improve or temporarily strengthen their emotional sense of self. Although stress-eating is deleterious in the long term, recognizing the role of interoception and the vagus nerve in strengthening a positive sense self could lead to effective treatment approaches for survivors of abuse and trauma. Promising interventions include noninvasive direct vagus nerve stimulation and mind-body modalities such as meditation, yoga, and massage, which can also improve vagus nerve function.

The link between history of abuse and impaired function of the anterior DMN likely provides an important mechanism by which emotional states are linked to obesity and health risks. Because the DMN links emotional states with autonomic and neuroendocrine (e.g., cortisol) function, the feelings of shame that are associated with abuse can drive dysregulation of the HPA axis and metabolic regulation. Indeed, in a sample of obese Black women who had experienced childhood violence/sex abuse, weight was only partly explained by health behaviors such as use of food in response to stress (Boynton-Jarrett, 2012) This suggests endocrine adaptions (e.g., cortisol system) can lead to increased fat storage and inflammation as a consequence of stress in childhood (Morais 2019). Stress may also directly induce insulin resistance, which could serve to increase appetite. Further, the dysregulation of cortisol receptors can also link obesity with inflammatory conditions, increasing likelihood of metabolic syndrome, irritable bowel syndrome, and mood disorders (Wiley 2016).

The effects of child abuse carry profound implications for lifelong social and emotional functioning. The maturation of the DMN is associated with the development of self-referential cognition and self-image, and is dependent upon social interactions, especially with parents during childhood and adolescence (Rebello 2019). Disordered relationships with caregivers can lead to impaired development of DMN connectivity, with implications for strength of self (self-box) and for increased risk of mood and other psychiatric disorders, pain conditions, and increased inflammation that follow from impaired DMN functioning. In this way, the intertwining of stress with metabolic programming towards obesity sets the stage for the vicious cycle of stress, poor diet, inflammation, and adverse health consequences.

Being Poor Predisposes to Overweight and Obesity

One paradox of obesity, which is assumed to follow from over-eating, is that low-income people are more likely to be obese than the general population (Richardson 2015). Indeed, food insecurity, defined as lack of availability or access to healthy food because of insufficient financial resources, is closely linked to obesity in developed countries, especially among women (Hernandez 2017, Van der velde 2018). One obvious explanation for this situation is that poor communities tend to be *obesogenic environments* (Sinha 2013). Many low-income rural and inner-city areas lack access to nutritious food, a condition referred to as a *food desert*. In food deserts, available food is typically low in nutritional value, highly processed, and calorie-dense. Furthermore, economic stress is linked to social stress, in that being relatively poor is associated with having lower social status. Barriers to eating healthfully may be insurmountable when one is poor or lives in an obesogenic environment. The inability to eat healthfully despite intent can lead not only to poor health consequent to diet, but also a damaged sense of self and self-efficacy. This experience of lack of control can further contribute to dysregulation of HPA axis function and elevated inflammation.

The link between severe obesity and stress among low-income women in the US seems to be somewhat independent from eating behaviors, again suggesting that the biological (e.g., cortisol) effects of stress on metabolism or lifestyle are important (Richardson 2015). The mechanisms may be similar to those that increase risk of obesity consequent to abuse. This suggests a mind-body interaction such that "the more you worry about food availability, the fatter you get." Since the purpose of stored fat in adipose tissue is to provide energy in case of food shortages, economic insecurity may drive psychological and endocrine processes that favor storage of fuel (Dhurandhar 2016). Socioeconomic stress may drive more fuel storage as an adaption to meet the challenges of unsecure, unsafe environments.

The Special Challenge of Minority Status

The most pernicious stressors in our society stem from social and economic disparities experienced by minority populations. Persons with minority status are more likely to have low-wage jobs, live in unsafe neighborhoods (e.g., higher crime rates or in polluted environments), and suffer stigma and discrimination. All of these can represent threats to the social self, and thus it is not surprising that people of color in the United States suffer from overweight and obesity, as well as the consequent diabetes, cardiometabolic syndrome, and hypertension at much higher rates than do Whites (Cuevas 2020, Wang 2018).

Social context is likely the most important contributor to racial differences in obesity, as opposed to physiological differences associated with ethnicity or race (Bleich 2010). Using a national dataset, a study compared Black and White obesity rates and health conditions in a low-income integrated neighborhood, where everyone was the same SES. In contrast to the national data set where racial differences were observed, no racial disparities in weight were found in the low-income integrated neighborhood. Thus, the findings support the idea that health disparities follow from social environmental factors. When social environmental factors are the same, racial differences in weight do not occur. Adverse social or environmental conditions may act as threats to the social self and predispose towards dysregulated HPA axis function and inflammation, and thus higher disease loads.

A complexity, however, concerns the different relationships of weight and SES between White and Black women (Ciciurkaite 2021). SES accounts for much of the differences in rates of obesity across populations of White women, among whom higher SES is associated with lower weight. In contrast, Black women with higher SES tend to weigh more than those at lower SES.

The reasons for this difference are not established but might conceivably relate to the unique stressors associated with minority status that are not improved by higher SES (Ciciurkaite 2021). For instance, many women struggle with workplace stress, especially family-work conflict, which could be accentuated in the context of minority status. There are also differences in cultural attitudes towards weight among Black and White women, such that higher weights are viewed more negatively among White women than Black women, and thus Black women may be less motivated to worry about their weight (Circiurkaite 2021). But given the fact that obesity is associated with co-occurring conditions that influence both the mind and body (e.g., cardiometabolic disease, mood disorders) and that people with minority status suffer at higher rates from these co-occurring conditions, barriers to achieving healthy weight need to be addressed.

Shame and Fat Stigma

In addition to the physiological consequences of weight, overweight and obese people face additional challenges related to their weight (Hilbert 2015, Tomiyama, 2014, 2019). *Weight stigma* describes the experience of being discriminated against, shunned, or bullied due to being overweight or obese. Weight stigma may be the most common type of stigma, and is prevalent in all aspects of our society, from the media to interpersonal relationships and even healthcare (Tomiyama 2014). This has serious practical implications for overweight or obese people in that weight stigma can impair career advancement, influence hiring, promotion, and firing, and reduce access to education, especially for women (Tomiyama 2019). Because minority populations are more likely to be overweight or obese, they experience additional stigma (Cuevas 2020). In addition to the effects of stress on the development of obesity, the experience of obesity itself can be stressful. Indeed, because stigma is an overt expression of disapproval, it can be thought of as a "poster child" for social-self stressors. Discriminatory attitudes and experiences with other people can lead to internalized negative stereotypes, or *self-stigma*, which markedly impairs quality of life, affecting mood and behavior (Hilbert 2015). Further, this self-shame increases risks for elevated inflammation and its consequences. For example, perceived weight discrimination is associated with atherosclerosis, diabetes, myocardial infarction and other heart conditions, gastric ulcers, and arthritis (Udo 2016).

In addition to the risk of serious physical health conditions, the psychological and behavioral consequences of weight stigma are considerable. Weight-related abuse and stigma is associated with disordered eating, especially binge eating. Weight stigma can encourage passive coping such as *weight-related experiential avoidance*, associated with unhealthy eating behavior and weight (Palmeira 2018). Unfortunately, weight stigma actually reduces the likelihood that someone will lose weight and can even contribute to further weight gain (Tomiyama 2019, Vartanian 2016). Social stress and shame, especially, have been reported to be linked to increased eating. For instance, experimental social exclusion, typically simulated in studies of people who believe they are playing a cooperative computer game, leads to increased cookie-eating after the session. Thus, inducing social stress can increase eating (Vartanian 2016). For children, the shame and bullying that can be associated with weight carries particularly dangerous implications, as they are associated with lifetime risks of disordered eating and other weight-related issues. Girls who were teased about their weight were more likely to gain weight or engage in disordered eating, especially bulimia, stress-eating, and restrictive eating (Vartanian 2016). These same effects can occur in boys.

The stress associated with stigma has worrisome physiological consequences. For instance, experiments inducing weight stigma increase cortisol levels in subjects who self-identified as heavy, even if they had a normal BMI. This suggests that weight stigma is so pervasive in our society that even people who are normal weight are susceptible to it. These experiments demonstrate the direct link between social stressors and cortisol reactivity. Perceived weight stigma by people who are overweight or obese is associated with elevated levels of cortisol and indicators of oxidative stress, increasing the risk for inflammation and chronic disease (Tomiyama 2014). Notably, although abdominal obesity, which as we will see accounts for much of the inflammation associated with obesity, was associated with higher cortisol and oxidative stress, this effect was accentuated among people who experienced weight stigma.

Given the effects of cortisol on appetite and fat storage, these findings provide a mechanistic link between weight stigma and increasing weight gain. Together this science reinforces the importance of addressing weight stigma in our society.

More women are overweight than men, and thus may experience more fat stigma (Circiurkaite 2021). Higher rates of overweight in women may stem from endocrine differences, in that estrogens tend to favor deposition of fat. As described above, women may also experience additional social stress given social and economic inequities in current American society. Among the genetic and environmental factors that drive the development of obesity, stress is a more important influence for women than for men (Cotter 2018). The basis for this difference has not been established, but given that cultural perceptions of beauty in women tend to focus on body weight, media images of female body types that are considered beautiful may have an impact on self-image for women who do not fit the ideal. In this way, body image and weight can be more relevant to social selves of women than men. Certainly, self-esteem seems to be linked to body weight more for women than for men (Weinberger 2016).

Nonetheless, both women and men experience fat stigma, and internalized stigma is associated with depression and disordered eating in men as well as women. Men who report fat stigma also report worse self-rated health that could not be accounted for by BMI or behaviors such as smoking or drinking (Himmelstein 2019). Thus, the experience of fat stigma exerts profound effects on how overweight or obese men feel.

Stress, Visceral Fat, and Inflammation Set Up the Vicious Cycle

Evidence shows that societal disparities and social stigmas impact health, in part, via effects on eating and obesity, which lead to concomitant inflammation. Some of the elevated inflammation likely follows from consumption of high energy/low-nutrition Western diet foods, as we shall see. But the combined effects of overeating with social stress-induced dysregulation of the cortisol system also drives the accumulation of pro-inflammatory fat.

Fat is an organ that functions to store fuel and release hormones *(adipokines* such as leptin) that control metabolism and influence appetite. Under certain circumstances fat can drive inflammation. Fat exists in two compartments: subcutaneous and visceral. Subcutaneous fat is found under the skin; visceral fat exists within the connective tissue around visceral organs, or on organs in the abdominal cavity. Visceral fat is sometimes called *abdominal fat*. The two compartments seem to serve different functions. Subcutaneous fat mostly stores lipid as an energy reserve in case of food shortage or illness. Visceral fat is more metabolically active, in that it releases fatty acids and very low-density lipoproteins (VLDL) into the circulation (Neeland 2020, Trim 2021, Uranga 2019). Some of these lipids are pro-inflammatory. For this reason, visceral fat is considered the more significant contribution to the increased risk of obesity co-morbidities, such as hyperlipidemia, atherosclerosis, and metabolic syndrome.

While the adaptive function of subcutaneous fat in storing energy substrates seems intuitively obvious, the normal role of visceral fat is less clear. Subcutaneous fat contains mostly adipocytes (fat cells), but up to 40% of the cells in visceral fat are pro-inflammatory immune cells. These immune cells release adipokines that contribute to low-grade systemic inflammation (Grant 2015, Trim 2012). Adipokines are cell-signaling molecules, or cytokines, given a special name when released by non-adipose tissue immune cells. But why does visceral fat contain so many immune cells? One possibility is that the normal role of visceral fat is to support immune function of the gut and serve as a reservoir for immune cells in case of infection.

In the context of over-nutrition/obesity, however, the fat tissue becomes overgrown. This overgrowth may exceed the vasculature's ability to supply it, and sections of the fat can become anoxic (Grant 2015, Neeland 2020). Anoxic fat releases damage signals, which further drives inflammation, as we will see in the next section (Grant 2015). In this way, the already inflamed state of fat increases inflammation. These inflammatory mediators (adipokines) induce inflammation in other tissues when released into the circulation. Such inflammation may occur in the pancreas and liver. Indeed, visceral adipose tissue is closely linked to the development of non-alcoholic fatty liver disease. Non-alcoholic fatty liver disease is currently the most common liver condition in the United States. One of the consequences of inflammation is to induce resistance to the hormone insulin, leading to further metabolic dysregulation (Petersen 2018). Obesity is a risk factor for immune dysregulation, including serious life-threatening response to infection, such as the *cytokine storm* sometimes seen in COVID-19 infection. It is thought that the already elevated and probably dysregulated inflammation is a major contributor to this increased risk (Butler 2020). Visceral adipose tissue has been specifically linked to severe Covid-19 (Petersen 2018, Deng 2020).

What predisposes to the growth of pro-inflammatory visceral fat? In general, the amount of visceral adipose tissue is correlated with the level of adiposity overall, such that with greater BMI there is more visceral fat (Agbim 2019). On the other hand, based initially on observations of people with Cushing's disease, in whom overproduction of cortisol is associated with marked expansion of visceral adipose tissue, chronic psychosocial stress leading to dysregulation of the HPA axis is an important contributor. Indeed, people with chronic stress are more likely to have increased visceral fat, possibly as a function of overeating combined with increased cortisol levels or dysregulation of the cortisol system (Lee 2018). Further, chronic stress along with impulsive risk-taking is also associated with increased visceral fat (Mason 2018). Impulsive risk taking itself is an indicator of impaired interoception linked to difficulty making healthy food choices. Thus, chronic stress is linked to visceral adiposity via multiple mechanisms.

Given the link between visceral adiposity and adverse health outcomes, it is important to note that the amount of visceral fat at a given BMI varies among ethnic groups. That is, at the same BMI, people of Asian or Hispanic/LatinX descent have greater amounts of visceral fat than do Black/African American, White/European American, or Native/Indigenous/Aboriginal Americans (Agbim 2019, Lear 2007). These differences imply that people of Asian or Hispanic/Latin background may need to be screened for visceral adipose tissue at lower BMIs. They may experience increased health risks at lower body weights. Nonetheless, even though some groups of people are vulnerable to excess visceral fat, all will develop excess visceral fat with excessive weight gain.

Overall, whereas obesity *per se* may not lead to metabolic disorders, a poor diet combined with chronic stress can lead to excess visceral fat, and thus inflammation. Ethnic differences can moderate the tendency to produce excess visceral fat. Because substantial, chronic stress is associated with both poor diet and increased weight, it should not be surprising that people of color and/or poverty have higher rates of chronic metabolic and cardio-metabolic disease.

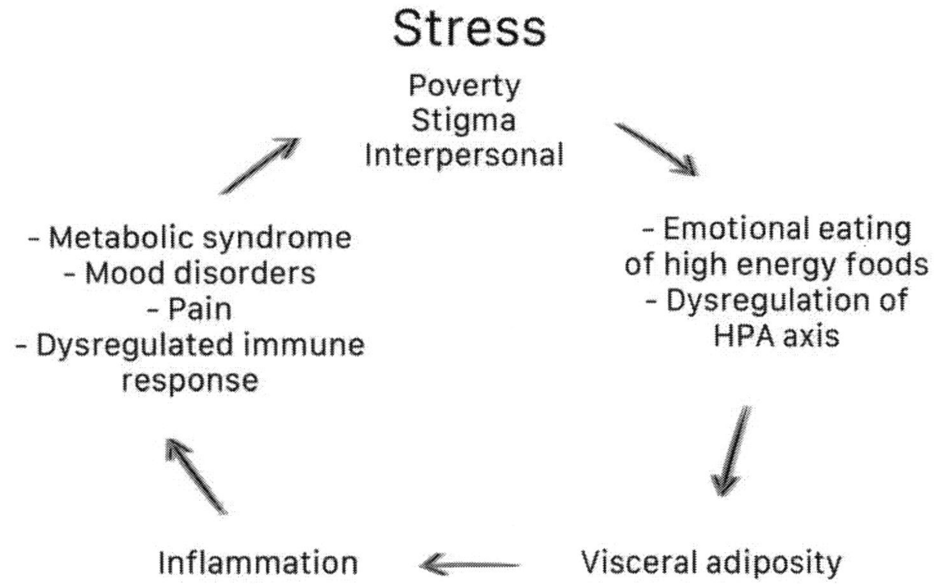

Figure Legend: Stress can encourage emotional eating of junk foods and changes in metabolic regulation that contribute to development of belly fat. This visceral fat contributes to inflammation, which increases risk of metabolic, mood, pain, and immune disorders. These illnesses may themselves cause stress, encouraging worsening of this cycle. Changing how we respond to stress and how we eat can help break this cycle.

How Does Inflammatory Fat Contribute to How We Feel?

An alarming consequence of socio-economic and social-self stress is an increase in *deaths of despair*: suicide, drug overdoses, and mortality from preventable diseases due to the stress and heavy reliance on Western diet foods that drive obesity and inflammation (Stokes 2020, Christ 2018, Jena 2018, Wieckowska-Gacek 2021). As we will see in upcoming chapters, inflammation is also closely linked with pain and mood disorders, and especially depression. Current trends of increasing pain and suicide, along with self-reported reductions in mental and physical health, track with trends of increasing weight (Stokes 2020).

Obesity is strongly associated with chronic pain, which can lead to functional limitation, depression, anxiety, and suicide (Stokes 2020). Indeed, it has been suggested that obesity trends may be driving recent increases in chronic pain. Both pain and obesity have increased concomitantly from the 1990s to 2016. Among middle-aged Americans, rates of chronic pain have increased from 17% to 28% in women and 13% to 22% in men, while rates of being overweight or obese have increased from 71-83% in women and 61-

75% in men. Further, the severity of reported pain correlates with increased weight (Shiri 2010, Stokes 2020). It is important to note that relationships between weight and pain are likely to be complex. For example, stress associated with pain may increase motivation for high-energy *mood foods* that contribute to both weight gain and inflammation, which can drive further pain.

Not all fat contributes to low grade inflammation and thus directly to pain. But extra weight can increase wear and tear on joints, such as the knees and spine, leading to osteoarthritis, inflammation, and pain (Moroni 2020). Indeed, both overweight and obesity increase the risk of experiencing low back pain, and the risk increases with increasing weight (Shiri 2010). The impact of obesity on musculoskeletal conditions, including osteoarthritis, can lead to loss of ability to work, impaired quality of life, and the need for help, including home care in older adults (Corica 2015).

Weight-related inflammation can exacerbate other chronic pain conditions such as fibromyalgia. Fibromyalgia is a chronic pain condition characterized by low-grade inflammation, mood, fatigue, and cognitive problems, and is highly co-morbid with obesity (Gota 2015. Pagliai 2020, Coskun Benliday 2019, Ursini 2011). Although weight loss does help reduce inflammation and improve fibromyalgia symptoms, pain can be a barrier to life-style modifications that can help reduce weight (Pagliai 2020, Narouz 2015, Kaleth 2018). Further, extra weight may make fatigue associated with fibromyalgia worse, and weight-associated inflammation can increase symptoms of pain, mood, and cognitive fuzziness.

Like obesity and pain, depression and obesity seem to have a bi-directional relationship, in that suffering from depression raises risks for obesity, and being obese raises risks for depression (Marazziti 2014, Milaneschi 2019). Severe obesity especially increases risk for depression (Milaneschi 2019). Dysregulation of the HPA axis is common in both conditions, as well as inflammation and measures of oxidative stress (Marazziti 2014). Notably, the links between depression and obesity are stronger in the context of abdominal/visceral adiposity. Inflammation contributes to mechanisms of insulin resistance, and brain insulin resistance has been associated with depression (Petersen 2018, Hamer 2019). Taken together, these observations are consistent with a mechanistic role for inflammation in linking obesity, and particularly visceral obesity, with depression. Further, interoceptive networks in brain that link eating behavior to emotion also respond to inflammation, integrating mood, stress, nutritional status, and immune function. Unfortunately, consumption of high-energy Western diet foods such as sweets and fats is common among people with depression, perhaps because of their convenience and rewarding properties (Marazziti 2014). These low-nutrition foods can ultimately worsen symptoms, and the emotional rewards of certain high-energy food, especially sweet foods, may render them difficult to give up.

Body Weight is "Defended"

Given that the risks of obesity are widely known, and indeed stigmatized, why are obesity rates rising? Even people who succeed at weight loss often find it difficult to keep the weight off. As many of us know too well, temporary and drastic calorie reduction does not usually lead to longer-term lower weight (Uranga, 2019) Only around 20% of people who lose significant amounts of weight are able to maintain that loss. Rather, once we spend some time at an elevated weight, the body seems to decide that it is the "new normal" and defends the new weight. This new normal is sometimes called a *set point* or *settling point*. Although this phenomenon is well-documented, the details of the mechanisms that underlie it are not established (Schwartz 2017). In general terms, however, defense of body weight set point is achieved by increasing appetite and by reducing metabolic rate and caloric expenditure, making us more efficient and more likely to store extra calories (Melby 2017).

As weight drops below the set/settling point, appetite increases. This is in part because ghrelin levels rise, increasing drive for foods, and especially high-energy foods. Notably, stress can also increase ghrelin, further complicating motivation to reduce food intake. In addition, part of the defense of the higher weight may involve the dysregulation of the hormone leptin (Izquierdo 2019). Leptin is made in fat cells and provides a signal related to metabolic status of these cells. In general, the higher the fat content and volume of food ingested, the more leptin will be released by fat cells. Conversely, if food is restricted for 2 or 3 days, such as during a diet, leptin levels fall drastically (Woods 2016). Leptin acts to decrease appetite, so it serves as a homeostatic brake on how much food we eat. Leptin levels drop when dieting, thus releasing the hormonal brake on appetite just when we need it most. This may be one of the ways that the body defends weight, even if that weight is at a higher level than is healthy. Further, in obesity, when there are chronically high levels of leptin, the leptin receptors can become resistant, analogous to insulin resistance in Type 2 diabetes, and glucocorticoid resistance in chronic stress. The loss of leptin's appetite-limiting effect leaves the obese person with one less restraint on their appetite. Overall, dieting and stress are associated with increased appetite, and dieting and obesity are associated with loss of a functional brake on appetite.

One recent finding in the factors driving overweight and obesity involves gut microbes. Obese people exhibit different gut microbe populations than lean people. Interestingly, when one reduces body weight, for instance after bariatric surgery, populations of microbes change dramatically, and this change is hypothesized to contribute to the beneficial effects of weight loss and bariatric surgery on measures of metabolism, such as glucose sensitivity (Meijnikman 2018). The most important determinant of microbe population identity is diet (Meijnikman 2018). Diets containing a variety of foods, especially fresh vegetables, fruits and whole/intact grains support a healthy, diverse population of microbes. The Western diet is associated with a much lower diversity of microbes. Low diversity in microbe populations is linked to a wide variety of disease conditions, including metabolic syndrome (Asnicar 2021). Importantly, a recent study linked diet and microbial composition to visceral fat specifically, which could also provide a connection between diet, visceral fat, and inflammation (Asnicar 2021). This is issue is discussed in more detail in Chapter 17.

As yet, the relationship between gut microbes and weight is a developing area of research, but there are several possible, and perhaps interacting, ways by which microbes could affect weight. One possibility is that some microbe species contribute to the obese condition, possibly by increasing the ability of our body to absorb food (Meijnikman 2018). In addition, microbes, probably via substances they release and by their interactions with the immune system, interact with the interoceptive pathways that influence our mood, cognition, and stress responses. Stress may modify microbe populations as well, by affecting diet and immune function. Because diet is the single most important factor in the composition of gut microbe populations, these findings provide a potential additional link between diet, weight, inflammation, and challenges to losing weight.

Finally, social environments can conspire to make it hard to adopt the behavior changes needed to support weight loss. Living in a food desert makes it that much harder to stick to a healthy diet. Media images don't help. Our natural tendencies to use food to regulate emotions, such as stress eating, are encouraged by advertisements, sometimes directly, for example, with the slogan "Milky Way—Comfort in every bite!" (Tomiyama 2019).

Improving Interoceptive Awareness and Stress Effects on Eating: Mindful and Intuitive Eating

Although losing weight and keeping it off is a serious challenge, it is worth doing.

Weight loss can reduce inflammation and stress, the risk of arthritis and back pain, fibromyalgia, and depression, as well as social stigma associated with weight (Moroni 2020, Pagliai 2020, Milaneschi 2019, Narouza 2015). However, any efficacious weight loss strategy needs to address the intertwining of neurological, physiological, psychosocial, and societal factors. Thus, controlling appetite requires achieving a balance between habit systems driving cravings for rewarding food and interoceptive systems detecting cues related to energy or nutritional needs and satiety.

What perceived cues are most important for stopping eating? Satiety factors reduce motivation for food and can be subtle. If food quickly is eaten quickly, or for hedonic or emotional reasons, we may find ourselves relying on the feeling of being overfull or stuffed as the critical signal that our drive to eat has been satisfied. But that stuffed feeling is supposed to be the gut's emergency signal, a last chance attempt to get us to stop eating. The small intestine secretes satiety hormones, such as cholecystokinin, serotonin, and GLP1 that let us know that if we are still eating, we should stop now. Unfortunately, it can take 20-30 minutes for ingested food to get to the small intestine to activate these satiety factors. If we are eating fast, we can get a lot of food down in that time. Thus, a key to eating an appropriate amount of food in a meal is slowing down and paying attention to these gut factors that signal when the gut thinks we have had enough.

But what about when that stuffed feeling is the goal? Feeling stuffed can be associated with safety or positive experiences, such as feasts, holidays, or social meals. The close relationship of eating, interoception, and emotion means that stress, including lifetime stress, can compromise attempts to regulate appetite. Failures in regulating appetite can lead to self-stigma and shame, which can increase stress and inflammation, further compromising attempts to regulate appetite. Thus, successful appetite management needs to include active awareness of one's personal emotional interpretations of food.

From the foregoing, it is evident that approaches to manage appetite and maintain a healthy weight need to address regulation of emotions and promote resilience to stress, in addition to enhancing interoceptive awareness of meal-related cues from the gut. Mindfulness or acceptance interventions, which are helpful for many stress-related conditions, target improving interoceptive awareness and promote non-judgmental observation of emotions as a way to help regulate them. Can *mindful eating*, or a similar approach called *intuitive eating,* help overcome barriers to adopting a healthy diet and maintaining healthy stable weight?

Mindful eating applies mindfulness principles such as non-judgmental awareness to the experience of eating (Dunn 2018, Warren 2017, Mason 2016). This involves actively noticing sensory and emotional features of food, as well as the emotional context of the meal. Is the food crunchy, salty, tangy, or sweet? Is it pleasurable or boring? Am I eating because I am hungry, or because I feel unrewarded, stressed, or empty? This process takes several seconds, so it can effectively slow down a meal, and may also relieve emotional pressure to fill up fast. Part of the awareness includes being mindful of the gut factors that can serve to support satiety. By paying attention to the sensory and rewarding aspects of the food, *mindful eating* also can help satisfy the cognitive factors and cravings that so often drive overeating. In this way, *mindful eating* can provide a sense of control regarding eating that translates to eating less. *Intuitive eating*, while similar to *mindful eating*, specifically involves rejection of diets, or labelling foods as bad (Cadena-Schlam 2015). The emphasis is on rejecting external influences that may induce negative emotions, and instead working with own's mind and body to establish healthy eating patterns. People following *intuitive eating* are encouraged to honor their hunger, and to experience satisfaction with foods. Both *mindful* and *intuitive eating* focus on internal awareness of food-related cues. Thus, the overall objectives of these two approaches are to help improve awareness of interoceptive signals and regulate emotional aspects of eating.

From personal experience of practicing mindful eating, I have found that paying close attention to what I eat encourages me to choose high-quality, colorful antioxidant foods. These foods turn out to be extremely healthful, as we will learn later. These foods turn out to be more rewarding and interesting to eat compared to the typical high-energy habit foods such as potato chips, white pasta, and plain mashed potatoes that are often preferred during stress. It is worth noting that the first bite of food is the most rewarding. Knowing this while paying attention to tastiness can help encourage eating smaller amounts of things like brownies, that while delicious, are not particularly nutritious. In this way, mindful eating exploits both gut factors and head factors to facilitate healthy food choices.

Over the course of several months of practicing mindful eating, I lost at least 40 pounds, without dieting or feeling deprived. In fact, I felt and continue to feel that I was enjoying food much more than previously. Like many lifestyle changes, however, old habits can creep back into one's life. After several years, I regained 20 pounds, at which point I had to interrogate myself as to which emotional factors were contributing to being less mindful about food. I noticed that I probably do have a Salience Network that is oversensitive to hunger signals, which may have resulted from a long history of food insecurity. I realized I need to think about my actual level of hunger, and any emotional triggers that might drive my appetite or a need to indulge. Indulging for me is, for instance, a larger portion of food because it is palatable, or an extra glass of wine, and I need to be aware of a tendency to allow occasional indulgences to become habits. After becoming more mindful, I have lost 10 of those pounds. Thus, over 8 years I have maintained a weight loss of about 30 pounds, or nearly 20% of my body weight.

From these experiences I can say that mindful eating is a safe and effective way to lose appreciable amounts of weight and keep it off. It leads to a slow and realistic weight loss. I will never be thin again but am able to eat a healthy diet and remain in the lower end of the overweight category. While I still struggle with internalized weight stigma, I find the mindfulness approach does help manage negative emotions and self-criticism. There are not many clinical trials of mindful eating reported, but early studies support my experience that slowing meals down does lead to greater awareness and appreciation of food, perception of interoceptive signals related to food, and a greater feeling of control over eating (Warren 2017). In addition, mindful and intuitive eating approaches can help prevent binge eating, reduce cravings and weight, and prevent weight gain (Dunn 2018, Warren 2017, Fuentas Artiles 2019).

Importantly, mindful and intuitive eating approaches provide a framework for addressing lifestyle and emotional factors that contribute to over-eating. The emphasis on self-compassion and rejection of external negative messages can help reduce self-stigma, shame, self-criticism, and promote resilience (Palmiera 2019, Hilbert 2015). Indeed, in studies of mindful and intuitive eating, participants report less depression, pain, stress, and anxiety, concomitant with success with weight loss.

Finally, mindful eating can improve awareness of longstanding eating habits. For instance, anecdotal accounts indicate that mindful eating may be particularly helpful for overweight or obese men. Many men establish eating habits when they are teenagers, which usually involves a growth spurt and a dramatic increase in appetite. I remember when my brother was a teenager, we had no leftovers in the house. Ever. He ate everything. If that pattern is carried into adulthood, the resulting weight gain can lead to serious health risks such as cardiometabolic syndrome. Mindful eating can help increase awareness of excessive food intake, spurring weight loss. Indeed, as one woman told me, "Mindful eating saved my partner's life."

Further Issues That Still Need To Be Addressed

Whereas recent progress in understanding the complexities of food, emotion, and weight is heartening, several important issues remain. For instance, what is a healthy weight? The general rule is that a BMI of less than 25 is normal weight, but this may be difficult to achieve or maintain for people with a history of obesity. Thus, specific target weights may need to be individualized to ensure adequate nutrition for people whose bodies may tend to defend higher weights.

Unfortunately, modern diet guidelines do not necessarily address individual differences in needs for macronutrients such as carbohydrates (Teichotz 2019). Guidelines can be critical and dismissive of ethnic cuisines, while ignoring the cultural impacts of foods (Krishna 2020). Components of some regional American diets, such as the Southern diet of sugary foods and processed meats, may indeed predispose to disease, but emotional attachments and social pressure may make such foods difficult to give up. Ethnic or traditional diets typically are based on whole foods, such as greens, spices, grains and beans, or wild-caught fish (such as the Okinawan diet of Japan or rural African diets) and can be shaped to support nutrition as well as cultural and emotional needs. Given the impact of obesity on communities of color, it seems imperative to provide diet guidelines and advice that are culturally sensitive.

Finally, the rates of overweight and obesity among children are alarming, given the fact that overweight children almost always grow up to be overweight or obese adults, with corresponding lifetime risks for type 2 diabetes, metabolic syndrome, mood disorders, and other inflammation-related conditions (Lee, 2018, Deal 2021). Currently there are neither well-developed resources nor a clear evidence base for interventions for weight-related problems in children and adolescents. For instance, there is some evidence that mindfulness interventions may help teenagers, but interventions may need to be tailored to overcome barriers to their adoption or use (Omiwole 2019). On the other hand, gardening and cooking programs can improve diets for children and adolescents, possibly by enhancing resilience and self-efficacy (Ruiz 2020). An additional advantage of such programs is that they can provide a basis for healthful lifestyle habits.

Key Points

- The increase in obesity rates observed over the last several decades has occurred for several different reasons, including changes in the quality of our food, and changes in society that have led to increased stress and weakened social ties.
- In the context of obesity, brain networks that control appetite and emotion become weakened in the presence of palatable, immediately rewarding foods, making it harder to control impulsivity and make good decisions about what to eat and when.
- Food and hunger seem to exert particularly strong influences on the brain's Salience Network. This means that food can be hard to ignore, and bottom-up signals of hunger are given particular attention compared to other interoceptive signals or factors that normally control food intake.
- Because a major objective of the challenge response is to provide sufficient metabolic fuels for managing challenges, the stress of unmet challenges can increase the drive for high-energy comfort foods.
- Stress can bias food preferences towards high-energy Western diet foods and impair normal restraints on appetite, and is therefore a very important risk factor for the development of overweight and obesity.
- Social stress, such as stigma, minority status, and poverty, is a pernicious type of stress that is most closely linked to overweight and obesity.
- Unlike most other tissues, overgrown fat tissue releases signals that produce pro-inflammatory responses, increasing inflammation in other tissues, and contributing to chronic pain and mood disorders.
- Obesity is associated with increased risk of cardiovascular and metabolic disease. Carrying excess weight also challenges joints, increasing the risk of osteoarthritis which can lead mobility impairments later in life.
- One surprising way that high-energy Western diet foods can influence body weight and mental and physical health is by influencing the populations of gut microbes.
- Eating a healthy amount of food and avoiding over-eating requires satisfying both *head factors* related to emotions and rewards and the *gut factors* that signal the status of physiological needs. Behavioral approaches, particularly mindful eating and intuitive eating techniques, can facilitate awareness of emotions, eating behavior and the sensory aspects of food. This can slow down eating behavior and allow awareness of gut-related satiety signals.

References

Agbim A, Carr RM, Pickett-Blakely O. Dagogo-Jack S. Ethnic Disparities in Adiposity: Focus on Nonalcoholic Fatty Liver Disease, Visceral, and Generalized Obesity. Obesity Reports, 8:243-254, 2019.

Alhalal E. Obesity in women who have experienced intimate partner violence. Journal of Advanced Nursing, 74:2785-2797, 2018.

Asnicar F, Berry SE, Valdes AM et al. Microbiome connections with host metabolism and habitual diet from 1,098 deeply phenotyped individuals. Nature Medicine, 27:321-332, 2021.

Bartlett BA, Iverson KM, Mitchell KS. Intimate partner violence and disordered eating among male and female veterans. Psychiatry Research, 260:98-104, 2018.

Bertone-Johnson ER, Whitcomb BW, Missmer SA, Karlson EW, Rich-Edwards JW. Inflammation and early-life abuse in women. American Journal of Preventative Medicine, 43:611-620, 2012.

Bleich SN, Thorpe Jr RJ, Sharif-Harris H, Fesahazion R, LaVeist TA. Social context explains race disparities in obesity among women. Journal of Epidemiology and Community Health, 64: 465–469. 2010.

Borowitz MA, Yokum S, Duval ER, Gearhardt AN. Weight-related differences in salience, default mode, and executive function network connectivity in adolescents. Obesity, 28:1438-1446, 2020.

Boynton-Jarrett R, Rosenberg L, Palmer JR, Boggs DA, Wise LA. Child and adolescent abuse in relation to obesity in adulthood: the Black Women's Health Study. Pediatrics, 130: 245-53, 2012.

Butler MJ, Barrientos RM. The impact of nutrition on COVID-19 susceptibility and long-term consequences. Brain, Behavior, and Immunity, 87:53-54, 2020.

Cadena- Schlam L, Lopez-Guimera G. Intuitive eating: An emerging approach to eating behavior. Nutricion Hospitalaria, 31:995-1102, 2015.

Christ A, Gunther P, Lauterbach MAR, Duewell P, Biswas D, Pelka K, et al. Western diet triggers NLRP3-dependent innate immune reprogramming. Cell, 172:162-175, 2018.

Chung YC, Ding C, Magkos F. The epidemiology of Obesity. Metabolism Clinical and Experimental, 92:6-10, 2019.

Ciciurkaite G. Race/ethnicity, gender and the SES gradient in BMI: The diminishing returns of SES for racial/ethnic minorities. Sociology of Health and Illness, 00:1-20, 2021.

Corica F, Bianch G, Corsonello A, Mazzella N, Lattanzio F, Marchesini G. Obesity in the context of aging: quality of life considerations. PharmacoEconomics, 33:655-672, 2015.

Coskun Benlidayi I. Role of inflammation in the pathogenesis and treatment of fibromyalgia. Rheumatology International, 39:781–79, 2019.

Cotter EW, Kelly NR. Stress-related eating, mindfulness, and obesity. Health Psychology, 37:516-525, 2018.

Cuevas AG, Chen R, Slopen N, Thurber KA, Wilson N, Economos C, Williams DR. Assessing the role of health behaviors, socioeconomic status, and cumulative stress for racial/ethnic disparities in obesity. Obesity, 161-170, 2020.

Davies R, Lehman E, Perry A, McCall-Hosenfeld, JS. Association of intimate partner violence (IPV) and healthcare provider-identified obesity. Women Health, 56:561-575, 2016.

Deal BJ, Huffman MD, Binns H, Stone NJ. Perspective: Childhood obesity requires new strategies for prevention. Advances in Nutrition, 11:1071-1078, 2020.

Deng M, Qi Y, Deng L, Wang H, XuY, Li Z, et al. Obesity as a potential predictor of disease severity in young COVID-19 patients: A retrospective study. Obesity, 28:1815-1825, 2020.

Dhurandhar EJ. The Food-Insecurity Obesity Paradox: A Resource Scarcity Hypothesis. Physiology and Behavior, 162:88-92, 2016.

Dickerson SS, Gruenewald TL, Kemeny ME. When the social self is threatened: Shame, physiology, and health. Journal of Personality, 72:1191-1216, 2004.

Ding Y, Ji G, Li G, Zhang W, Hu Y, Lio L, et al. Altered interactions among resting-state networks in individuals with obesity. Obesity, 28:601-608, 2020.

Donofry SD, Stillman CM, Erickson KI. A review of the relationship between eating behavior, obesity and functional brain network organization. Social Cognitive and Affective Neuroscience, 15:1157-1181, 2020.

Dunn C, Haubenreiser M, Johnson M, Nordby K, Aggarwal S, Myer S, Thomas C. Mindfulness approaches and weight loss, weight maintenance, and weight regain. Current Obesity Reports, 7:37-49, 2018.

Engin AB. Adipocyte-macrophage crosstalk in obesity. (AB Engin, A Engin, eds) Advances in Experimental Medicine and Biology, 960, 327-343, 2017.

Fang J, Rong P, Hong Y, Fan Y, Lui J, Wang H et al. Transcutaneous vagus nerve stimulation modulates default mode network in Major Depressive Disorder. Biological Psychiatry, 79:266-273, 2016.

Farr OM, Li CR, Mantzoros CS. Central nervous system regulation of eating: Insights from human brain imaging. Metabolism, 65: 699-713, 2016.

Fuentes Artiles R, Staub K, Aldakak L, Eppenberger P, Ruhli F, Bender N. Mindful eating and common diet programs lower body weight similarly: Systematic review and meta-analysis. Obesity Reviews, 20:1619-1627, 2019.

Gluck ME, Viswanath, P, Stinson EJ. Obesity, appetite, and the prefrontal cortex. Current Obesity Reports, 6:380-388, 2017.

Goodarzi M. Genetics of obesity: what genetic association studies have taught us about the biology of obesity and its complications. Lancet Diabetes and Endocrinology, 6:223-236, 2018.

Gota CE, Kaouk S, Wilke WS. Fibromyalgia and Obesity: The Association Between Body Mass Index and Disability, Depression, History of Abuse, Medications, and Comorbidities. Journal of Clinical Rheumatology, 21:289-295, 2015.

Grant RW, Dixit VD. Adipose tissue as an immunological organ. Obesity, 23:512-518. 2015.

Hamer JA, Testani D, Mansur RB, Lee Y, Subramaniapillai M, McIntyre RS. Brain insulin resistance: A treatment target for cognitive impairment and anhedonia in depression. Experimental Neurology, 315:1-8, 2019.

Herhaus B, Petrowski K. Cortisol stress reactivity to the Trier Social Stress Rest in obese adults. Obesity Facts, 11:491-500, 2018.

Nemmingsson E, Johansson K, Reynisdottir S. Effects of childhood abuse on obesity: a systematic review and meta-analysis. Obesity Reviews, 15:882-893, 2014.

Hernandez DC, Reesor LM, Murillo R. Food insecurity and adult overweight/obesity: Gender and race/ethnic disparities. Appetite, 117:373-378, 2017.

Hilbert A, Braehler E, Schmidt R, Löwe B, Häuser W, Zenger M. Self-Compassion as a Resource in the Self-Stigma Process of Overweight and Obese Individuals. Obesity Facts, 8:293-301, 2015.

Himmelstein MS, Puhl RM, Quinn DM. Overlooked and understudied: Health consequences of weight stigma in men. Obesity, 27:1598-16-5, 2019.

Hotamisligil GS. Inflammation, metaflammation and immunometabolic disorders. Nature, 542:177-185, 2017.

Izquierdo AG, Crujeiras AB, Casanueva FF, Carreira MC. Leptin, obesity, and leptin resistance: Where are we 25 years later? Nutrients, 11:2704, 2019.

Jena PK, Sheng L, Di Lucente J, Jin L-W, Maezawa I, Wan Y-J Y. Dysregulated bile acid synthesis and dysbiosis are implicated in Western diet-induced systemic inflammation, microglial activation, and reduced neuroplasticity. FASEB Journal, 32:2866-2877, 2018.

Jung FU, Bae YJ, Kratzsch J, Riedel-Heller SG, Luck-Sikorski C. Internalized weight bias and cortisol reactivity to social stress. Cognitive, Affective, & Behavioral Neuroscience, 20:49–58, 2020.

Kaleth AS, Slaven JE, Ang DC. Obesity Moderates the Effects of Motivational Interviewing Treatment Outcomes in Fibromyalgia. Clinical Journal of Pain, 34:75-81, 2018.

Krishna, P. Is American Dietetics a White-Bread World? These Dietitians Think So. The New York Times, available at: https://nyti.ms/36QBJpF, December 7, 2020.

Lanius RA, Terpou BA, McKinnon MC. The sense of self in the aftermath of trauma: lessons from the default mode network in posttraumatic stress disorder. European Journal of Psychotraumatology, 11: 1807703, 2020.

Lear SA, Humphries KH, Kohli S, Chockalingam A, Frolich JJ, Birmingham CL. Visceral adipose tissue accumulation differs according to ethnic background: results of the Multicultural Community Health Assessment Trial (M-CHAT). American Journal of Clinical Nutrition, 86:353-359, 2007.

Lee EY, Yoon K-H. Epidemic obesity in children and adolescents: Risk factors and prevention. Frontiers in Medicine, doi.org/10.1007/s1684-118-0640-1, 2018.

Marazziti D, Grazia Rutigliano G, Baroni S, Landi P, Dell'Osso L. Metabolic syndrome and major depression. CNS Spectrums, 19:293–304, 2014.

Martinez KB, Leone V, Chang EB. Western diets, gut dysbiosis, and metabolic diseases: Are they linked? Gut Microbes, 8:130-142, 2017.

Mason AE, Epel ES, Aschbacher K, Lustig RH, Acree M, Kristeller J et al. Reduced reward-driven eating accounts for the impact of a mindfulness-based diet and exercise intervention on weight loss: data from the SHINE randomized controlled trial. Appetite, 100:86-93, 2016.

Mason AE, Samantha Schleicher S, Coccia C, Epel ES, Aschbacher K. Chronic stress and impulsive risk-taking predict increases in visceral fat over 18 months. Obesity, 26:869-876, 2018.

Meijnikman AS, Gerdes VE, Nieuwdorp M, Herrema H. Evaluating causality of gut microbiota in obesity and diabetes. Endocrine Reviews, 39:133-153, 2018.

Melby CL, Paris HL, Foright RM, Peth J. Attenuating the Biologic Drive for Weight Regain Following Weight Loss: Must What Goes Down Always Go Back Up? Nutrients, 9:468, 2017.

Milaneschi Y, Simmons WK, van Rossum EFC, Penninx BWJH. Depression and obesity: evidence of shared biological mechanisms. Molecular Psychiatry, 24:18-33, 2019.

Morais JBS, Severo JS, Beserra JB, de Oiveira ARS, Cruz KJC, Melo SRS, do Nascimento GVR, de Macedo GFS, Marreiro DdN. Association Between Cortisol, Insulin Resistance and Zinc in Obesity: a Mini-Review. Biological Trace Element Research, 191:323-330, 2019.

Moroni L, Farina N, Dagna L. Obesity and its role in management of rheumatoid and psoriatic arthritis. Clinical Rheumatology, 39:1039-1047, 2020.

Morris EE, Smith JC, Yonus Farooqui S, Suris AM. Unseen battles: The recognition, assessment, and treatment issues of men with military sexual trauma (MST). Trauma, Violence and Abuse, 15:94-101, 2013.

Narouze S, Souzdalnitski D. Obesity and Chronic Pain: Systematic Review of Prevalence and Implications for Pain Practice. BMF Regional Anesthesia and Pain Medicine, 40:91-111, 2015.

Neeland IJ, Boone SC, Mook-Kanamori DO, Ayers C, Smit RAJ, Tzouli I, et al. Metabolomics profiling of visceral adipose tissue: results from MESA and the NEO study. Journal of the American Heart Association, 8: e010810, 2019.

Omiwole M, Richardson C, Huniewicz P, Dettmer E, Paslakis G. Review of mindfulness-related interventions to modify eating behaviors in adolescents. Nutrients, 11:2917, 2019.

Pagliai G, Ilaria Giangrandi I, Monica Dinu M, Francesco Sofi F, Colombini B. Nutritional Interventions in the Management of Fibromyalgia Syndrome. Nutrients, 12:2525, 2020.

Palmeira L, Cunha M, Pinto-Gouveia J. Processes of change in quality of life, weight self-stigma, body mass index and emotional eating after an acceptance-, mindfulness- and compassion-based group intervention (Kg-Free) for women with overweight and obesity. Journal of Health Psychology, 8:1056-1069, 2019.

Pandey N, Ashfaq SN, Dauterive ED, MacCarthy AA, Copeland LA. Military sexual trauma and obesity among women veterans. Journal of Women's Health, 27, 306-310, 2018.

Petersen MC, Shulman GI. Mechanisms of insulin action and insulin resistance. Physiological Reviews, 98:2133-2223, 2018.

Raichle ME. The brain's default mode network. Annual Review of Neuroscience, 38:433-447, 2015.

Rebello K, Moura LM, Xavier G, Spindola LM, Carvalho CM, Queiroz Hoexter M, et al. Association between spontaneous activity of the default mode network hubs and leukocyte telomere length in late childhood and adolescence. Journal of Psychosomatic Research, 127:109864, 2019.

Reddon H, Patel Y, Turcotte M, Pigeyre M, Meyre D. Revisiting the evolutionary origins of obesity: lazy versus peppy-thrifty genotype hypothesis. Obesity Reviews, 19:1525-1543, 2018.

Rich EL, Stoll FM, Rudebeck PH. Linking dynamic patterns of neural activity in orbitofrontal cortex with decision making. Current Opinion in Neurobiology, 49:24-32, 2018.

Richardson AS, Arsenault JE, Cates SC, Muth MK. Perceived stress, unhealthy eating behaviors, and severe obesity in low-income women. Nutrition Journal, 14:122, 2015.

Ross CA. Psychodynamics of Eating Disorder Behavior in Sexual Abuse Survivors. American Journal of Psychotherapy, 63:211-226, 2009.

Ruiz LD, Zuelch ML, Dimitratos SM, Scherr RE. Adolescent Obesity: Diet Quality, Psychosocial Health, and Cardiometabolic Risk Factors. Nutrients:12, 43, 2020.

Seabrook LT, Borgland SL. The orbitofrontal cortex, food intake and obesity. Journal of Psychiatry and Neuroscience, 45:304-312, 2020.

Soares JM, Marques P, Magalhaes R, Santos NC, Sousa N. The association between stress and mood across the adult lifespan on default mode network. Brain Structure and Function, 222:101-112, 2017.

Schwartz MW, Seeley RJ, Zeltser LM, Drewnowski A, Ravussin E, Redman LM, Leibel RL. Obesity Pathogenesis: An Endocrine Society Scientific Statement. Endocrine Reviews, 38:267-296, 2017.

Shiri R, Karppinen J, Leino-Arjas P, Solovieva S, Viikari-Juntura, E.The Association Between Obesity and Low Back Pain: A Meta-Analysis. American Journal of Epidemiology, 171:135-154, 2010.

Simmons WK, DeVille DC. Interoceptive Contributions to Healthy Eating and Obesity. Current Opinion in Psychology, 17:106-112, 2017.

Sinha R, Jastreboff AN. Stress as a common risk factor for obesity and addiction. Biological Psychiatry, 73: 827–835, 2013.

Smith HA, Markovic N, Danielson ME, Alicia Matthews A, Youk A, Talbott EO, Larkby C, Hughes T. Sexual Abuse, Sexual Orientation, and Obesity in Women. Journal of Women's Health, 19:1525-1532, 2010.

Stokes AC, Xie W, Lundberg DJ, Hempstead K, Zajacova A, Zimmer Z, Glei DA, Meara E, Preston SH. Increases in BMI and chronic pain for US adults in midlife, 1992 to 2016. SSM-Population Health, 12:100644, 2020.

Teicholz N. Diets are not one-size-fits-all. So why do we treat dietary guidelines that way? The Washington Post, May 2, 2019.

Tomiyama AJ, Epel ES, McClatchey TM, Poelke G, Kemeny ME, McCoy SK, Daubenmier J. Associations of weight stigma with cortisol and oxidative stress independent of adiposity. Health Psychology, 33:862-867, 2014.

Tomiyama AJ. Stress and Obesity. Annual Review of Psychology, 70:703-718, 2019.

Trim WV, Lynch L. Immune and non-immune functions of adipose tissue leukocytes. Nature Reviews Immunology, DOI 10.1038/s41577-021-00635-7. Online ahead of print. 2021.

Udo T, Purcell K, Grilo CM. Perceived weight discrimination and chronic medical conditions in adults with overweight and obesity. International Journal of Clinical Practice, 70:1003-1011, 2016.

Uranga RM, Keller JN. The Complex Interactions Between Obesity, Metabolism and the Brain. Frontiers in Neuroscience, 13: article 513, 2019.

Ursini F, Naty S, Grembiale RD. Fibromyalgia and obesity: the hidden link. Rheumatology International, 31:1403-1408, 2011.

van der Valk ES, Savas M, van Rossum EFC. Stress and Obesity: Are There More Susceptible Individuals? Current Obesity Reports, 7:193-203, 2018.

Vartanian LR, Porter AM, Weight stigma and eating behavior: A review of the literature. Appetite, 102:3-14, 2016.

Wang T, He C. Pro-inflammatory cytokines: The link between obesity and osteoarthritis. Cytokine and Growth Factor Reviews, 44:38-50, 2018.

Wang Y, Beydoun M. The obesity epidemic in the United States- gender, age, socioeconomic, racial/ethnic, and geographical characteristics: a systematic review and meta-regression analysis. Epidemiologic Reviews, 29:6-28, 2007.

Warren JM, Smith N, Ashwell M. A structured literature review on the role of mindfulness, mindful eating and intuitive eating in changing eating behaviours: effectiveness and associated potential mechanisms. Nutrition Research Reviews, 30:272-283, 2017.

Wieckowska-Gacek A, Mietelska-Porowska A, Wydrych M, Wijda U. Western diet as a trigger of Alzheimer's Disease: From metabolic syndrome and systemic inflammation to neuroinflammation and neurodegeneration. Aging Research Reviews, 70:101290, 2021.

Weinberger N-A, Kersting A, Reidel-Heller SG, Luck-Sikorski C. Body dissatisfaction in individuals with obesity compared to normal-weight individuals: A systematic review and meta-analysis. Obesity Facts, 9:424-441, 2016.

Wittbrodt MT, Gurel NZ, Nye JA, Ladd S, Shandhi MH, Huang M, et al. Non-invasive vagal nerve stimulation decreases brain activity during trauma scripts. Brain Stimulation, 13:1333-1348, 2020.

Wiley JW, Higgins GA, Athey BD. Stress and glucocorticoid receptor transcriptional programming in time and space: Implications for the brain–gut axis. Neurogastroenterology and Motility, 28:12-25, 2016.

Woods SC, Begg DP. Regulation of the motivation to eat. Current Topics in Behavioral Neuroscience, 27:15-34, 2016.

Zhu Z, Guo Y, Shi H, Liu C-L, Panganiban RA, Chung W, O'Connor LJ, Himes BE, Gazal S, Hasegawa K, Camargo CA, Lu Qi L, Moffatt MF, Hu FB, Lu Q, Cookson WOC, Liang L. Shared genetic and experimental links between obesity-related traits and asthma subtypes in UK Biobank. Journal of Allergy and Clinical Immunology, 145:537-549, 2020.

Further Reading

Food Addicts in Recovery. Available from FoodAddicts.org

CHAPTER 7: INFLAMMATION: WHAT IS IT, AND WHEN DO WE NEED TO WORRY ABOUT IT?

- WHAT IS INFLAMMATION?

- OVERVIEW

- CAST OF CHARACTERS THAT ORCHESTRATE INFLAMMATION

- PATHOGEN-ASSOCIATED MOLECULAR PATTERNS (PAMPS): SIGNALS OF INFECTION

- COMMENSAL MICROBE-ASSOCIATED MOLECULAR PATTERNS (MAMPS): COMMENSAL MICROBE INFLUENCE ON THE IMMUNE SYSTEM

- PATTERN RECOGNITION RECEPTORS (PRRS): SENSORY RECEPTORS OF THE IMMUNE SYSTEM

- NUCLEAR FACTOR KAPPA B (NFKB): A MASTER REGULATOR OF THE IMMUNE RESPONSE

- INFLAMMASOMES: FACTORIES FOR INFLAMMATION

- MITOCHONDRIA: POWERHOUSES OF THE CELL

- REACTIVE OXYGEN AND NITROGEN SPECIES (ROS & RNS): BOTH KILLERS AND MESSENGERS

- CYTOKINES: IMPORTANT HORMONE-LIKE MESSENGERS OF THE IMMUNE SYSTEM

- WHAT HAPPENS DURING INFLAMMATION?

- THE WELL-REGULATED MILITIA: BALANCE BETWEEN PRO-INFLAMMATORY AND ANTI-INFLAMMATORY MECHANISMS

- PROSTAGLANDINS: REGULATORS OF INFLAMMATION

- CORTISOL LINKS CHALLENGE RESPONSES WITH METABOLISM AND INFLAMMATION

- KEY POINTS

The mechanism that links stress, diet and quality of life is inflammation. As a collaboration between the immune system and the nervous system, inflammation serves to defend against dangerous microbes and toxins. This defense can lead to collateral damage, but inflammation also coordinates tissue repair and healing.

Like other responses to challenges, inflammation must be well-regulated. Unconstrained inflammation damages tissues and disrupts their function. Indeed, unregulated inflammation is at the root of virtually all chronic diseases. Inflammation has a particularly deleterious effect on the brain. Low grade inflammation in the brain drives neurodegenerative diseases and depression, as well the *sickness syndrome* of fatigue, brain fog, low mood and anxiety, sleep problems, and anhedonia, or lack of ability to feel pleasure (Heneka 2018, Meyer 2020, Dantzer 2008). These symptoms are common companions of most chronic disease (Friedman 2019). Because they compromise brain function, including cognition, they impair the ability to manage challenges, thereby causing stress.

Both stress and diet can induce inflammation in the absence of actual pathogens, or damage to the body. Thus, inflammation is truly a pivotal node in the vicious cycle of stress, poor diet, and disease (Christ 2019). To understand how lifestyle, especially diet, affects health, we must understand what exactly happens during inflammation, and specifically how lifestyle can help regulate inflammation, or make it much worse. Although the exact mechanisms of inflammation may seem arcane, how a food affects the immune system is a major part of whether the food is healthy or not. Therefore, to make informed choices about specific foods, it is necessary to understand the basics of inflammation, and how foods can keep inflammation well-regulated, or not.

What is Inflammation?

Inflammation is the immune system's first response to a threat, which can be a pathogen, such as a microbe or toxin, or damage to body tissue (Hernandez-Lemus 2018, Medzhitov 2010, Rossi 2021). For example, if we sustain a cut to the skin, immune cells in the skin recruit other cells to the area to help fight any microorganisms that might be dangerous. Blood vessels in the area become leaky, giving rise to the familiar swelling and redness we associate with inflammation. The area can also feel painful. Immune cells arrive at the wound site and release chemicals that kill pathogens; some cells (macrophages) actually "eat" or engulf microbes or toxins and digest them. This phase of the immune system response is called *pro-inflammatory* or *Type 1 inflammation*. When the infection is cleared, the immune system switches to an anti-inflammatory, pro-growth healing phase, called *Type 2* inflammation, which cleans up cellular debris and rebuilds damaged tissue. In this way, the immune system is rather like the military, in that it fights disease, but also can repair and rebuild.

The immune system is very effective at killing pathogens, but the chemicals it uses (e.g., hydrogen peroxide; other reactive oxygen and nitrogen species, which will be described in detail in the following section) can cause collateral damage to healthy tissues. For that reason, it is important that the inflammation is limited, and that the switch to the healing phase happens quickly. When that transition is not made, inflammation becomes chronic. There are many factors that can contribute to the development of chronic inflammation, including genetic predisposition, but stress and poor diet are the most important ones that we can control. To understand how to minimize chronic inflammation, we need to know what goes on during inflammation: how it is triggered, what steps activate immune cells, and how the response can be turned off.

Overview

To protect us against infections and monitor the condition of our bodies, the immune system has to be able to quickly determine whether or not a particular molecule or microbe is dangerous. In this way, the immune system functions as a sensory system (Goehler 2000, Sun 2019, Veiga-Fernades 2017). Once danger is detected, the immune system must mount a rapid and coordinated response. This response involves the release of hormone-like mediators that recruit other cells and release toxic molecules that neutralize the threat. When the threat has been managed, the response is turned off and a healing phase ensues (Medzhitov 2010, Rossi 2021).

CAST OF CHARACTERS THAT ORCHESTRATE INFLAMMATION

Inflammation is carried out by many kinds of molecules that work together to fight pathogens or repair damage. These characters will be showing up repeatedly when we talk about how food affects the body and mind and how diet can modify disease.

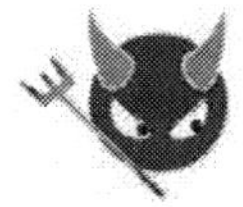

Pathogen-Associated Molecular Patterns (PAMPs): Signals of Infection

PAMPs are parts of pathogens, such as cell wall or genetic material, that can't easily hide from the immune system by changing their form or mutating. The immune system uses them as a signal of the presence of microbes or toxins that could be dangerous (Medzhitov 2010, Kaur 2019). Because they are essential structures of bacteria and viruses, the pathogen can't change these PAMPs without serious consequences for its survival. PAMPs therefore make good cues for the immune system because the pathogens can't evade surveillance through mutation. Some examples of PAMPs include genetic material such as DNA, and bacterial cell wall components such as lipopolysaccharide (LPS). PAMPs can be present in food, for instance bacteria or parasites in uncooked or undercooked meats, or in fruits or vegetables grown in unclean conditions. The immune system also reacts to herbicides, such as glyphosate, or pesticides, which can persist on vegetables and grains as PAMPs. This an important way that poor-quality diets can drive inflammation. We depict PAMPs as little demons because they signal the presence of potentially harmful invaders.

Commensal Microbe-Associated Molecular Patterns (MAMPs): Commensal Microbe Influence on the Immune System

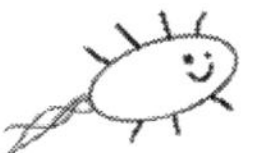

Commensal Microbes are bacteria, viruses and fungi that normally live in the gut. They do not cause disease, and many have beneficial actions, such as producing vitamins and fuel. Many of these benign creatures live in your gut and play a role in immune health. We depict them as the happy microbe above.

Microbe-Associated Molecular Patterns (**MAMPs**) are products of the commenal microbes that normally live in and on us. The products include short-chain fatty acids (butyrate, acetate, propionate) or bacterial products that can induce both immune tolerance or inflammation (Maslanik 2012, Knudsen 2018, Langgartnter 2019, Stilling 2016).

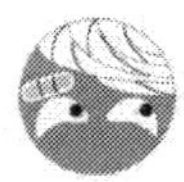

Damage-Associated Molecular Patterns (DAMPs) Signal Damaged Cells

Damage-Associated Molecular Patterns (**DAMPs**), also called *alarmins,* are signals that our own cells generate when they are damaged (Medzhitov 2010, Zindel 2020). Some of these molecules are actively displayed by the damaged cell and function as "eat me" signals to attract scavenging immune cells. Other

DAMPs are parts of cells that belong inside the cell, such as DNA. If these internal cell components are exposed to the immune system, they alert the immune system to tissue damage or stress. (Gong 2020, Zindel 2020). The immune system must destroy the damaged cells or they can transform into cancer cells. In addition, some lipids and proteins that either circulate in the blood or form part of our cell membranes can become DAMPS when oxidized. DAMPs can be produced in food that is cooked at high temperatures or during other kinds of processing (Smith 2017). This may be a reason processed foods increase risk of conditions such as diabetes and even food allergies (Sergi 2021, Smith 2017). We depict DAMPs as sad and injured to reflect their role in signaling cell damage.

Pattern Recognition Receptors (PRRs): Sensory Receptors of the Immune System

How does the immune system sense pathogens? It does so by using its own special set of sensory receptors. Specifically, immune cells detect the danger signals provided by PAMPs and the damage signals provided by DAMPs using pattern recognition receptors (PRRs). Using a strategy of recognizing common patterns associated with types of dangerous microbes, cell damage, and other threats helps enable the immune system to respond to new threats with intelligence gained from prior experience. Immune cells expose these PRRs on their own cell membranes to detect PAMPs and DAMPs, signs of danger and damage (Kaur 2019). There are many of these PRRs. Some are known to be relevant to dietary influences on inflammation. For example, TOLL-like receptor 4 (TLR4) is a PRR that detects both pathogens and toxins. Receptors for glycated proteins, abbreviated RAGE, are PRRs that detect proteins that have reacted with excess sugar. Another example is LOX1, a PRR that detects oxidized lipids, which are fats that have been changed through reaction with oxygen. These will be discussed shortly in the context of how diet induces inflammation.

When a danger signal PAMP or a damage signal DAMP binds to a pattern recognition receptor, such as TLR4, it activates a sequence of signals inside the cell that leads to an inflammatory response.

Nuclear Factor kappa B (NFkB): A Master Regulator of the Immune Response 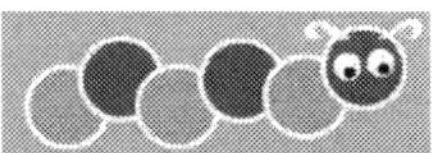

NFkB is a protein that turns on or off selected genes to act as a master regulator of the immune response. Inflammation is complex, and proper host defense requires a prompt and coordinated response to infection or damage. This response is initiated and amplified by special proteins such as NFkB (Mitchell 2016, Zhang 2017). These proteins normally live in the cell cytoplasm. When PRRs detect danger or damage as PAMPs and/or DAMPs, this generates a signal inside the cells that spurs these proteins to move into the cell nucleus. Within the nucleus, they bind to DNA and induce the expression of many proteins that carry out the inflammatory response. These induced proteins include the *inflammasomes,* discussed below. This cellular response connects the detection of danger to the inflammatory response.

Because NFkB serves a critical function in inflammation, it is a key target of biologics, or biological anti-inflammatory drugs. Some biological drugs for autoimmune conditions target NFkB to limit its effects. Many foods found to have anti-inflammatory ingredients, such as curcumin and quercetin, act to inhibit the activation of NFkB (Li 2016, Malaguarnera 2019).

Because inflammation can be life-saving or life-threatening, we have used a caterpillar to depict NFkB. By regulating inflammation, NFkB can promote life as a pollenating butterfly, or damage life around it as a hungry insect.

Inflammasomes: Factories for Inflammation 

Inflammasomes are complexes of proteins within cells that manufacture substances that drive inflammation (Iwata 2013, Wei 2019). One way they do this is by triggering the release of cytokines that serve to activate other cells, including blood vessel cells, other immune cells, and cells of the nervous system. In this way, they act like factories that produce and coordinate the weapons of the immune system.

Because of this powerful role, inflammasome functions must be well-regulated, Indeed, gene-linkage studies, which correlate gene varieties with specific diseases, implicate genes that make up the inflammasome in several diseases (Ahmed 2017). Inflammasome activity seems to be a critical link between stress and inflammation and associated cognitive disfunction and neurodegenerative diseases (Iwata 2013, Wei 2017). Thus, differences in inflammasome structure and function may contribute to individual differences in susceptibility to disease.

Mitochondria: Powerhouses of the Cell 

Mitochondria provide energy for cells by breaking down substances such as glucose or ketone bodies. Mitochondria transfer energy from this metabolism into the bonds of other molecules. These molecules are then transported to other places in the cell where energy is needed. This process provides ready to use energy for the cell, but also causes the formation of reactive oxygen species (ROS) as a byproduct. During inflammation, inflammasomes signal mitochondria to increase production of ROS, because ROS are effective weapons (Mills 2017). Here, elevated metabolism and ROS production help with the immune response to challenges. When blood sugar is high, especially in the context of a high-sugar diet, the extra energy from the sugar causes mitochondria to produce excessive ROS. Here, the ROS are not needed to fight pathogens, and thus can damage healthy cells instead. Excessive ROS produced from extra glucose is one mechanism by which high-sugar diets induce inflammation (Luc 2019).

Reactive Oxygen and Nitrogen Species (ROS & RNS): Both Killers and Messengers 

***Reactive Oxygen and Nitrogen Species* (ROS & RNS)** play several roles in the body (Pacher 2007). They provide signals reporting metabolic activity and damage to DNA. Some even act as neurotransmitters. They are effective weapons, because they *oxidize* proteins and lipids, thus impairing their function and causing damage. This is a very efficient way of killing things. Unfortunately, reactive oxygen species are not specific in what they damage, and unregulated oxidation of our healthy cells is a major way that inflammation contributes to disease. Indeed, oxidation of foods is the major reason for spoilage. Oxidized versions of certain foods, and especially fats, can increase or cause inflammation.

In addition to serving as powerful weapons in host defense, ROS and RNS have "day jobs." For instance, one RNS, nitric oxide, serves as a neurotransmitter and is critically important for regulation of vascular tone and blood pressure (Pacher 2007). Another RNS, nitrate, signals that DNA has been damaged, and induces cells to repair the damage. So, even though it is tempting to think of these molecules as dangerous, and that it might be important to keep them suppressed, in fact the better goal is to keep their formation and activity well regulated.

Cytokines: Important Hormone-like Messengers of the Immune System

Cytokines are proteins that serve to signal damage or danger. They are made mostly by immune cells, including T-cells, which coordinate different aspects of immune function. There are many different cytokines, as well as functional related molecules, such as *chemokines*. Cytokines are conceptually grouped into two categories based generally on function.

Pro-inflammatory Cytokines Instigate and Sustain Inflammation 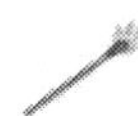

When immune cells detect damage or danger, they release "pro-inflammatory" cytokines such as Tumor Necrosis Factor (TNF), Interleukin-1 (IL-1), interferon and others. The cytokines activate pattern recognition receptors on cells (PRRs), which trigger activation of NFkB. This can activate inflammation or serve to keep it going. Many different cells express receptors for pro-inflammatory cytokines, including neurons and other cells of the nervous system (Dantzer 2007). Indeed, pro-inflammatory cytokines play pivotal roles in the induction and maintenance of chronic pain conditions, and in fatigue, brain fog, and mood alterations during sickness or inflammation (Matsuda 2019, Dantzer 2007, D'Mello 2017).

Pro-inflammatory cytokines are sometimes called *Type 1* cytokines. Type 1 cytokines get their name from the immune cells, called T-helper type 1 (TH1), that were the first cells found to release these cytokines. TH1 cells, and other cells including, monocytes and macrophages, that release type 1 cytokines are critical for killing bacteria, viruses, and cancer cells. They are part of a first line of defense against pathogens termed *innate immunity* (Kauer 2019). Innate immune cytokine responses tend to be specialized according to infection type (Medzhitov 2010). For instance, the cytokine IL-1 is particularly important for inducing responses to pathogenic bacteria, whereas type 1 interferons are critical for antiviral activity (Mayer-Barber 2017). This difference is important for developing effective interventions for diseases involving type 1 inflammation, such as viral infection.

Anti-Inflammatory Cytokines: The Brakes on Inflammation 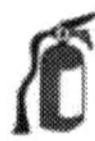

Similarly, type 2 cytokines get their name from the T-cells that release them: T-helper type 2 (TH2) cells. Type 2 cytokines such as interleukin-4 (IL-4) and interleukin-10 (IL-10) serve to turn off the pro-inflammatory phase (Allen 2014, Gieseck 2018). They have powerful inhibitory effects on the release of type 1 cytokines. In addition, they initiate and help coordinate healing and tissue re-modeling (Allen 2014, Gieseck 2018). For example, type 2 cytokines act during pregnancy to reduce inflammation and the risk of rejecting the fetus, and help the uterus and cervix prepare for delivery (Schminky 2014).

Type 2 cytokines do play a role in host defense, however, and are particularly important for fighting parasites (Allen 2014). If a pathogen, such as a worm, is too big or complex to kill, type 2 cytokines build a wall of fibrous tissue around it to form a cyst. This isolates the parasite and prevents it from inflicting damage while also cutting off its access to nutrients.

Like all components of the immune system, type 2 responses must be well-regulated and balanced with type 1 systems. For instance, overactive type 2 responses are associated with multiple conditions, such as fibrosis, allergies, and asthma (Gieseck 2018). In addition, because type 2 cytokines can powerfully inhibit type 1 responses, an immune system skewed toward type 2 response is associated with increased risk of infection and cancer (Wan 2020, Rossi 2021).

The simplified illustrations show below depict how inflammation can be initiated and terminated.

What Happens During Inflammation?

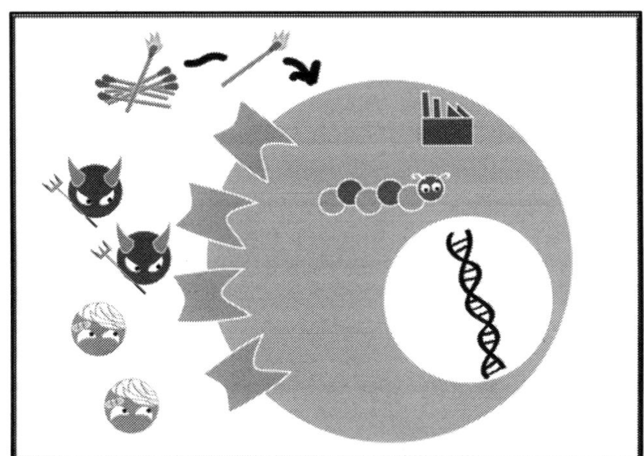

Infection, tissue damage, or ongoing inflammation generates PAMPs, DAMPs, and pro-inflammatory cytokines.

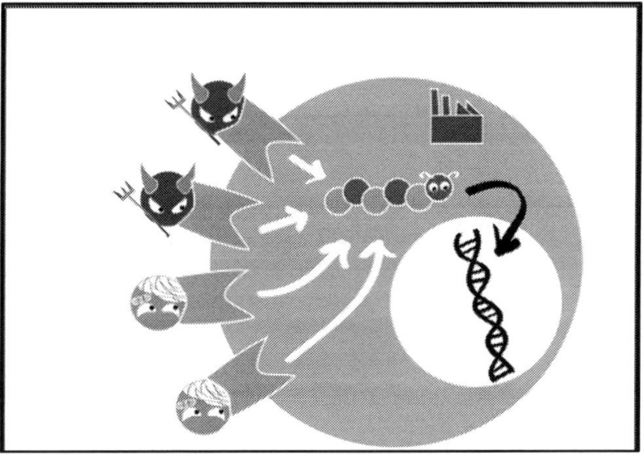

The PAMPs, DAMPs or pro-inflammatory cytokines bind to receptors (PRRs) on immune cells. Activation of the receptors causes NFkB to move to the nucleus, where it can interact with DNA.

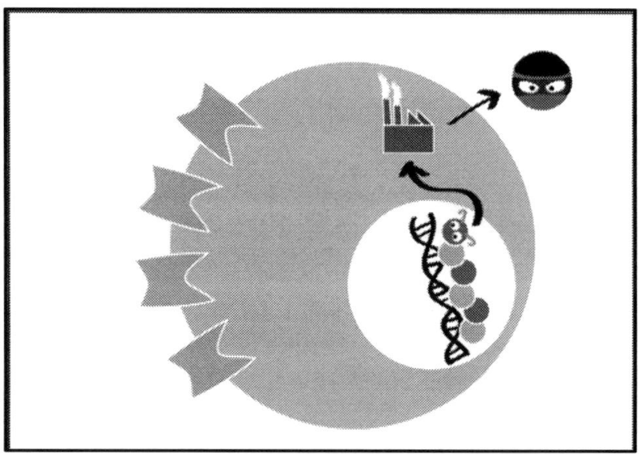

NFkB activates inflammasomes, which cause increased production and release of cytokines and reactive oxygen and nitrogen species.

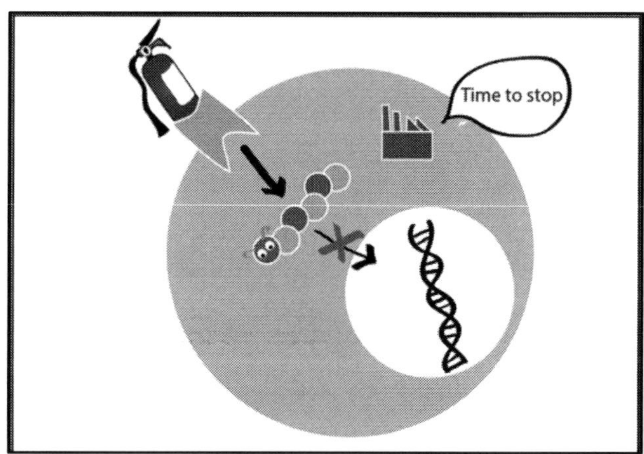

When the inflammation is ready to resolve and the healing phase can begin, anti-inflammatory cytokines signal inflammasomes to stop producing pro-inflammatory mediators.

The Well-Regulated Militia: Balance Between Pro-Inflammatory and Anti-Inflammatory Mechanisms

Because inflammation is critical for fighting infection and for supporting recovery, we don't want it to be suppressed too much. Indeed, the main danger of powerful anti-inflammatory drugs is that they render people susceptible to potentially fatal infections (Rossi 2021). Further, inflammation's function in removing cellular debris and other byproducts of normal cell function is key to maintaining health. Inflammation also plays a role in learning, through remodeling neural connections in the brain. Anything, such as sleep loss, that prevents this sort of immune cell activity can damage tissue and cause dysfunction (Besedovsky 2019, Shimba 2020). Inflammation must be well regulated to maintain a balance between tissue-damaging actions, and healing and growth functions.

For this reason, T-cells, macrophages, and dendritic cells, which detect injury or infection and coordinate inflammation and other immune responses, adopt *phenotypes* or functional identities associated with promoting inflammation or regulating it. For instance, in the gut, host-defense capability is regulated by pro-inflammatory T-helper type 17 (TH17) cells, and this is restrained by the activity of regulatory T-cells (Tregs). An imbalance in favor of TH17 cells in the gut is associated with inflammatory bowel disease and food allergies. On the other hand, an imbalance in favor of Tregs has been associated with cancer susceptibility (Tanaka 2019).

Prostaglandins: Regulators of Inflammation

Inflammation proceeds as a cascade of chemical mediators subsequent to detection of PAMPs and DAMPs, These initiate a sequence of signaling leading to inflammation (Ricciotti 2011). At the top of this cascade are prostaglandins, which are among the earliest signals generated by immune and other cells that sense damage or pathogens. Prostaglandins are the principal target of the non-steroidal anti-inflammatory drugs (NSAIDs; aspirin, ibuprofen, naproxen, etc.). NSAIDs are highly effective at controlling inflammation because inhibiting prostaglandins prevents or reduces the activation of NFkB and other downstream inflammatory pathways. Notably, dietary anti-inflammatory agents, such as curcumin, quercetin, and resveratrol, have anti-prostaglandin actions (Li 2016, Pirola 2008, Yu 2018).

Although the best characterized prostaglandins, such as prostaglandin E2 (PGE2) are potently pro-inflammatory, other prostaglandins function to regulate inflammation and trigger healing. Further, pro-inflammatory prostaglandins, such as PGE2 also support normal physiological functions. For instance, PGE2 contributes to maintenance of the gut barrier. This role explains why gastrointestinal bleeding can be a side effect of NSAID use. Risk for gastrointestinal bleeding varies depending on the specific drug, and risk is low for over-the-counter doses (Moore 2018).

Prostaglandins are synthesized from omega-6 polyunsaturated fatty acids (PUFAs; linoleic acid). This is one of the reasons that omega-6 PUFAs are hypothesized to contribute to inflammation, with the assumption being that the more omega-6 PUFAs in the diet, the more pro-inflammatory prostaglandins will be generated (Fritsche 2014). However, the synthesis of prostaglandins does not seem to be substrate-driven. In other words, it doesn't depend on the amount of omega-6 PUFAs consumed. Instead, it depends on activation of the enzymes in the context of danger signals, such as pathogens, toxins, tissue damage, or ongoing inflammation. Thus, pro-inflammatory effects of omega-6 PUFAs are more likely to derive from other factors, such as their vulnerability to oxidation. Oxidation may be facilitated by the excessive processing in manufactured Western diet foods.

Cortisol links Challenge Responses with Metabolism and Inflammation

One of the principal and best-known functions of cortisol is to restrain inflammation. Indeed, cortisol and analogs of it are widely used clinically for this purpose. Activation of cortisol receptors, which are transcription factors like NFkB, serves to down-regulate the expression of pro-inflammatory mediators, including cytokines. In this way, cortisol functions as a signal to "flip the switch" from inflammation to healing.

A lesser appreciated but important function of cortisol is to ensure that the immune system is provided with sufficient metabolic fuel to mount effective responses to infection or other challenges. Indeed, innate immunity is closely linked to metabolism (Weichhart 2015). One of the first physical responses to infection is a rapid release of cortisol (Straub 2016). Thus, cortisol responses are bi-phasic: early responses mobilize metabolic substrates to support pro-inflammatory immune function, whereas later releases of cortisol serve to help wind down the inflammatory response (Dhabhar 2014).

The inhibitory effects of cortisol on the expression of pro-inflammatory mediators such as cytokines implies that stress, which results in increased cortisol release, should be anti-inflammatory. Indeed, during acute stressors, high levels of cortisol are released and cortisol does seem to be anti-inflammatory. Cortisol or drugs that act like it are widely used as anti-inflammatory agents. Examples of this sort of acute stressor would include physical stressors such as a car accident. In contrast, however, chronic stress characterized by cortisol levels that are chronically elevated is associated with *increased* inflammation. How can this happen?

Normally, cortisol levels rise and fall during the day at predictable times in a *cortisol rhythm*, and many cells are dependent on that rhythm. Cortisol is important for regulating many aspects of metabolism, and for restraining activity of the immune system. Because cortisol tends to inhibit immune cell activity such as remodeling tissue and removing cellular debris, these functions occur mostly at night, when cortisol levels are normally low (Dhabhar 2014).

When stress is chronic, however, and basal levels of cortisol are elevated, cells can become resistant to cortisol, or *glucocorticoid-resistant*. This may help in maintaining housekeeping functions, but glucocorticoid resistance can make regulating inflammation much harder (Nikkheslat 2015). Further, stress also leads to permanent or semi-permanent epigenetic changes in the expression of genes for pro-inflammatory cytokines, such as IL-6 (Dudek 2021, Palma-Gudiel 2021). These epigenetic changes make it even harder to regulate inflammation.

Whereas chronically elevated cortisol levels serve to dysregulate immune functions, they can also directly *induce* inflammation (Bauer 2019). Recent studies have shown that cortisol also seems to act as a DAMP (Frank 2013). Cortisol can bind to PRRs and therefore directly drive inflammation, priming microglia, macrophages, activating inflammasomes, and especially driving neuroinflammation (Frank 2013). Thus, stress is a pathological condition that the immune system treats as a potential threat. The immune system assumes that chronic stress is a signal of damage. In this way, inflammation can be a consequence of chronic stress. Indeed, this tight connection between inflammation and stress constitutes one of the major ways that stress predisposes for disease, and exacerbates ongoing inflammatory conditions such as chronic pain and depression (Bauer 2019).

Key Points

- Inflammation is an immune-directed process, that when well-regulated, saves our lives when we have infections.
- Immune cells that are involved in inflammation have important other jobs related to healing, growth, and even learning.
- When inflammation is not properly regulated, it becomes chronic, damaging cells and leading to disease conditions including cardiovascular, metabolic, and neurodegenerative disease, as well as chronic pain, mood and gastrointestinal disorders, and autoimmune conditions.
- Inflammation is initiated by molecules that signal the presence of pathogens (PAMPs) and/or damage to tissues (DAMPs). These signals are detected by pattern-recognition receptors (PRRs) that activate inflammatory responses by the cell. In this way, the immune system acts like a sensory system.

- The tendency toward developing chronic inflammation often results from inheriting genes that make regulation of inflammation more difficult. Healthy lifestyles, including diet, can mitigate the effects of genetics.
- The brain plays an important role in regulating inflammation, in part by controlling cortisol. This underlies how things like stress can make us more susceptible to illness and inflammation, but also enables positive emotional states, and mind-body modalities such as meditation, to regulate inflammation.

References

Ahmed Nasef N, Mehta S, Ferguson LR. Susceptibility to chronic inflammation: an update. Archives of Toxicology, 91:1131-1141, 2017.

Allen JE, Sutherland TE. Host protective roles of type 2 immunity: Parasite killing and tissue repair, flip sides of the same coin. Seminars in Immunology. 26:329-340, 2014.

Bauer ME, Teixeira AL. Inflammation in psychiatric disorders: what comes first? Annals of the New York Academy of Sciences, 1437:57-67, 2019.

Besedovsky L, Lange T, Haack M. The sleep-immune crosstalk in health and disease. Physiological Reviews, 99:1325-1380, 2019.

Christ A, Latz E. The Western lifestyle has lasting effects on metaflammation. Nature Reviews Immunology, 19:267-268, 2019.

Dantzer R, O'Connor JC, Freund GG, Johnson RW, Kelley KW. From inflammation to sickness and depression: when the immune system subjugates the brain. Nature Neuroscience Reviews, 9:46-56, 2008.

Dhabhar FS. The effects of stress on immune function: the good, the bad, and the beautiful. Immunology Research, 58:193-210, 2014.

D'Mello C, Swain MG. Immune-to-brain communication pathways in inflammation-associated sickness and depression. Current Topics in Behavioral Neuroscience, 31:73-94, 2017.

Dudek KA, Kaufmann FN, Lavoie O, Menard C. Central and peripheral stress-induced epigenetic mechanisms of resilience. Current Opinion in Psychiatry, 34: 1-9, 2021.

Frank MG, Watkins LR, Maier SF. Glucocorticoids as a neuroendocrine alarm signal of danger. Brain, Behavior, and Immunity, 33:1-6, 2013.

Friedman E, Shorey C. Inflammation in multimorbidity and disability: An integrative review. Health Psychology, 38:791-801, 2019.

Fritsche K L. Linoleic acid, vegetable oils, and inflammation. Missouri Medicine, 111:4143, 2014.

Goehler LE, Gaykema RP, Hansen MK, Maier SF, Watkins LR. Vagal immune-to-brain communication: a visceral chemosensory pathway. Autonomic Neuroscience Basic and Clinical, 85:49-59, 2000.

Heneka MT, McManus RM, Latz E. Inflammasome signalling in brain function and neurodegenerative disease. Nature Reviews Neuroscience, 19:610-621,2018.

Hernández-Lemus E, Soto ME, Rosales C. Editorial: Integrative Approaches to the Molecular Physiology of Inflammation. Frontiers in Physiology, 9:1825, doi: 10.3389/fphys.2018.01825 2018.

Iwata M, Ota KT, Duman RS. The inflammasome: Pathways linking psychological stress, depression and systemic illnesses. Brain, Behavior, and Immunity, 31: 105-14, 2013.

Kaur BP, Secord, E. Innate Immunity. Pediatric Clinics of North America, 66: 905–911, 2019.

Knudsen KEB, Laerke HN, Hedemann MS, Neilsen TS, Ingerslev AK, Nielsen DSG, et al. Impact of diet-modulated butyrate production on intestinal barrier function and inflammation. Nutrients, 10:1499, 2018.

Langgartner D, Lowry CA, Reber SO. Old Friends, immunoregulation, and stress resilience. Pflügers Archive - European Journal of Physiology, 471:237–269, 2019.

Li Y, Yao J, Han C, Yang J, Chaudhry MT, Wang S, et al. Quercetin, inflammation, and immunity. Nutrients, 8:167, 2016.

Luc K, Schramm-Luc A, GUzik TJ, Mikolajczyk RP. Oxidative stress and inflammatory markers in prediabetes and diabetes. Journal of Physiology and Pharmacology, 70:809-824, 2019.

Malaguarnera L. Influence of resveratrol on the immune response. Nutrients, 11:956, 2019.

Maslanik T, Tannura K, Mahaffey L, Loughridge AB, Bennison L, Ursell L et al. Commensal bacteria and MAMPs are necessary for stress-induced increases in I-1b and IL-18 but not IL-6, IL10 or MCP-1. PLOS One, 7: e50636, 2012.

Matsuda M, Huh Y, Ji R-R. Roles of inflammation, neurogenic inflammation, and neuroinflammation in pain. Journal of Anesthesia, 33:131-139, 2019.

Meyer JH, Cervenka S, Kim, M-J, Kreisel WC, Henter ID, Innis RB. Neuroinflammation in psychiatric disorders: PET imaging and promising new targets. Lancet Psychiatry, 7:1064-1074, 2020.

Medzhitov R. Inflammation 2010: new adventures of an old flame. Cell, 140:771-776, 2010.

Mills EL, Kelly B, O'Neill LAJ. Mitochondria are the powerhouses of immunity. Nature Immunology, 18:488-498, 2017.

Mitchell S, Vargas J, Hoffmann A. Signaling via the NFkB system. Wiley Interdisciplinary Reviews in Systems Biology and Medicine. 8:227-241, 2016.

Moore N, Scheiman JM. Gastrointestinal safety and tolerability of oral non-aspirin over-the-counter analgesics. Postgraduate Medicine, 130:188-199, 2018.

Nikkhesalt N, Zunszain PQ, Horowitz MA, Barbosa IG, Parker JA, Myint A-M et al. Insufficient glucocorticoid signaling and elevated inflammation in coronary artery disease patient with comorbid depression, Brain, Behavior, and Immunity, 48:8-18, 2015.

Pacher P, Beckman JS, Liaudet L. Nitric oxide and peroxynitrite in health and disease. Physiology Reviews, 87:315-424, 2007.

Palma-Gudiel H, Prather AA, Lin J, Oxendine JD, Guintivano J, Xia K, et al. HPA axis regulation and epigenetic programming of immune-related genes in chronically stressed and non-stressed mid-life women. Brain, Behavior, and Immunity, 92:49-56, 2021.

Pirola L, Frojdo S. Resveratrol: One molecule, many targets. IUMB Life, 60:323-332, 2008.

Ricciotti E, FitzGerald GA. Prostaglandins and Inflammation. Arteriosclerosis Thrombosis and Vascular Biology, 31:986–1000, 2011.

Rossi J-F, Lu ZY, Massart C, Levon K. Dynamic immune/inflammation precision medicine: The good and the bad inflammation in infection and cancer. Frontiers in Immunology, 12:595722, 2021.

Schminkey DL, Groer M. Imitating a stress response: A new hypothesis about the innate immune system's role in pregnancy. Medical Hypotheses, 82:721-729, 2014.

Sergi D, Boulestin H, Campbell FM, Williams LM. The role of dietary advanced glycation end-products in metabolic dysfunction. Molecular Nutrition and Food Research, 65: e1900934, 2021.

Shimba A, Ikuta K. Glucocorticoids regulate circadian rhythm of innate and adaptive immunity. Frontiers in Immunology, 11:2143, 2020.

Smith PK, Masilamani M, Li X-M, Sampson HA. The false alarm hypothesis: Food allergy is associated with high dietary advanced glycation end-products and proglycating dietary sugars that mimic alarmins. Journal of Allergy and Clinical Immunology, 139:429-437, 2017.

Speckmann B, Steinbrenner H, Grune T, Klotz L-O. Peroxynitrite: From interception to signaling. Archives of Biochemistry and Biophysics, 595:153-160, 2016.

Straub RH, Cutolo M. Glucocorticoids and chronic inflammation. Rheumatology, 55:ii6-ii14, 2016.

Stillin RM, van de Wouw M, Clarke G, Stanton C, Dinan TG, Cryan JF. The neuropharmacology of butyrate: The bread and butter of the microbiota-gut-brain axis. Neurochemistry International, 99:110-132, 2016.

Sun H, Sun C, Aiao W, Sun R. Tissue-resident lymphocytes: from adaptive to innate immunity. Cellular and Molecular Immunology, 16:2015-215, 2019.

Tanaka A, Sakaguchi S. Targeting Treg cells in cancer immunotherapy. European Journal of Immunology, 49:1140-1146, 2019.

Veiga-Ferdandes H, Freitas A. The Sensory Immune System Theory. Trends in Immunology, 38:777-788, 2017.

Wan J, Cai W, Wang H, Cheng J, Su Z, Wang S, Xu H. Role of type 2 innate lymphoid cell and its related cytokines in tumor immunity. Journal of Cellular Physiology, 35:3249-3257, 2020.

Wei P, Yang F, Zheng Q, Tang W, Li J. The Potential Role of the NLRP3 Inflammasome activation as a link between mitochondria ROS generation and neuroinflammation in postoperative cognitive dysfunction. Frontiers in Cellular Neuroscience, 13:73, 2019.

Weichhart T, Hengstschläger M, Linke M. Regulation of innate immune cell function by mTOR. Nature Immunology Reviews, 15:599-614, 2015.

Yu Y, Shen Q, Lai Y, Park SY, Ou X, Lin D et al. Anti-inflammatory effects of curcumin in microglial cells. Frontiers in Pharmacology, 9:386, 2018.

Zhang Q, Lenardo MJ, Baltimore D. 30 years of NFkB: A blossoming of relevance to human pathobiology. Cell, 168:37-57, 2017.

Zindel J, Kubes P. DAMPs, PAMPs, and LAMPs in immunity and sterile inflammation. Annual Review of Pathology, 15:493-518, 2020.

- HOW THE IMMUNE SYSTEM SIGNALS THE BRAIN
- NEURAL INTEROCEPTIVE IMMUNE-TO-BRAIN PATHWAYS
- CYTOKINES CAN ALSO CIRCULATE IN BLOOD: HUMORAL IMMUNE-TO-BRAIN SIGNALING
- THE IMMUNE SYSTEM IN THE BRAIN
- CYTOKINES CAN MAKE YOU STUPID: NEUROINFLAMMATION AND COGNITION
- INFLAMMATION AND "HOW WE FEEL"
- DIET CAN CONTRIBUTE TO THE SICKNESS SYNDROME
- BIDIRECTIONAL EFFECTS OF IMMUNE-TO-BRAIN COMMUNICATION: ATTITUDES AFFECT INFLAMMATION
- NEGATIVE ATTITUDES, SOCIAL STRESS, AND LONELINESS ARE PRO-INFLAMMATORY
- KEY POINTS

Over the past fifteen years or so I have encountered many people who relate a now-familiar story of co-occurring symptoms. They have gastrointestinal problems, such as celiac disease, food sensitivities, acid reflux, irritable bowel syndrome, or inflammatory bowel disease. They are on proton pump inhibitors, such as Prilosec, for reflux. They have mood disturbances, such as depression, anxiety, or both. They are taking medications for mood disorders. They often have fatigue and cognitive "fuzziness." They have problems sleeping. They have a pain condition, such as migraine headache, fibromyalgia, or pain associated with irritable bowel. Often their physicians and other practitioners can't explain the symptoms, but their clinicians usually insist they can't be related. For instance, people are often told that gluten allergy can't affect the brain. This leaves people feeling frustrated, helpless, and a little scared.

I recognize this pattern of symptoms instantly as the hallmark of *sickness syndrome*, which results from activation of the immune system in the context of an infection or during inflammation (Mechanic 1962). This syndrome is well-known to be induced by pro-inflammatory cytokines associated with inflammation (Dantzer 2007, Watkins 1995, Goehler 2000, Konsman 2000, Quan 2007, Shattuck 2016) and symptoms are mediated by the brain. However, the level of inflammation needed to induce these symptoms does not need to be high, and it may not seem evident to practitioners that there is anything wrong. But if the syndrome is not recognized, the underlying cause of the inflammation will not be addressed, leading to prolonged suffering, or even death if the inflammation is being caused by cancer or a serious infection.

In a normal situation involving inflammation, the infection is resolved, healing begins, and the sickness syndrome resolves. However, if the condition becomes chronic, the symptoms of sickness can persist. Sickness syndrome is often seen in chronic disease conditions such as diabetes, heart disease, autoimmune disease, chronic pain, and cancer, or with chemotherapy for cancer.

How the Immune System Signals the Brain

When the immune system is activated by infection, after detecting PAMPs, or damage, after detecting DAMPs, cytokines are released by immune cells that amplify inflammation by signaling other cells. Part of the body's initial response involves signaling the brain, because some of the responses necessary to fight infection involve coordination by the brain (Dantzer 2007, Watkins 1995, Goehler 2000). Such responses include fever and release of cortisol, followed by the fatigue, cognitive fuzziness, and low mood that are the classic symptoms of sickness syndrome. These responses are considered to be beneficial during infection (Saper 2012), because elevated body temperature during infection slows the growth of bacteria or viruses, and the immune system works more effectively at higher temperatures. Behavioral changes, such as fatigue, sleepiness, low mood, and cognitive fuzziness encourage conservation of energy to fight the infection, and social isolation reduces the risk of spreading the infection to other people.

This immune-to-brain communication forms an important channel of interoception, the system that senses the condition of the body. Infection and inflammation are challenges that can be life-threatening, thus, several pathways convey immune-related information to the brain (Quan 2007). This seeming redundancy ensures the integrity of these critical signals to the brain.

Neural Interoceptive Immune-to-Brain Pathways

Inflammation consequent to infection or tissue damage induces cytokines and other mediators, such as prostaglandins, from local immune cells in the affected tissues. The vagus nerve and the sympathetic nervous system have receptors for these inflammatory mediators, and they signal the presence of inflammation within these tissues to the brain.

The vagus nerve collects information from the tissues it innervates and conveys signals to the brainstem relay stations. Specifically, the vagus sends signals from heart, lung, gastrointestinal tract, liver, pancreas, and some lymph nodes to the dorsal vagal complex. The dorsal vagal complex is a collection of brain centers that integrate information for the autonomic nervous system. From there, several different pathways forward the information to brain networks that manage different aspects of response to challenges (Gaykema 2011 Marvel 2004). One follows the classic interoception pathway, which ascends through the midbrain to the thalamus, and then to the insula. This is part of the Salience Network (SN). Another pathway targets the hypothalamus, which organizes neuroendocrine and sympathetic nervous system responses, including cortisol release and regulation of blood pressure and blood glucose. Still another pathway signals the amygdala, which helps organize autonomic responses and integrate them with emotions. These pathways activate the SN and anterior Default Mode Network (DMN), giving rise to our experience of illness. Along the way, brain regions that function in arousal and motivation are also targeted (Felger 2017, Harrison 2016). These regions include the raphe nuclei that signal using serotonin, the ventral tegmental areas that signal using dopamine, and hypothalamic areas that signal using histamine. The influence of inflammatory activation on these areas likely contributes to the effects on alertness/fatigue and motivation (Gaykema 2011, Felger 2017, Quadt 2018).

Sensory nerves of the sympathetic system mostly run along blood vessels to supply every tissue of the body. In addition to detecting inflammation in visceral tissues, these nerves can also detect inflammation in skin, joints, blood vessels, as well as the sinuses, mouth, scalp and so forth. In general, these nerves signal pain, and they activate pathways that ascend the spinal cord and follow the interoceptive pain pathways that ultimately target the insula and prefrontal cortex (Quadt 2018).

Cytokines can also Circulate in Blood: Humoral Immune-to-Brain Signaling

In the context of severe local inflammation or systemic inflammation, cytokines can spill over into the circulation, or they can be released from immune cells in the blood. These blood-borne cytokines propagate the signal to the brain by binding to receptors at the brain barrier areas, such as the meninges, circumventricular organs, and blood vessels (Banks 2015, Quan 2017). They can also be actively transported into the brain, particularly in certain interoceptive areas like the hypothalamus and hippocampus, where they bind to receptors (Banks 2015). Neuronal and glial cells express receptors for cytokines. Activation of the cytokine receptors and activate inflammation within the brain, or neuroinflammation, which can disrupt functions such as learning and memory (Dantzer 2007, DiSabato 2016). Signals transduced at brain barrier areas activate the same drive on neural networks as do vagally-transduced inflammatory signals. These also produce similar sickness syndrome symptoms.

The Immune System IN the Brain

Until recently, the brain was thought to be an "immunoprivileged" organ that has little interaction with the immune system. It was believed that immune cells normally did not enter the brain. We now know the brain has a close, collaborative, and bidirectional relationship with the immune system (Quan 2007). In fact, the brain has its own set of immune cells, mostly comprised of *microglia* (Korin 2017). Microglia are similar to macrophages, monocytes, and dendritic cells found in the rest of the body (Barr 2019). In addition, many other types of immune cells live in the brain's barrier regions, including the meninges and blood vessels. These include macrophages, dendritic cells, mast cells, and T cells.

Although microglia are similar in function to the monocyte family of immune cells, unlike these cells, they do not develop from bone marrow. Rather, they differentiate very early in development in the embryonic yolk sac, then migrate to the fetal liver, and then into the developing brain (Barr 2019). Once there, microglia secrete growth factors and help the new brain cells survive, migrate, and establish connections with each other. Conditions associated with microglial dysfunction include autism and other neurodevelopmental disorders.

Like peripheral immune cells, microglia tend to be polarized in function: they support pro-inflammatory Type 1 or anti-inflammatory and regulatory Type 2 functions (Li 2020). In healthy, younger brains, microglia are more polarized to the Type 2 phenotype (DiSabato 2016). This makes sense because the brain is particularly sensitive to the deleterious effects of inflammation. Microglia functioning in a type 2 mode provides growth factors and continues to facilitate synaptogenesis and neuroplasticity. They also remove cellular debris, helping to "take out the garbage." These functions are considered *neuroprotective* (DiSabato 2016).

During chronic inflammation, such as seen in neurodegenerative diseases, aging, or chronic stress, microglia change their shapes and function (DiSabato 2106, Ward 2015). They shift away from releasing growth factors to releasing pro-inflammatory cytokines, including IL-1, IL6, or TNF (Di Sabato 2016, Ward 2015). This phenomenon is termed neuroinflammation. Neuroinflammation a key pathophysiological feature of neurodegenerative diseases such as Alzheimer's disease and multiple sclerosis, and neuropsychiatric conditions including depression, schizophrenia, autism spectrum, and bipolar disorder (Paper 2019).

Cytokines Can Make You Stupid: Neuroinflammation and Cognition

The neuroprotective actions of microglia include modulation of learning and memory. This involves low levels of cytokines including IL-1 and TNF (Bourgognon 2020, DiSabato 2016). However, in the context of severe illness, such as COVID-19 infection or neurodegenerative disease, high levels of these cytokines in the brain can act to impair learning and memory (Rahman 2021, Bourgognon 2020). In addition, microglial release of reactive oxygen and nitrogen species can damage brain tissues and exacerbate cognitive dysfunction.

Notably, neuroinflammation can be triggered by inflammation in the body, or by damage or pathogens within the brain (Andonegui 2018, Di Sabato 2016). This is likely a mechanism underlying the association between chronic disease or damage to the body, and neurological conditions such as dementia, that are characterized by neuroinflammation (Behl 2021, Flores-Aguilar 2021). Two examples of cognitive impairment due to inflammation are the "fibro fog" associated with fibromyalgia and "chemo brain" linked with chemotherapy. Neuroinflammation is also seen in psychiatric illness, particularly severe depression and post-traumatic stress disorder (PTSD), which can also involve cognitive impairment.

Inflammation and "How We Feel"

The idea that immune system-related signals such as cytokines can cause mood and cognitive symptoms is supported by neuroimaging studies of humans treated with a PAMP to induce experimental inflammation (Lasselin 2016). Studies where humans are treated with lipopolysaccharide from gram-negative bacteria, thus exposing the subjects to a PAMP in the absence of the pathogen, have shown subsequent development of anxiety, depression, and memory impairment (Yirmiya 2000, Lasselin 2016). This finding reinforces the link between inflammation and depression (Miller 2009). Other studies have reported that inflammation biases the brain toward experience of increased negative emotions (Harrison, 2016, Quadt 2020). In depressed people, inflammation is associated with anhedonia and fatigue (Felger 2017, Chaves-Filho 2019). These findings provide a direct link from inflammation to the kinds of experiences associated with not feeling "well."

Diet Can Contribute to the Sickness Syndrome

People with poor diet, including prepared or fast foods, are more likely than those with a healthy diet to report symptoms of fatigue, mood disorders, chronic pain, and sleep problems, which are hallmarks of sickness syndrome (Bramorska 2021, Firth 2019, Lopez-Taboada 2020). These symptoms imply that inflammation is present. But how could these diets be causing inflammation?

As we will see in the upcoming chapters, diets that are high in processed foods and refined carbohydrates often contain additives or toxin residues that can act like PAMPs or DAMPs, and induce dysbiosis or inflammation in the gut and/or liver (Herieka 2016, Barnett 2020, Faraj 2019). Glyphosate, the main component of Roundup®, is one example of such a residue found on crops (Barnett 2020). Further, a diet poor in micronutrients or good quality protein may not provide the necessary nutrients to keep cells healthy, leading to release of damage signals like DAMPs, which also drive inflammation. Further, a poor diet generally does not support a healthy gut microbial population. A healthy gut microbial population is also important for regulating inflammation and healthy brain function (Langgartner 2019, Valles-Colover 2019). The inflammation associated with a poor diet can drive sickness symptoms, and a poor diet can exacerbate sickness symptoms associated with chronic disease. Thus, inflammation directly links diet with how we feel.

Bidirectional Effects of Immune-to-Brain Communication: Attitudes Affect Inflammation

Our social lives and attitudes also influence inflammation. People who have positive attitudes, and active supportive social lives with meaningful activities or hobbies, have less inflammation and disease than do people who are lonely and/or have negative attitudes (Eisenberger 2016). They also tend to live longer healthier lives (Yang 2016). Just as what is going on in the immune system influences brain functions, what is going on the brain influences immune function.

This bidirectional interaction is carried out by peripheral autonomic nerves, and hormones such as cortisol, that are under control of the brain. The effects of the nerve signals and hormones can either be pro- or anti-inflammatory. Emotions affect the output of certain cortical brain regions and the hypothalamus. These outputs determine the pattern of neuronal activity and their influence on immune function, as well as blood pressure and blood sugar levels. Negative emotions, such as anger or stress, lead to elevated levels of cortisol and sympathetic activation (Lampert 2010, Hackett 2015, Pauly 2021, Viana Machado 2021). Chronic hypercortisolemia and sympathetic activation lead to inflammation, hypertension, and hyperglycemia. These can drive chronic disease and mechanistically link negative emotional states with disease (Rohlender 2014). In contrast, positive emotions engage brain circuits, including parts of the anterior Default Mode Network (DMN) that activate the vagus nerve (Alexander 2021). Vagus nerve activity reduces blood pressure and inflammation, helping to shift the body into a healing, homeostatic mode instead of stress (Bonaz 2016, Zila 2017).

Negative Attitudes, Social Stress and Loneliness are Pro-Inflammatory

The idea that personality can influence health derived from findings from the Framingham Heart Study, a large prospective study which began in the 1950's. It was designed to assess many possible risks for heart disease, including health behaviors such as smoking, family history, and attitudes. By the 1970's, it was clear that a pattern of behavior, termed *Type A Personality*, conferred a significant risk for heart disease (Haynes 1980). Type A Personality was characterized by feelings of time pressure, competitiveness, cynical and/or hostile attitudes, and impatience (American Psychological Association, 2022). In the years since the findings were reported, further studies have shown that cynicism and hostility were the main features that conferred the increased risk of heart disease, as well as other conditions (Janicki-Deverts 2009). But what is meant by *cynicism* and *hostility*?

For the purposes of research, cynicism is defined as a tendency to be disparaging or distrustful of the motives of other people (Michel 2014). People who score high in cynicism will agree with statements such as "most people behave only in their own self-interest," and "most people are likely to take advantage of you, if you let them." Hostility is considered to reflect hypervigilant behavior towards threats, and aggressive response to threats. Concerns about dominance and retribution for perceived slights is also associated with hostility (Michel 2014). This combination of behaviors is reflected in enhanced psychophysiological arousal, and increased levels of inflammation or inflammatory markers, such as increased pro-inflammatory cytokines (Marsland 2008).

The demonstration that attitudes can affect health spurred other researchers to ask whether other patterns of attitudes could predict disease. It has since been shown that people with a passive coping style, pessimistic and depressive attitudes, and a tendency towards *social inhibition* are also at higher risk for metabolic disease and increased inflammation (Janicki-Deverts 2010, Jandackova 2017). This cluster of attitudes and behavior patterns have been termed Type D personality. Taken together, these findings underline the fact that if we want to feel better, and experience a good quality of life, we must address our attitudes and coping styles, and develop positive approaches to challenges.

While attitudes that drive negative emotions can induce or increase inflammation, social experiences such as being excluded or bullied, or feeling lonely, also influence inflammation (Eisenberger 2010, Kiecolt-Glaser 2010, Quadt 2020). People who report feeling lonely have higher levels of pro-inflammatory cytokines in their blood than other people. Moreover, laboratory studies show that non-lonely volunteers involved in social exclusion experiments show short-term increases in circulating pro-inflammatory cytokines, concomitant with their reports of lower mood following the experience.

The link between loneliness, mood, and inflammation is particularly important in the context of mental illness. It has been appreciated for many years that psychological stress worsens symptoms of depression and schizophrenia (Howes 2017). Social stress, in particular loneliness, turns out to be the main factor accounting for this effect (Slavich 2010). Negative attitudes are associated with lower functioning in schizophrenia, but social skills training and other interventions that promote self-efficacy are associated with functional improvement (Ventura 2014, Javed 2018, Turner 2018). The association of inflammation with schizophrenia, autism, and depression is increasingly evident (Howes 2017, Prata 2017, Savitz 2018). The mechanisms that underlie the association are unclear, but the links between social stress and inflammation suggest that interventions that can help support positive attitudes and coping and improve social skills may ameliorate effects of inflammation of the neuropsychiatric symptoms associated with these disorders.

Key Points

- Inflammation affects how we feel by activating interoceptive immune-to-brain communication pathways that induce sickness symptoms of fatigue, low mood, anxiety, and cognitive "fuzziness".

- Inflammation in the body can lead to inflammation in the brain, called neuroinflammation. Neuroinflammation is associated with mood symptoms, cognitive impairment, and risk for neurodegenerative diseases.
- This immune-to-brain communication is a major mechanism by which diet influences how we feel.
- Immune-to-brain communication is bi-directional such that what is going on in the brain, such as attitudes, response to challenges or stress, how connected we feel to other people, and mood states such as depression, influence the condition of our bodies via influence on the HPA axis, cortisol levels, and the autonomic nervous system.
- Social relationships play an outsized role in health. People who are lonely and/or feel disconnected from society experience higher levels of inflammation and risk of many diseases. Similarly, good social integration can protect people at risk from the deleterious effects of socio-economic stress.

References

Alexander R, Aragon O, Bookwala, Cherbuin N, Batt JM, Kahrilas IJ, et al. The neuroscience of positive emotions and affect: Implications for cultivating happiness and well-being. Neuroscience and Biobehavioral Reviews, 121:220-247, 2021.

American Psychological Association. APA Dictionary of Psychology, available at: dictionary.apa.org/type-a-personality, accessed on June 20, 2022.

Andonegui G, Zelinski EL, Schubert CL, Knight D, Craig LA, Winston BW, et al. Targeting inflammatory monocytes in sepsis-associated encephalopathy and long-term cognitive impairment. JCI Insight, 3: e99364, 2018.

Banks WA. The blood-brain barrier in neuroimmunology: Tales of separation and assimilation. Brain, Behavior, and Immunity, 44:1-8, 2015.

Barnett JA, Gibson DL. Separating the empirical wheat from the pseudoscientific chaff: A critical review of the literature surrounding glyphosate, dysbiosis and wheat sensitivity. Frontiers in Microbiology, 11:556729, 2020.

Barr E, Barak B. Microglia roles in synaptic plasticity and myelination in homeostatic conditions and neurodevelopmental disorders. Glia, 67:2125-2141, 2019.

Behl T, Makkar R, Sehgal A, Singh S Sharma N, Zengin G, et al. Current trends in neurodegeneration: Cross talks between oxidative stress, cell death, and inflammation. International Journal of Molecular Sciences, 22:7432, 2021.

Bonaz B, Sinniger V, Pellissier S. Anti-inflammatory properties of the vagus nerve: potential therapeutic implications of vagus nerve stimulation. Journal of Physiology, 594:5781-5790, 2016.

Bourgognon J-M, Cavanaugh J. The role of cytokines in modulating learning and memory and brain plasticity. Brain and Neuroscience Advances, 4:1-13, 2020.

Bramorska, A, Zarzycka, W, Podolecka, W, Kuc, K, Brzezicka, A. Age-Related Cognitive Decline May Be Moderated by Frequency of Specific Food Products Consumption. Nutrients, 13:2504. 2021.

Chaves-Filho AJM, Macedo DS, Freitas de Lucena D, Maes M. Shared microglial mechanisms underpinning depression and chronic fatigue syndrome and their comorbidities. Behavioral Brain Research, 372:111975, 2019.

Dantzer R, O'Connor JC, Freund GG, Johnson RW, Kelley KW. From inflammation to sickness and depression: when the immune system subjugates the brain. Nature Reviews Neuroscience, 9: 46-56, 2008.

DiSabato D, Quan N, Godbout JP. Neuroinflammation: The Devil is in the Details. Journal of Neurochemistry, 139:136-153, 2016.

Ditzen B, Heinrichs M. Psychobiology of social support: The social dimension of stress buffering. Restorative Neurology and Neuroscience, 32:149-162, 2014.

Eisenberger NI, Inagaki TK, Mashal NM, Irwin MR. Inflammation and social experience: An inflammatory challenge induces feelings of social disconnection in addition to depressed mood. Brain Behavior and Immunity, 24:558-563, 2010.

Eisenberger NI, Moieni M, Inagaki TK, Muscatell KA, Irwin MR. In sickness and in health: the co-regulation of inflammation and social behavior. Neuropsychopharmacology, 2016.

Faraj TA, Stover C, Erridge C. Dietary Toll-like receptor stimulants promote hepatic inflammation and impair reverse cholesterol transport in mice via macrophage-dependent interleukin-1 production. Frontiers in Immunology, 10:1404, 2019.

Felger JC, Treadway MT, Inflammation effects on motivation and motor activity: role of dopamine. Neuropsychopharmacology Review, 42:216–241, 2017.

Firth J, Veronese N, Cotter J, Shivappa N, Hebert JR, Ee C, et al. What is the role of dietary inflammation in severe mental illness? A review of observational and experimental findings. Frontiers in Psychiatry, 10:350, 2019.

Flores-Aguilar L, Iolita MF, Orciani C, Tanna N Yang J, Bennett DA, Cuello AC. Cognitive and brain cytokine profile of non-demented individuals with cerebral amyloid-beta deposition. Journal of Neuroinflammation, 18:147, 2021.

Gaykema RP, Goehler LE. Ascending caudal medullary catecholamine pathways drive sickness-induced deficits in exploratory behavior: brain substrates for fatigue? Brain Behavior and Immunity. 25:443-60, 2011.

Goehler LE, Gaykema RP, Hansen MK, Anderson K, Maier SF, Watkins LR. Vagal immune-to-brain communication: a visceral chemosensory pathway. Autonomic Neuroscience, 85:49-59, 2000.

Hackett RA, Lazzarino AI, Carvalho LA, Hamer M, Steptoe A. Hostility and Physiological Responses to Acute Stress in People with Type 2 Diabetes. Psychosomatic Medicine, 77:458-466, 2015.

Harrison NA, Voon V, Cercigniani M, Cooper EA, Pessiglione M, Critchley HD. A neurocomputational account of how inflammation enhances sensitivity to punishments versus rewards. Biological Psychiatry, 80:73-81, 2016.

Haynes S, Feinleib M, Kannel WB. The relationship of psychosocial factors to coronary heart disease in the Framingham study III. Eight-year incidence of coronary heart disease. American Journal of Epidemiology, 111:37-58, 1980.

Herieka M, Faraj TA, Erridge C. Reduced dietary intake of pro-inflammatory Toll-like receptor stimulants favorably modifies markers of cardiometabolic risk in healthy men. Nutrition, Metabolism and Cardiovascular Diseases, 26:194-200, 2016.

Howes OD, McCutcheon R. Inflammation and the neural diasthesis-stress hypothesis of schizophrenia: a reconceptualization. Translational Psychiatry, 7: e1024, 2017.

Jandackova VK, Julian Koenig J, Jarczok MN, Fischer J, Thayer JF. Potential biological pathways linking Type-D personality and poor health: A cross-sectional Investigation. PLoS One, 12(4): e0176014, 2017.

Janicki-Deverts D, Cohen S, Doyle WJ. Cynical Hostility and Stimulated Th1 and Th2 Cytokine Production. Brain Behavior and Immunity, 24: 58-63, 2010.

Javed A, Charles A. The importance of social cognition in improving functional outcomes in schizophrenia. Frontiers in Psychiatry, 9 article 157, 2018.

Kiecolt-Glaser JK, Close relationships, inflammation, and health. Neuroscience and Biobehavioral Reviews, 35:33-38, 2010.

Konsman JP, Luheshi GN, Bluthe R-M, Dantzer R. The vagus nerve mediates behavioural depression, but not fever, in response to peripheral immune signals; a functional anatomical analysis. European Journal of Neuroscience, 12: 4434-4446, 2000.

Korin B, Ben-Shaanan TL, Schiller M, Dubovik T, Azulay-Debby H, Boshnak NT, Koren T, Rolls A. High-dimensional, single-cell characterization of the brain's immune compartment. Nature Neuroscience, 20:1300-1311, 2017.

Langgartner D, Lowry CA, Reber SO. Old Friends, immunoregulation, and stress resilience. Pflügers Archive - European Journal of Physiology, 471:237–269, 2019.

Lampert R. Anger and ventricular arrhythmias. Current Opinion in Cardiology, 25:46-52, 2010.

Lasselin J, Elsenbruch S, Lekander M, Axelsson J, Karshikoff B, Grigoleit J-S, Engler H, Schedlowski M, Benson S. Mood disturbance during experimental endotoxemia: Predictors of state anxiety as a psychological component of sickness behavior. Brain Behavior and Immunity, 57:30-37, 2016.

Li N, Stewart T, Sheng L, Shi M, Cilento EM We Y, et al. Immunoregulation of microglial polarization: an unrecognized physiological function of ⊡-synuclein. Journal of Neuroinflammation, 17:272, 2020.

Lopez-Taboada I, Gonalez-Pardo H, Conejo NM. Western diet: Implications for brain function and behavior. Frontiers in Psychology, 11:564413, 2020.

Marsland AL, Prather AA, Petersen KL, Cohen S, Manuck SB. Antagonistic characteristics are positively associated with inflammatory markers independently of trait negative emotionality. Brain, Behavior, and Immunity, 22:753-761, 2008.

Marvel FA, Chen CC, Badr N, Gaykema RP, Goehler LE. Reversible inactivation of the dorsal vagal complex blocks lipopolysaccharide-induced social withdrawal and c-Fos expression in central autonomic nuclei, 18:123-34, 2004.

Mechanic D. The concept of illness behavior. Journal of Chronic Diseases, 15:189-194, 1962.

Michel JS, Pace VL, Edun A, Sawhney E, Thomas J. Development of and validation of an explicit aggressive beliefs and attitude scale. Journal of Personality Assessment, 96:327-338, 2014.

Miller AH, Maletic V, Raison CL. Inflammation and its discontents: The role of cytokines in the pathophysiology of depression. Biological Psychiatry, 65:732-741, 2009.

Pape K, Tamouza R, Leboyer M, Zipp F. Immunoneuropsychiatry - novel perspectives on brain disorders. Nature Reviews Neurology, 2019.

Prata J, Santos S, Almeida MI, Coehlo R, Barbosa MA. Bridging autism spectrum disorders and schizophrenia through inflammation and biomarkers - pre-clinical and clinical investigations. Journal of Neuroinflammation, 14:170, 2017.

Pauly T, Drewelies J, Kolodziejczak K, Katzorreck M, Lucke AJ, Schilling OK, et al. Positive and negative affect are associated with salivary cortisol in the everyday life of older adults: A quantitative synthesis of four aging studies. Psychoneuroendocrinology, 133, 105403, 2021.

Quadt L, Critchley HD, Garfinkel SN. The neurobiology of interoception in health and disease. Annals of the New York Academy of Sciences, 1428:112-128, 2018.

Quadt L, Esposito G, Critchley HD, Garfinkel SN. Brain-body interactions underlying the association of loneliness with mental and physical health. Neuroscience and Biobehavioral Reviews, 116:283-300, 2020.

Quan N, Banks WA. Brain-immune communication pathways. Brain, Behavior, and Immunity, 21: 727-735, 2007.

Rahman MA, Islam K, Rahman S, Alamin M. Neurobiological cross-talk between COVID-19 and Alzheimer's Disease. Molecular Neurobiology, 58:1017-1023, 2021.

Rohleder N. Stimulation of systemic low-grade inflammation by psychosocial stress. Psychosomatic Medicine, 76:181-189, 2014.

Saper CB, Romanovsky AA, Scammell TE. Neural circuitry engaged by prostaglandins during sickness syndrome. Nature Neuroscience, 8:1088-1095, 2012.

Savitz J, Harrison NA. Interoception and Inflammation in psychiatric disorders. Biological Psychiatry: Neuroscience and Neuroimaging, 2018.

Shattuck EC, Muehlenbein MP. Towards an integrative picture of human sickness behavior. Brain Behavior and Immunity, 57:255-262, 2016.

Slavich GM, O'Donovan A, Epel ES, Kemeny ME. Black Sheep Get the Blues: A Psychobiological Model of Social Rejection and Depression. Neuroscience and Biobehavioral Reviews, 35: 39-45, 2010.

Sturgeon JA, Zautra AJ, Social pain and physical pain: shared paths to resilience. Pain Management, 6:63-74, 2016.

Turner DT, McGlanaghy E, Cuijpers P, van der Gaag M, Karyotaki E, MacBeth A. A Meta-analysis of social skills training and related interventions for psychosis. Schizophrenia Bulletin, 44:475-491, 2018.

Valles-Colomer M, Falony G, Darzi Y, Tigchelaar EF, Wang J, Tito RY, Schiweck C, Kurilshikov A, Joossens M, Wijmenga C, Claes S, Van Oudenhove L, Zhernakova A, Vieira-Silva S. The neuroactive potential of the human gut microbiota in quality of life and depression. Nature Microbiology, 2019.

Ventura J, Subotnik KL, Ered A, Gretchen-Doorly D, Hellemann GS, Vaskinn A, Nuechterlein K. The relationship of attitudinal beliefs to negative symptoms, neurocognition, and daily functioning in recent-onset schizophrenia. Schizophrenia Bulletin, 40:1308-1318, 2014.

Viana Machado A, Garcia Pereira M, Souza GGL, Xavier M, Aguiar C, de Oliveira L, Mocaiber I. Association between distinct coping styles and heart rate variability changes to an acute psychosocial stress task. Science Reports, 11:24025, 2021.

Ward RJ, Dexter DT, Crighton RR. Aging, neuroinflammation and neurodegeneration. Frontiers in Bioscience, 7:189-204, 2015.

Watkins LR, Maier SF, Goehler LE. Immune activation: the role of pro-inflammatory cytokines in inflammation, illness responses and pathological pain states. Pain, 63:289-302, 1995.

Yang, CY, Boen C, Gerken K, Li T, Schorpp K, Harris, KM, Social relationships and physiological determinants of longevity across the human life span. Proceedings of the National Academy of Science, 113:578-583, 2016.

Yirmiya R, Pollak Y, Morag M, Reichenberg A, Barak O, Avitsur R, Shavit Y, et al. Illness, cytokines and depression. Annals of the New York Academy of Sciences, 917:478-487, 2000.

Zila I, Mokra D, Kopincova J, Kolomaznik M, Javorka M, Calkovska A. Vagal-immune interactions in cholinergic anti-inflammatory pathway. Physiology Research, 66: S139-S135, 2017.

- GENES AND INFLAMMATION

- THE IMMUNE SYSTEM, FOOD, AND INFLAMMATION IN EARLY LIFE

- ADVERSE CHILDHOOD EXPERIENCES PROGRAM INFLAMMATION IN ADULTHOOD

- DOES CHILDHOOD OBESITY LEAD TO INCREASED RISK OF DISEASE IN ADULTHOOD?

- INFLAMMATION AS WE AGE: INFLAMMAGING

- INFLAMMATION, AGING, AND NEURODEGENERATIVE DISEASES

- LIFESTYLE AFFECTS INFLAMMATION AS WE AGE

- KEY POINTS

Immune system function changes over our lives, from the time we are born to when we are elderly. One key factor that affects these changes is diet. What we eat as children affects how well we grow, and poor diets can increase the risk of obesity and/or inflammation later in life. The many individual differences in how healthy we stay depend upon interactions between the genes we inherit and our lifestyles. As we age, our diets can influence our risk of cognitive impairment, and other disorders related to inflammation.

Genes and Inflammation

There is tremendous variation in vulnerability to disease across different individuals. Some people can eat junk food and live sedentary lives and remain fairly healthy into middle age. Others are highly conscientious about the food they eat, stay physically active, and try to manage their stress, but struggle nevertheless with inflammatory conditions such as autoimmune, gastrointestinal, pain, and allergic conditions. What accounts for these differences? In general, disease risk follows from interactions of inherited gene variants with epigenetic changes that result from life experiences and lifestyle, including stress and diet. Many of the genes associated with risk for inflammatory conditions are involved with the inflammasomes, cytokines, and pathogen-sensing systems (Ahola-Olli 2017, Kanchan 2021, Ribeiro 2020). Variants in these genes can cause dysregulation of inflammation, leading to an effective pro-inflammatory phase response to pathogens, but difficulty in transitioning from inflammation into the healing phase.

Gene-linkage studies identify gene variants that are associated with specific diseases and thus may play a role in causing them. Gene-linkage studies have revealed a possible link between immune-related genes and a wide variety of conditions, including heart disease, diabetes, inflammatory bowel disease (IBD), schizophrenia, autism, and neurodegenerative diseases, including Parkinson's disease and Alzheimer's disease (Ahola-Olli 2017). Some of these immune-related genes are targets of *epigenetic modifications* that can impair proper immune function (Sancesario 2018). For example, some immune-related genes may be modified in response to stress (Zannas 2019). Therefore, lifestyle factors such as diet and stress management are likely to influence disease risk by interacting with genetic susceptibilities. For example,

IBD is associated with specific genes involved in pathogen-sensing, which likely leads to impaired regulation of inflammation (Ahola-Olli 2017, Rubin 2012). When people with these gene variants develop an imbalance in microbes, severe and sometimes life-threatening inflammation is triggered at the gut barrier (Rubin 2012). In this way, genes interact with life experiences to induce disease.

The Immune System, Food, and Inflammation in Early Life

Our immune systems are essentially naïve when we are born. A major goal of immune system development is to learn what kinds of foreign things, like food, are dangerous and should be attacked and destroyed, and which things are safe or beneficial and should be tolerated (Kucuksezer 2020, Nowak-Wegrzyn 2017). When applied to food, this process is called *oral tolerance* and involves the active inhibition of immune responses to food.

There seems to be a critical period during the first year or so of infancy, when the immune system actively learns tolerance (Peters 2016). Although the details of this critical period are not well understood, current recommendations are that infants start on solid foods around 4 months of age, so that they can properly develop oral tolerance.

When oral tolerance does not develop properly, the immune system treats harmless food items, such as peanuts or gluten, as dangerous. This leads to food sensitivities and allergies. Why this happens in some children but not others is not entirely clear. Food allergies do run in families, implying genetic components (Kanchan 2021). Many children with food allergies, especially to peanuts, also suffer from atopic skin conditions such as eczema (Kanchan 2021, Nowak-Wegrzyn 2017). It has been suggested that if skin creams containing peanut oil are used on broken skin, they may sensitize the immune system to peanuts (Peters 2016).

Another key factor in the development and course of food allergy concerns the gut microbiome (Marrs 2018, Bunyavanich 2019). As we will see in Chapter 17, gut microbes play critical roles in modulating the gut immune system. Recent studies have shown that people with food allergies have different populations of gut microbes than people who have healthy food tolerances. Moreover, disturbed microbe populations (i.e., dysbiosis) often precede food allergy development (Bunyavanish 2019).

Experience with different kinds of foods during early childhood seems to teach tolerance. For instance, early experience with peanuts reduces the risk of developing peanut allergies later in childhood. However, this effect has not yet been demonstrated for other food allergies (Peters 2016). When introducing new foods to babies, whole foods such as eggs, appear to be safer and less antigenic (immune-stimulating) than processed foods, such as pasteurized egg protein powder. Similarly, hypoallergenic baby formula, which contains processed, partially digested components, has not actually been found to be less allergenic (Peters 2016).

Adverse Childhood Experiences Program Inflammation in Adulthood and Increase Risk of Obesity and Chronic Disease

Not only does stress, neglect, trauma, or abuse in childhood predispose children to psychological and neuroendocrine problems, but these Adverse Childhood Experiences (ACE) lead to increased levels of inflammation, as early as young adulthood (Felitti 2019, Danese 2017, Gonzalez 2013). ACE in early childhood particularly increases risk of these negative health consequences. Increased inflammation in those with ACE has been linked to epigenetic changes in the regulation of genes that control inflammation and the HPA axis (Gonzalez 2013). Increased inflammation dramatically increases the risk for chronic pain conditions such as fibromyalgia and irritable bowel syndrome, and metabolic disease and psychiatric conditions, particularly depression (Groenewald 2020, Olivieri 2012, Park 2016, Campbell 2018, Danese 2017). People who experience ACE also experience higher risk for aging-related cognitive impairment, quite possibly related to the increased long-term experience of inflammation (Lin 2021).

ACE lead to a much higher risk of obesity throughout the lifespan, from childhood through old age (Ernst 2019, Feely 2019, Gustafson 2004, McKelvey 201). Some of this increased risk for obesity may follow from the fact that many children who experience trauma or neglect are from low-income families and have a poor diet, even as adults (Goldstein 2021, Aquilina 2021). Diets high in refined carbohydrates, and especially sugars such as fructose, are associated with increased inflammation, even in children and adolescents. This increased inflammation can be expected to exacerbate mood and stress-related neuroendocrine dysregulation. Together these may contribute to difficulty regulating emotions. An impaired ability to regulate emotions is a key component of eating disorders and emotional eating. Emotional eating typically involves preference for high-carbohydrate, sugary foods that can induce inflammation (van Strien 2013). In this way, mood symptoms arising from adverse childhood experiences are worsened by a poor diet, which can further drive mood symptoms and emotional eating.

Sexual abuse, experienced in either childhood or adulthood, is particularly associated with eating disorders, obesity, and metabolic syndrome (Almuneef 2021, Grilo 2001, Levine 2016). Sexual abuse in ACE survivors may be complicated by shame and secrecy that accompanies the abuse. This secrecy may be demanded by the perpetrators and often follows the victims into adulthood. Unfortunately, the shame and secrecy of sexual abuse often prevent help-seeking. If the emotional damage from the abuse is not addressed, it can be hard to develop a healthy relationship with food. Further, obesity has been suggested to serve an adaptive function by attenuating or hiding features that may attract further sexual attention. Although the burdens of the abuse can be lifted with psychotherapy, shame and other psychological consequences of the abuse may prevent a victim from admitting the experience. However, if primary care practitioners could regularly inquire of their obese patients whether they have experienced unwanted sexual experiences, it could provide an opportunity for the survivors to finally unburden themselves and take the first steps towards emotional healing and addressing their weight issues.

Does Childhood Obesity Lead to Increased Risk of Disease in Adulthood?

The number of children who are overweight or obese has increased dramatically in the last two decades. Being overweight or obese in childhood dramatically increases the risk of being obese as an adult

(Simmons 2016). Because obesity contributes to many chronic diseases in adulthood, there is considerable concern that the epidemic of childhood obesity could lead to worsening of the metabolic disease epidemic in adulthood, as well as other diseases (Deal 2020, Smith 2016).

A major worry related to childhood obesity is that it is associated with increased inflammation, thus incurring a susceptibility to disease conditions later in life (Smith 2016). There are as yet few studies that have addressed this issue, partly because the children at the beginning of the epidemic are still young adults. Studies addressing the health of overweight and obese children, however, have shown marked increases in the rate of type 2 diabetes and non-alcoholic fatty liver disease (Nier 2018). These two diseases were previously very rare in children. Although metabolic disorders in children are typically associated with obesity, high-sugar diets are a risk factor for these disorders and for inflammation in normal-weight children as well (Nier 2019). In contrast, overweight teenagers who eat lots of vegetables and legumes have less inflammation than those who do not (Cabral 2018). Thus, diet is a key factor related to the consequences of overweight and obesity, and an important target for intervention.

Inflammation As We Age: *Inflammaging*

Immune system functions change when we hit mid-life (Weiskopf 2009). The most obvious experience of this is increased, low-grade inflammation called *inflammaging* (Calder 2017, Teissier 2019). As we age, we may find ourselves feeling stiff in the morning or more sensitive to pain. Older adults may experience low moods or have less energy than when they were younger. This is due in large part to increased inflammation. The fact that inflammation plays a critical role in the pathophysiology of chronic disease helps explain the relationship of age to the increased incidence of cancer, cardiovascular and kidney disease, metabolic diseases, and neurodegenerative diseases such as Alzheimer's disease and Parkinson's disease, and others.

How does this happen? Wear and tear on the body, injury, illness, and poor diet can damage cells. The resulting inflammation activates immune cells by the generation and release of DAMPs from the damaged cells, which then signal immune cells such as macrophages or microglia. This immune cell activation *primes* these cells, which means that they respond faster and with more inflammatory mediators the next time we become ill, are injured, or continue to eat a poor diet (Glass 2015). This can be considered a type of immune system learning, rather like practice effects wherein we get better at doing things if we do them often. But in this case, we are getting better at becoming inflamed!

Aging, Inflammation, and Neurodegenerative Diseases

Brain function is exquisitely sensitive to inflammation (Flores-Aguilar 2021). Increased inflammation and microglial priming over the lifespan is associated with the development of neurodegenerative diseases such as Alzheimer's disease and Parkinson's disease (Li 2018). Increased inflammation may be the result of accumulated damage over time due to disease, especially cardiovascular or metabolic disease, or poor diet. Indeed, aging is the most reliable risk factor for developing neurodegenerative diseases (Hou 2019). Although the factors that initiate the neurodegenerative process have yet to be established, and may vary from case to case, inflammation is clearly involved early on, and is not simply a by-product of the disease process (Heneka 2018). Inflammation may well be the critical mechanistic link between genetic and environmental risk factors for neurodegenerative diseases. This emphasizes the importance of regulating inflammation for healthy brain function. Neurodegenerative processes begin well before symptoms appear. Once symptoms are apparent the process is irreversible, at least with current medical technology. Thus, there is considerable interest in identifying modifiable risk factors that could serve as targets for early or mid-life intervention strategies.

Lifestyle Affects Inflammation As We Age

Some people seem to be more affected by age-related inflammation than others. Inborn factors, including gene variants for inflammatory mediators and their receptors, and proteins of the inflammasome can confer either a tendency for effective regulation of inflammation, or increase the risk of inflammation and disease susceptibility. As noted above, early life experiences also influence inflammation, as do lifestyle factors such as diet and exercise (Augusto-Oliveira 2021). For instance, it has been estimated that one third of all Alzheimer's disease cases are attributable to lifestyle habits, including physical inactivity, stress, poor diet, poor sleep, and low level of social and cognitive activity.

The lifestyle risks associated with mild cognitive impairment and Alzheimer's disease are well-documented to drive inflammation. A diet high in refined carbohydrates, especially sugar, induces inflammation in a variety of ways. A high-sugar diet can lead to Type 2 diabetes and hypertension, which are also risk factors for Alzheimer's disease (Wieckowska-Gacek 2021). Lifetime psychological stress is also associated with increased risk of dementia (Sindi 2017, Sutin 2018). This is likely due in part to the effects of chronic stress on inflammation and diet. Poor sleep, defined as less than 6 hours a night, is a stressor that results in chronic low-grade inflammation, and is also associated with increased risk of cognitive impairment and dementia (Mattis 2016). Poor sleep seems to impair the ability of microglia, the brain's immune cells, to support neuronal function, thus increasing wear and tear and neuroinflammation. Sleep disturbance also seems to increase inflammation in the body, raising risks for conditions such as depression and metabolic syndrome that can be linked to cognitive impairment over time (Irwin 2016).

The ability to retain good cognitive function as we age depends on how active we keep our brains. New learning requires the brain to remodel neuronal connectivity in the context of new experiences, an ability referred to as *neuroplasticity* (Sweatt 2016). Neuroplasticity involves a complex process that requires energy, protein synthesis, and changes in gene expression. If the brain is not stimulated by both physical and mental activity and new experiences, it gradually loses neuroplasticity, leading to mild cognitive impairment (Augusto-Oliveira 2021). Loss of neuroplasticity can be prevented or ameliorated by physical activity, which seems to help protect the brain from oxidative stress and stimulates brain activity. Thus, regular exercise seems to be protective against *brain aging* and other age-related chronic diseases (McGurran 2019). Frequent and varied social interactions, along with staying intellectually active, supports neuroplasticity as well (Phillips 2017). These can protect against age-related cognitive impairment.

Key Points

- Immune system function changes throughout the lifespan, such that we are more prone to excessive inflammation as we get older. This is called *inflammaging*.

- During early life, our immune systems are learning the difference between things in the environment, such as food or microbes, that are safe and beneficial and should be tolerated, versus things that are dangerous and must be avoided.
- Immune system function can be dramatically influenced by Adverse Childhood Experiences (ACE). These can permanently bias the immune system towards inflammation. This *developmental programming* can influence risk of disease and inflammation throughout the lifespan.
- As we age, our immune systems tend to become primed to respond with inflammation. This pro-inflammatory tendency likely contributes to the greater incidence of chronic diseases among older people.
- We begin to age as soon as we are born. While many factors that determine our level of inflammation are genetic, lifestyle choices, especially when we are young, can help regulate inflammation.
- Healthy aging means maintaining well-regulated inflammation. This is aided by moderate exercise, regular sleep, and social and intellectual activity. A healthy diet is also key to healthy aging, and the factors that determine what makes a food healthy or not will be discussed in the next four chapters.

References

Augusto-Oliveira M, Verkhratsky A. Lifestyle-dependent microglial plasticity: training the brain guardians. Biology Direct, 16:12, 2021.

Ahola-Olli AV, Wirtz P, Haulinna AS, Aalto K, Pitkanen N, Lehtomaki T, et al. Genome-wide association study identifies 27 loci influencing concentrations of circulating cytokines and growth factors. The American Journal of Human Genetics, 100:40-50-2017.

Almuneef M. Long term consequences of child sexual abuse in Saudi Arabia: A report from national study. Child Abuse and Neglect, 166:103967, 2021.

Aquilina SR, Shrubsole MJ, Butt J, Sanderson M, Schlundt DG, Cook MC, Epplein M. Adverse childhood experiences and adult diet quality. Journal of Nutritional Science, 10: e95, 2021.

Bunyavanich S, Berin MC. Food allergy and the microbiome: Current understandings and future directions. Journal of Allergy and Clinical Immunology, 144:1468-1477, 2019.

Cabral M, Araujo J, Lopes C, Ramos E. Food intake and high-sensitivity C-reactive protein levels in adolescents. Nutrition, Metabolism, and Cardiovascular Diseases, 28:1067-1074, 2018.

Caldera PC, Bosco N, Bourdet-Sicard R, Capurone L, Delzenne N, Doré J, Franceschi C, Lehtinenj MJ, Recker T, Salvioli S, Visioli F. Health relevance of the modification of low grade inflammation in ageing (inflammaging) and the role of nutrition. Ageing Research Reviews, 40:95-199, 2017.

Campbell JA, Farmer GC, Nguyen-Rodriguez S, Walker R, Egede L. Relationship between individual categories of adverse childhood experiences and diabetes in adulthood in a sample of US adults: Does it differ by gender? Journal of Diabetes Complications, 32:139-143, 2018.

Danese A, Lewis SJ. Psychoneuroimmunology of early-life stress: The hidden wounds of childhood trauma. Neuropsychopharmacology Reviews, 42:99-114, 2017.

Deal BJ, Huffman MD, Binns H, Stone NJ. Perspective: Childhood obesity requires new strategies for prevention. Advances in Nutrition, 11:1071-1078, 2020.

Ernst M, Tibunos AN, Werner A, Beutel ME, Plener PL, Fergert JM, Brahler E. Sex-dependent associations of childhood neglect and bodyweight across the lifespan. Scientific Reports, 9:5080, 2019.

Felitti VJ, Anda RF, Nordenberg D, Williamson DF, Spitz AM, Edwards V, Koss MP, Marks JS. Relationship of childhood abuse and household dysfunction to many of the leading causes of death in adults: The Adverse Childhood Experiences (ACE) Study. American Journal of Preventative Medicine, 56:774-786, 2019.

Flores-Aguilar L, Iolita MF, Orciani C, Tanna N Yang J, Bennett DA, Cuello AC. Cognitive and brain cytokine profile of non-demented individuals with cerebral amyloid-beta deposition. Journal of Neuroinflammation, 18:147, 2021.

Gardner R, Feely A, Layte R, Williams J, McGavock J. Adverse childhood experiences are associated with an increased risk of obesity in early adolescence: a population-based prospective cohort study. Pediatric Research, 86: 522-528, 2019.

Glass CK, Natoli G. Molecular control of activation and priming in macrophages. Nature Immunology, 17:26-33, 2015.

Goldstein E, Topitzes J, Miller-Cribbs J, Brown RL. Influence of race/ethnicity and income on the link between adverse childhood experiences and child flourishing. Pediatric Research, 89:1861-1869, 2021.

Gonzalez A. The impact of childhood maltreatment on biological systems: Implications for clinical interventions. Paediatric and Child Health, 18:415-418, 2013.

Grilo CM, Masheb RM. Maltreatment in outpatients with binge eating disorder: Frequency and associations with gender, obesity and eating-related psychopathology. Obesity Research, 9:320-325, 2001.

Groenewald CB, Murray CB, Palermo TM. Adverse childhood experiences and chronic pain among children and adolescents in the United States. Pain Reports, 5: e839, 2020.

Gustafson TB, Sarwer DB. Childhood sex abuse and obesity. Obesity Reviews, 5:129-135, 2004.

Heneka MT, McManus RM, Latz E. Inflammasome signaling in brain function and neurodegenerative disease. Nature Reviews Neuroscience, 19:610-621, 2018.

Hou Y, Dam V, Babbar M, Weo Y, Hasselbach SG, Croteau DL, Bohr VA. Ageing as a risk factor for neurodegenerative disease. Nature Reviews Neurology, 15:565-581, 2019.

Irwin MR, Olmstead R, Carroll JE. Sleep disturbance, sleep duration, and inflammation: A systematic review and meta-analysis of cohort studies and experimental sleep deprivation. Biological Psychiatry, 80:40-52, 2016.

Kanchan K, Clay S, Irizar H, Bunyavanich S, Mathias RA. Current insights into the genetics of food allergy. Journal of Allergy and Clinical Immunology, 147:15-28, 2021.

Kucuksezer UC, Ozdemir C, Akdis M, Akdis CA. Influences of innate immunity on immune tolerance. Acta Medica Academica 49:164-180, 2020.

Levine JA, McCrady-Spitzer SK, Bighorse W. Obesity and sex abuse in American Indians and Alaska Natives. Journal of Obesity and Weight Loss Therapy, 6(4): e119, 2016.

Li J-W, Zong Y, Cao X-P Tan L, Tan L. Microglial priming in Alzheimer's disease. Annals of Translational Medicine, 6:176, 2018.

Lin Z, Chen X. Adverse childhood circumstances and cognitive function in middle-aged and older Chinese adults: Lower level or faster decline? SSM- Population Health, 14:100767, 2021.

Marrs T, Sim K. Demystifying dysbiosis: Can the gut microbiome promote oral tolerance over IgE-mediated food allergy? Current Pediatric Reviews, 14:156-163, 2018.

Mattis J, Sehgal A. Circadian Rhythms, Sleep, and disorders of aging. Trends in Endocrinology and Metabolism, 27:192-203, 2016.

McGurran H, Glenn JM, Madero EN, Bott NT. Prevention and treatment of Alzheimer's Disease: Biological mechanisms of exercise. Journal of Alzheimer's Disease, 69:311-388, 2019.

McKelvey LM, Saccente JE, Swindle TM. Adverse childhood experiences in infancy and toddlerhood predict obesity and health outcomes in middle childhood. Childhood Obesity, 15:206-215, 2019.

Nier A, Brandt A, Conzelmann IB, Ozel Y, Bergheim I. Non-alcoholic fatty liver disease in overweight children: Role of fructose intake and dietary pattern. Nutrients, 10:1329, 2018.

Nier A, Brandt A, Baumann A, Conzelmann AB, Ozel Y, Berheim I. Metabolic abnormalities in normal weight children are associated with increased visceral fat accumulation, elevated plasma endotoxin levels and a higher monosaccharide intake. Nutrients, 11:652, 2019.

Nowak-Wegrzyn A, Chatchatee P. Mechanisms of tolerance induction. Annals of Nutrition and Metabolism, 70(suppl 2):7-24, 2017.

Olivieri P, Solitar B, Dubois M. Childhood risk factors for developing fibromyalgia. Open access Rheumatology: Research and Reviews, 4:109-114, 2012.

Park SH, Videlock EJ, Shih W, Presson AP, Mayer EA, Chang L. Adverse childhood experiences are associated with irritable bowel syndrome and gastrointestinal symptom severity. Neurogastroenterology and Motility, 28:1252-1260, 2016.

Peters RL, Dang TD, Allen KF. Specific oral tolerance induction in childhood. Pediatric Allergy and Immunology, 27:784-794, 2016.

Ribeiro RM., Graca L. Untangling the immune basis of disease susceptibility. eLife, 9:e56886, 2020.

Rubin DC, Shaker A, Levin MS. Chronic intestinal inflammation: inflammatory bowel disease and colitis-associated colon cancer. Frontiers in Immunology, 3:107, 2012.

Sancesario GM, Bernardini S, Alzheimer's Disease in the omics era. Clinical Biochemistry, 59:9-16, 2018.

Simmonds M, Llewellyn A, Owen CG, Woolacott N. Predicting adult obesity from childhood obesity: a systematic review and meta-analysis. Obesity Reviews, 17:95-107, 2016.

Sindi S, Hagman G, Hakansson K, Kulmala J, Nilsen C, Kareholt I, Soininen H, Solomon A, Kivipelto M. Mid-life work stress increases dementia risk in later life: The CAIDE 30-year study. Journal of Gerontology: Psychological Sciences Social Sciences, 72:1044-1053, 2017.

Smith KB, Smith MS. Obesity statistics. Primary Care Clinical Office Practice, 43:121-135, 2016.

Sutin AR, Stephan Y, Terracciano A. Psychological distress, self-beliefs, and risk of cognitive impairment and dementia. Journal of Alzheimer's Disease, 65:1041-1050, 2018.

Sweatt JD. Neural plasticity and behavior- sixty years of conceptual advances. Journal of Neurochemistry, 139:179-199, 2016.

Teissier T, Boulanger E. The receptor for advanced glycation end-products (RAGE) is an important pattern recognition receptor (PRR) for inflammaging. Biogerontology, 20:279–301, 2019.

Van Strien T, Cebolla A, Etchemendy E, Gutierrez-Maldonaldo M, Botell C, Banos R. Emotional eating and food intake after sadness and joy. Appetite, 66:20-25, 2013.

Weiskopf D, Weinberger B, Grubeck-Loebestein B. The aging of the immune system. Transplant International, 22:1041-1050, 2009.

Wieckowska-Gacek A, Mietelska-Porowska A, Wydrych M, Wojda U. Western diet as a trigger of Alzheimer's disease. From metabolic syndrome and systemic inflammation to neuroinflammation and neurodegeneration. Aging Research Reviews, 70:101397, 2021.

Zannas AS, Jia M, Hafner K, Baumert J, Wiechmann T, Pape, et al. Epigenetic upregulation of FKBP5 by aging and stress contributes to N-FkB-driven inflammation and cardiovascular risk. PNAS, 116:11370-11379, 2019.

CHAPTER 10: UNDERSTANDING OXIDATION AND ANTIOXIDANTS

- THE JANUS FACE OF OXIDATION: METABOLISM VS. OXIDATIVE STRESS
- REACTIVE OXYGEN SPECIES (ROS) AND REACTIVE NITROGEN SPECIES (RNS) ARE EFFECTIVE WEAPONS FOR THE IMMUNE SYSTEM
- EXAMPLE: LIPID OXIDATION
- HOW WE PREPARE FOODS AND STORE OILS CAN INFLUENCE LIPID OXIDATION
- KEY POINTS

Damage to cells and tissues during poorly regulated inflammation is caused by *oxidation* and *oxidative stress*. Oxidation causes damage to cells and tissues, which is called oxidative stress. For that reason the body has endogenous antioxidant systems that function to buffer the body from oxidation. Antioxidants can be found in foods as well, mostly in vegetables, fruits, and nuts. This is one of the important reasons why plant-based foods are considered part of a healthy diet. Conversely, some foods can be oxidized during production, processing, or cooking, producing PAMPs or DAMPs which can induce inflammation (Koh 2015, Roldan 2014, Tao 2015, Choi 2017, Losso 2021, Wetzels 2017). Food processing can also reduce the activity of protective ingredients such as antioxidant plant constituents (Al-Juhaimi 2018). The ability of food to influence inflammation positively or negatively is a main mechanism by which diet affects quality of life and overall health. Diet's impact on inflammation underlines the importance of making informed choices about food. Therefore, to understand and predict the effects of specific food items on health, it is imperative to be familiar with the mechanisms by which inflammation causes disease. Only when we understand how foods influence inflammation will we be able to discriminate between useful versus dangerous diet advice and make good choices about food. Because the major damage done to tissues during inflammation is caused by oxidative stress, we must understand how oxidative stress occurs.

The Janus Face of Oxidation: Metabolism versus Oxidative Stress

Janus was the Roman god of beginnings, transitions, and endings, and is usually shown with two faces: one facing the future, and one the past. Oxidation is also two-faced. On the one hand, oxidation has the potential to be lethal. It is one of the most important factors driving damage to cells, disease, and death. It is also a potent weapon of the immune system, employed to protect the body against pathogens. But on the other hand, oxidation provides the energy for complex life. Oxidation underlies the process by which mitochondria release energy for cellular functions (Papachristoforou 2020). Without the energy produced by mitochondria, cells would be significantly limited and unable to maintain function.

Glucose is a major fuel for mitochondria and is broken down in a process called *respiration*. Respiration involves oxidation of glucose, which while generating significant energy, necessarily generates reactive oxygen and nitrogen species. Excessive levels of these reactive oxygen and nitrogen species can damage the mitochondria and other parts of the cell, including genetic material (Butterfield 2019, Khan 2017, Luc

2019, Mota 2015, Valacchi 2018). As such, oxidation during respiration both fuels cells and puts them at risk of damage.

What exactly, is oxidation?

Reactive Oxygen Species (ROS) and Reactive Nitrogen Species (RNS) are Effective Weapons for the Immune System

One normal consequence of the inflammation cascade is the generation of molecules called reactive oxygen (ROS) and nitrogen (RNS) species. These ROS and RNS are examples of *radicals* or *free radicals"*, chemicals that have an unpaired electron and are thus highly reactive. These are highly effective weapons for killing pathogens because they damage molecules (Mills 2017).

Oxidation involves stealing electrons or protons (hydrogen atoms) from other molecules, and thereby *oxidizing* them. Basically, oxidation is being mugged of subatomic particles. Being mugged in this way is a problem because the structure of molecules determines their ability to perform specific functions. Oxidation changes the structure or shape of molecules, thus affecting their functions. There are other ways of changing the structure of molecules that can also trigger inflammation. RNS can *substitute* onto molecules, changing their structures by becoming part of the molecule.

Oxidized or otherwise damaged molecules, especially lipids, become sources of damage-related signals called DAMPs. DAMPs induce inflammation directly or can exacerbate ongoing inflammation. Unfortunately, the immune system's response to threats can be a bit of an one-size-fits-all solution. The presence of pathogen-related signals and DAMPs trigger an inflammatory response, even when the inflammation can actually prolong and worsen the problems.

Example: Lipid Oxidation

One of the most important consequences of chronic inflammation is the oxidation (sometimes called peroxidation) of lipids. Lipids play critical roles in the structures of cells, as well as in signaling between cells, and in metabolism. For example, cell membranes are made of lipids and their properties are crucial for signaling that occurs across these membranes. The brain is enriched in lipids, because they form much of the myelin sheath that insulates neuronal axons, which make up the brain's white matter. However, the lipids in cell membranes are vulnerable to oxidation, which damages them and can then lead to loss of function or even cell death (Stockwell 2017). Thus, inflammation in the brain has serious consequences for myelin and the cells that produce it (Haider 2011).

Fats are fairly simple molecules, made up of chains of carbon atoms bound to hydrogen atoms. Short-chain fatty acids have only a few carbons, and long-chain fatty acids have many. The carbon atoms in the "backbone" of fats need to bind to four other atoms to be stable. In a *saturated fat*, each carbon within the chain binds to the carbons on each side, and the other two bonds are made with hydrogen atoms. Sometimes there are not enough hydrogen atoms to go around, so the carbon atoms will form two bonds (i.e. a double bond) with one of the adjacent carbon atoms, one bond with the other adjacent carbon atom, and the last bond with a hydrogen. These fats are called *unsaturated fats because* they contain fewer than the maximum number of hydrogens. A carbon-carbon double bond makes it harder to hang

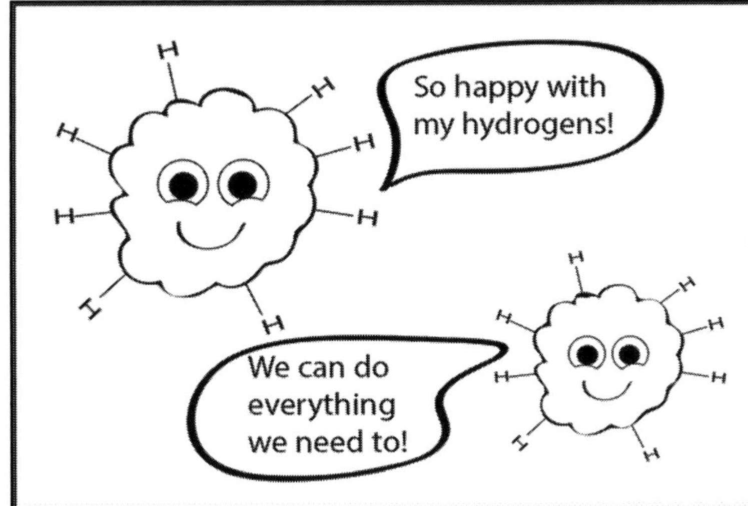

on to the single hydrogen, rendering unsaturated fats vulnerable to being mugged by reactive species (ROS or RNS).

One way to think of this process is to think of an atom as having hands that need to be holding something, e.g., the "hand" of another element. For example, a carbon atom would have four "hands." The hands of a chain of carbons in a fat are holding hands with either another carbon or a hydrogen. As long as everyone's hands are full, the molecule is stable and able to perform its normal functions. But if a fat becomes oxidized, one of its hydrogens is stolen and now has an empty hand. An empty hand makes the element, and the molecule it is part of, unstable and prone to react with other atoms. Having a free hand can impair the function of the molecule. The molecule is now motivated to fill its hand by stealing a hydrogen itself, usually from an adjacent fatty acid molecule.

This process of oxidizing lipids is called *lipid peroxidation* (Gianazza 2019). This process is particularly dangerous because oxidized lipids become *fatty acid radicals* with free hands. Those fatty acid radicals can go on to oxidize other lipids. This produces a propagation phase where the empty hands of one radicalized fatty acid steals from another molecule, creating a new empty-handed fatty acid. This propagation can amplify the damage from the initial oxidation. The process only stops when the oxidized lipid encounters another oxidized lipid, each providing a free hand to hold, or the oxidized lipid encounters an antioxidant.

Some of these fatty acid radicals become further processed into *reactive aldehydes* called Advanced Lipid End-products (ALES) (Gianazza 2019). These ALES also act as DAMPs, triggering or increasing inflammation (Busch 2017). ALEs bind to a Pattern Recognition Receptor (PRR) on immune cells called LOX1, which activates NFkB (Feng 2014). Some evidence indicates that ALEs also activate TLR4, another Pattern Recognition Receptor. TLR4 usually responds to microbial signals, but possibly also toxins, and can further boost inflammatory responses. Lipid oxidation contributes to inflammation in several conditions, especially cardiovascular disease, but also neurological conditions, gastrointestinal diseases, metabolic syndrome, and cancer (Gianazza 2019, Pirillo 2013, Faizo 2021, Keewan 2020, Haider 2011, McDonald 2018, Murdocca 2021, Reichert 2020, Sottero 2018, Stankova 2019).

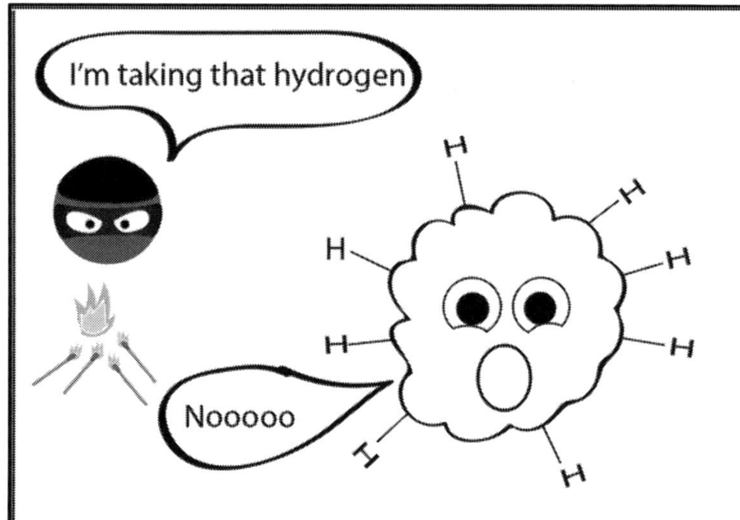

Molecules (such as lipids) need to have the right number of elements in a particular shape, to do their jobs. Inflammation can cause the release of reactive oxygen or nitrogen species, such as hydrogen peroxide, superoxide, or peroxynitrite. These can "steal" hydrogens or electrons from molecules such as lipids.

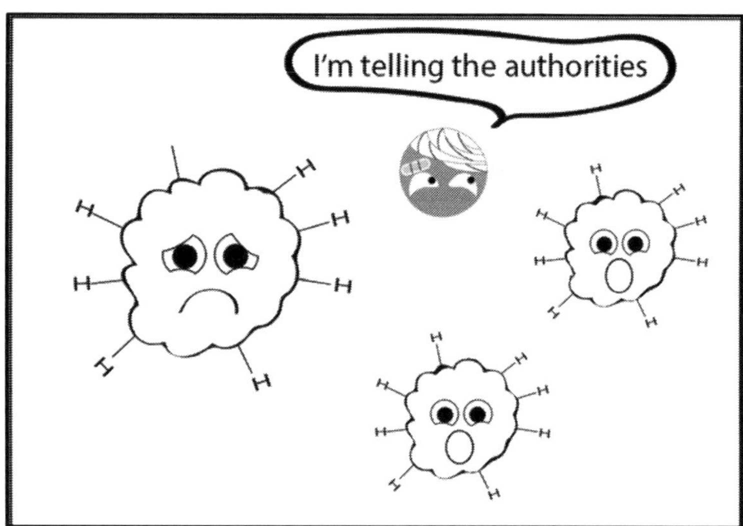

Damage to the lipids causes them to generate Advanced Lipid oxidation End-products (ALEs) that function as damage-associated molecular patterns (DAMPs).

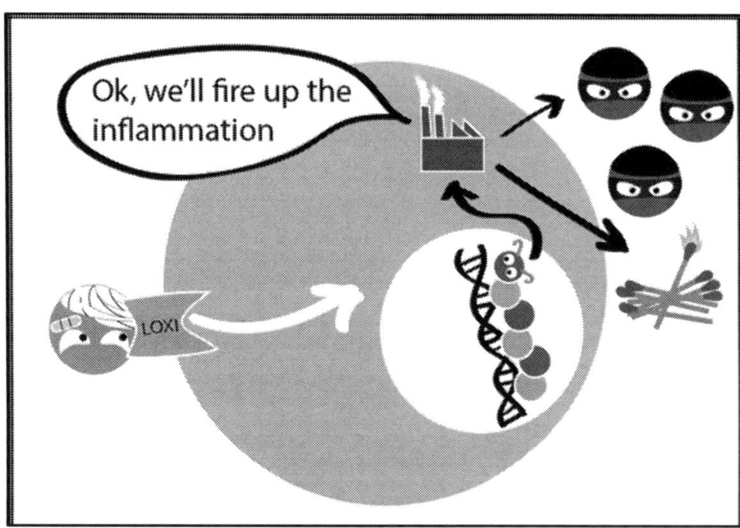

The DAMPs signal immune cells to begin the process of inflammation, which can involve the formation of more reactive oxygen and nitrogen species. The inflammatory response causes more damage to lipids.

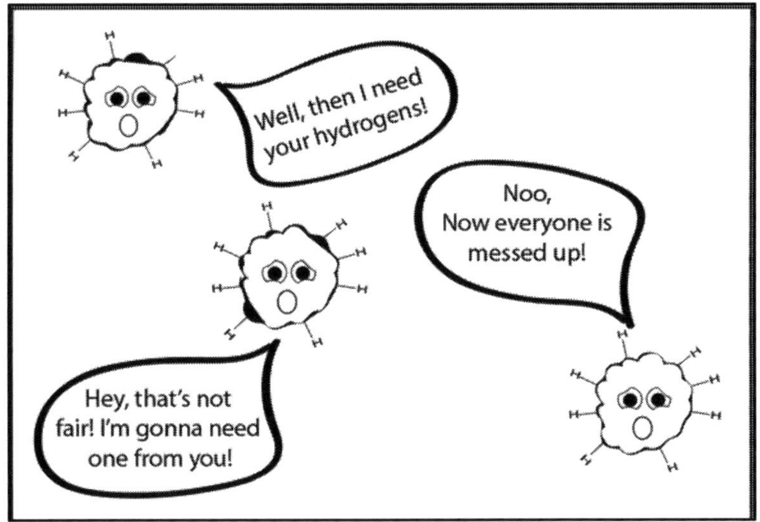

The damaged lipids then become reactive (i.e., they become fatty acid radicals) themselves and go on to steal hydrogens from their neighbors. The damaged neighbors then become reactive, propagating the damage throughout the cell membranes and tissue.

Propagation of oxidation through fatty acids is particularly troublesome for the brain, as it is enriched in the polyunsaturated fatty acids that are most vulnerable to oxidation. Propagation of oxidized lipids in neuronal membranes or myelin can contribute to damage in autoimmune conditions such as multiple sclerosis (Hu 2019). Further, damage to blood vessels and the build-up of oxidized lipids in arterial plaque drives inflammation and blockage, which contributes to infarcts and metabolic disturbances that lead to dementia (Shay 2013, Tsoupras 2018).

How We Prepare Foods and Store Oils can Influence Lipid Oxidation

When lipids in our bodies become oxidized, they can directly induce inflammation. In addition, dietary lipids or fats can also be oxidized during cooking or manufacturing. Can dietary fats drive inflammation? Evidence indicates that they can (Keewan 2020, Skinner 2021, Tao 2015, Vine 1997). Oxidized lipids in the diet are absorbed into the body and are incorporated into very low-density lipids (VLDL), the fraction of blood lipids associated with inflammation (Staprans 1996, Faizo 2021). Further, oxidized lipid in the diet drives inflammation in the gut, providing one mechanism by which Western diet foods can contribute to development of gastrointestinal disorders (Keewan 2020).

Which fats are most vulnerable to oxidation? Unsaturated fats, including mono- and polyunsaturated fatty acids (PUFAs) such as vegetable oils, are particularly vulnerable to oxidation because of their structure. Oxidation can occur in the absence of ROS or RNS, particularly if the fatty acids are exposed to oxygen or metals, light, or high temperature (Skinner 2021, Tao 2015). This is called auto-oxidation, and PUFAs are more easily auto-oxidized than other fats. Other fats can be auto-oxidized over time as well. Thus, food can be a source of pro-inflammatory fats.

For this reason, many unsaturated vegetable oils are considered less safe than saturated fats for cooking purposes such as frying or grilling. Unsaturated fats are vulnerable to oxidation when they are exposed to high temperatures and air in metal cooking vessels, especially for long periods of time (Koh 2015, Tao 2015). Therefore, saturated fats such as coconut oil, butter, or lard are recommended for frying or grilling, rather than unsaturated vegetable oils such as canola, corn, or nut oils. Fats should not be reused after frying, because the longer they are heated, the more oxidized they become and the more likely they will contain ALEs (Koh 2015). Polyunsaturated fats are best used uncooked for cold meals, such as dressing for salads. Light can oxidize oils as well, especially if the bottles have been opened and are thus exposed to oxygen. For that reason, oils should be stored in dark glass or plastic bottles in the cupboard or refrigerator.

The rate of oxidation of fats in the presence of heat and oxygen increases over time (Koh 2015). That is, the longer the heating process, the more fats become oxidized. This has practical implications for commercially fried foods, especially fast-food or cafeteria settings in which cooking oils are heated for hours, even days, without being replaced. This leads to oil oxidation. Food cooked in such oils, especially fish or vegetables that are rich in PUFAs, will also contain oxidized lipids (Koh 2015). Lipid oxidation can also lead to oxidation of other components of foods including proteins and carbohydrates, which is a concern for commercially produced and highly processed foods (Schaich 2012, Wang 2016). The link between oxidized lipids and inflammation is thus a contributing factor to the health risks of the Western diet (Keewan 2020, Skinner 2021).

Key Points

- Oxidation is a normal chemical process that mitochondria use to generate energy for cells to use.
- Oxidative stress occurs intentionally during times when inflammatory pathways are activated, because oxidation is a powerful weapon of the immune system's arsenal. See Chapter 3 on NFkB and the inflammasome for more detail.
- Reactive oxygen or nitrogen species oxidize molecules by stealing electrons or protons (hydrogens) from them. This damages the molecules. Some of the victims then become "radicalized" themselves and propagate the process, increasing the damage. Damaged molecules induce or increase inflammation, and unregulated oxidation is implicated in the pathology of most disease conditions.
- Food processing, storage, or preparation influences the amount of oxidized lipids in oils and oil-containing foods. Heat, light, and air increase the rate of auto-oxidation of lipids. Oxidized lipids in foods may account for the deleterious effects of high-fat diets for conditions such as atherosclerosis and metabolic syndrome.

References

Al-Juhaimi F, Ghafoor K, Ozcan MM, Jahurul MHA, Babiker EE, Jinap S, et al. Effect of various food processing and handling methods on preservation of natural antioxidants in fruits and vegetables. Journal of Food Sciences and Technology, 55:3872-3880, 2018.

Busch CJ, Binder CJ. Malondialdehyde epitopes as mediators of sterile inflammation. Biochimica et Biophysica Acta, 1862:398-406, 2017.

Butterfield DA, Halliwell B. Oxidative stress, dysfunctional glucose metabolism and Alzheimer disease. Nature Reviews Neuroscience, 20:148-160, 2019.

Choi S-H, Sviridov D, Miller YI. Oxidized cholesteryl esters and inflammation. Biochimica et Biophysica Acta, 1862:393–397, 2017.

Faizo N, Narasimhulu CA, Forsman A, Yooseph S. Peroxidized linolenic acid, 13-HPODE, alters gene expression profile in intestinal epithelial cells. Foods, 10:314, 2021.

Feng Y, Cai ZR, Tang Y, Hu G, Lu J, He D, Wang S. TLR4/NFkB signaling pathway-mediated and oxLDL-induced up-regulation of LOX-1, MCP-1, and VCAM-1 expression in human umbilical vein endothelial cells. Genetics and Molecular Research, 13:680-695, 2014.

Gianazza E, Brioschi M, Martinez Fernandez A, Banfi C. Lipoxidation in cardiovascular disease. Redox Biology, 23:101119, 2019.

Haider L, Fischer MT, Frischer JM, Bauer J, Hoftberger R, Botond G, Esterbauer H, Binder CJ, Witztum JL, Lassmann H. Oxidative damage in multiple sclerosis lesions. Brain, 134:1914-1924, 2011.

Hu C-L, Nydes M, Shanley KL, Morales Pantoja IE, Howard TA, Bizzozero OA. Reduced expression of the ferroptosis inhibitor GPx4 in multiple sclerosis and experimental autoimmune encephalomyelitis. Journal of Neurochemistry, 148: 426-439, 2019.

Keewan E, Narasimhulu CA, Rohr M, Hamid S, Parthasarathy S. Are fried foods unhealthy? The dietary peroxidized fatty acid, 13-HPODE, induces intestinal inflammation in vitro and in vivo. Antioxidants, 9:926, 2020.

Khan A, Alam K, Md. Zafaryab, Rizvi MA. Peroxynitrite modified histone as a pathophysiological biomarker in autoimmune disease. Biochimie, 140:1-9, 2017.

Koh E, Surh J. Food types and frying frequency affect the lipid oxidation of deep frying oil for the preparation of school meals in Korea. Food Chemistry, 174:467-472, 2015.

Losso JN. Food processing, dysbiosis, gastrointestinal inflammatory diseases, and antiangiogenic functional foods and beverages. Annual Review of Food Science Technology, 12:235-258, 2021.

Luc K, Schramm-Luc A, Guzik TJ, Mikolajczyk TP. Oxidative stress and inflammatory markers in prediabetes and diabetes. Journal of Physiology and Pharmacology, 70:809-824, 2019.

McDonald T, Puchowicz M, Borges K. Impairments in Oxidative Glucose Metabolism in Epilepsy and Metabolic Treatments Thereof. Frontiers in Cellular Neuroscience, 12:274, 2018.

Mills EL, Kelly B, O'Neill LAJ. Mitochondria are the powerhouses of immunity. Nature Immunology, 18:488-498, 2017.

Mota SI, Costa RO, Ferreira IL, Santana I, Caldeira GL, Padovano C, Fonseca AC, Baldeiras I, Cunha C, Letra L, Oliveira CR, Pereira CMF, Rego AC. Oxidative stress involving changes in Nrf2 and ER stress in early stages of Alzheimer's disease. Biochimica et Biophysica Acta, 1852:1428–1441, 2015.

Murdocca M, De Masi C, Pucci S, Mango R, Novelli G, Di Natale C, Sangiuolo F. LOX-1 and cancer: an indissoluble liaison. Cancer Gene Therapy, 28:1088-1098, 2021.

Papachristoforou E, Lambadiari V, Maratou E, Makrilakis K. Association of glycemic indices (Hyperglycemia, glucose variability, and hypoglycemia) with oxidative stress and diabetic complications. Journal of Diabetes Research, 220:7489795, 2020.

Pirillo A, Norata GD, Catapano AL. LOX-1, OxLDL, and atherosclerosis. Mediators of Inflammation, 1013:152786, 2013.

Reichert CO, de Feitas FA, Sampraio-Silva, Rokita-Roas L, de Lime Barros P, Levy D, Bydlowski. Ferroptosis mechanisms involved in neurodegenerative diseases. International Journal of Molecular Sciences, 21:8765, 2020.

Roldan M, Antequera T, Armenteros M, Ruiz J. Effect of different temperature–time combinations on lipid and protein oxidation of sous-vide cooked lamb loins. Food Chemistry, 149:29–136, 2014.

Schaich KM. Thinking outside the classical chain reaction box of lipid oxidation. Lipid Technology, 24:55-58, 2012.

Shah GN, Morofuji Y, Banks WA, Price TO. High Glucose-Induced Mitochondrial Respiration and Reactive Oxygen Species in Mouse Cerebral Pericytes is Reversed by Pharmacological Inhibition of Mitochondrial Carbonic Anhydrases: Implications for Cerebral Microvascular Disease in Diabetes. Biochemical and Biophysical Research Communications, 440: 354-358, 2013.

Sottero B, Rossin D, Poli G, Biasi F. Lipid oxidation products in the pathogenesis of inflammation-related gut diseases. Current Medicinal Chemistry, 25:13-11-1326, 2018.

Skinner J, Arora P, McMath N, Penumetcha M. Determination of oxidized lipids in commonly consumed foods and a preliminary analysis of their binding affinity to PPARg. Foods, 10:1702, 2021.

Stockwell BR, Angeli JPF, Bayir H, Bush A, Conrad M, Dixon S et al. Ferroptosis: a regulated cell death nexus linking metabolism, redox biology, and disease. Cell, 171-273-285, 2017.

Staprans I, Rapp JH, Pan X-M, Feingold KR. Oxidized lipids in the diet are incorporated by the liver into very low density lipoprotein in rats. Journal of Lipid Research, 37:420-430 1996.

Tao L. Oxidation of polyunsaturated fatty acids and its impact on food quality and human health. Advances in Food Technology and Nutritional Sciences Open Journal, 1(6): 135-142. 2015.

Tsoupras A, Ronan Lordan R, Zabetakis I. Inflammation, not cholesterol, is a cause of chronic disease. Nutrients, 10:604, 2018.

Valacchi G, Virgili F, Cervellati C, Pecorelli A. OxInflammation: From Subclinical Condition to Pathological Biomarker. Frontiers in Physiology, 9:858, 2018.

Vine DF, Croft KD, Beilin LJ, Mamo J.C.L. Absorption of Dietary Cholesterol Oxidation Products and Incorporation into Rat Lymph Chylomicrons. Lipids, 32:887-893, 1997.

Wang Y-J, Makela N, Maina NH, Lampi A-M, Sontag-Strohm. Lipid oxidation induced oxidative degradation of cereal beta-glucan. Food Chemistry, 197:13324-1330, 2016.

Wetzels S, Wouters K, Schalkwijk CG, Vanmierlo T, Hendriks JJA. Methylglyoxal-derived advanced glycation endproducts in Multiple Sclerosis. International Journal of Molecular Sciences, 18:421, 2017.

- ANTIOXIDANTS WORK IN SYSTEMS

- PROTECTING AGAINST OXIDATIVE STRESS: NRF2 AND THE ANTIOXIDANT RESPONSE

- METALLOTHIONEINS AND ZINC

- DIETARY ANTIOXIDANTS: VITAMINS AND POLYPHENOLS

- DIET VERSUS SUPPLEMENTS: WHAT IS THE BEST WAY TO INFLUENCE OXIDATIVE STRESS?

- BIOAVAILABILITY: WHAT GETS ABSORBED?

- ANTI-INFLAMMATORY DIETARY INGREDIENTS

- KEY POINTS

Oxidation crucially functions to extract energy from nutrients, and many of the reactive molecules generated in this process have important signaling roles in the body (Speckman 2016). However, too many reactive molecules, or *radicals*, can lead to oxidative stress, damage to tissues, and inflammation (Korkmas 2009). To protect against potential oxidative stress, the body produces many of its own endogenous antioxidants, including glutathione, superoxide dismutase (SOD), melatonin, and uric acid (He 2017). These antioxidants are particularly important when mitochondria are highly active and oxidizing. Examples of these high-activity periods are during inflammation, after hyperglycemia, and during other metabolic challenges.

Plants also produce antioxidants for the same reason, and therefore we can include these plants and their nuts in our diets to potentially boost our antioxidant capability. Consuming these extra antioxidants can be particularly important if we are under stress or eating foods that have been damaged by oxidation during cooking or commercial processing, as discussed in Chapter 10 (Keewan 2020, Koh 2015, Schaich 2012).

Antioxidants Work in Systems

Possibly the biggest challenge for the body in regulating the number of reactive species and safety of the oxidation process is the *redox conundrum*. During oxidation, a molecule loses an electron. This process is discussed in Chapter 10. That reaction may be part of metabolic processes, breaking down molecules to release energy, or the reaction may occur in the context of inflammation. To stabilize the molecule that has lost the electron, another molecule must donate an electron to replace it, typically by providing a hydrogen atom. Antioxidants play the role of the hydrogen donor. The redox conundrum refers to the fact that the donor molecule, or antioxidant, can become unstable or radicalized by losing its hydrogen atom, and will then require further proton or electron donation to return to a stable state.

This redox conundrum is usually prevented by the fact that antioxidants work in systems, where the antioxidant is recycled by another substance that donates an electron or proton/hydrogen. Many of the recycling molecules in these systems are enzymes, but they can also be other antioxidants. For example, Vitamin E is recycled by Vitamin C (Cobley 2015). This may explain findings that Vitamin E supplementation for conditions associated with oxidative stress is often more effective when combined with Vitamin C (Amini 2021, Hemila 2009). This may also explain why clinical trials have found that providing single antioxidant supplements rarely provides health benefits, but studies on the effects of eating whole foods containing multiple antioxidant systems have shown some small benefits. Similarly, clinical studies focused on whole foods have shown large effects for complex conditions, including cardiovascular and metabolic diseases and mood disorders, which are associated with oxidative stress (Billingsley 2018, Razavi Zade 2016, Huang 2019, Jacka 2017). The MIND (i.e., the Mediterranean-DASH Intervention for Neurodegenerative Delay) or other Mediterranean diets, which include a variety of whole foods containing many different antioxidants, are examples of diets that have shown benefits in clinical trials (Billingsley 2018, Cherian 2019).

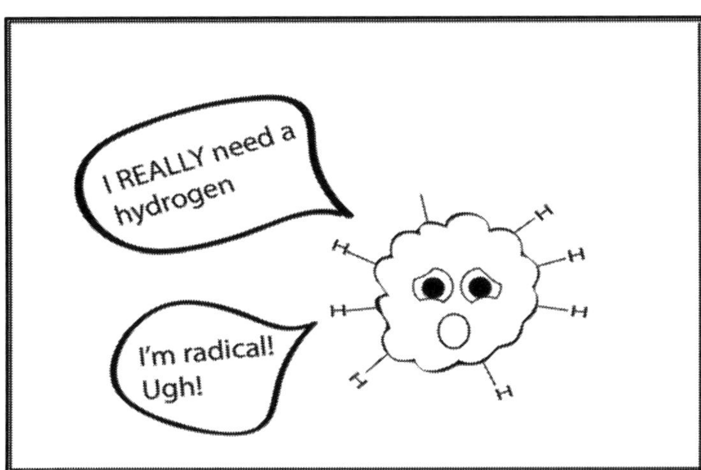

Lipids damaged by oxidation (losing an electron) can become Fatty Acid Radicals, which steal hydrogens from other lipids.

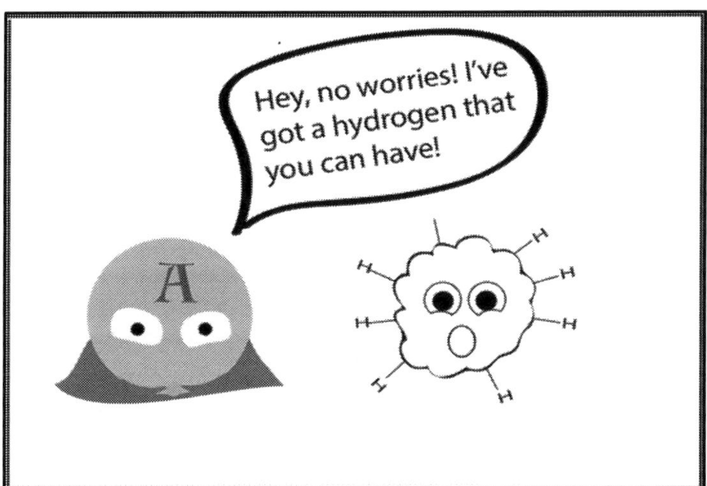

Antioxidants work by donating hydrogens or electrons to molecules that have been oxidized.

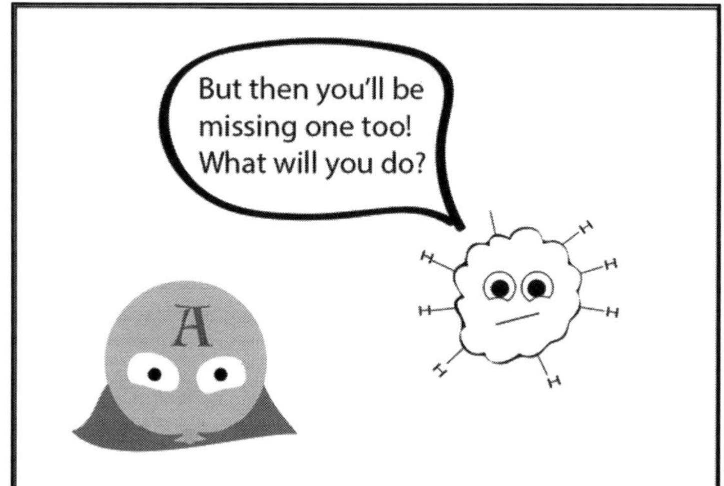

The problem is that now the antioxidant is missing a hydrogen or electron and can become reactive itself (the redox conundrum).

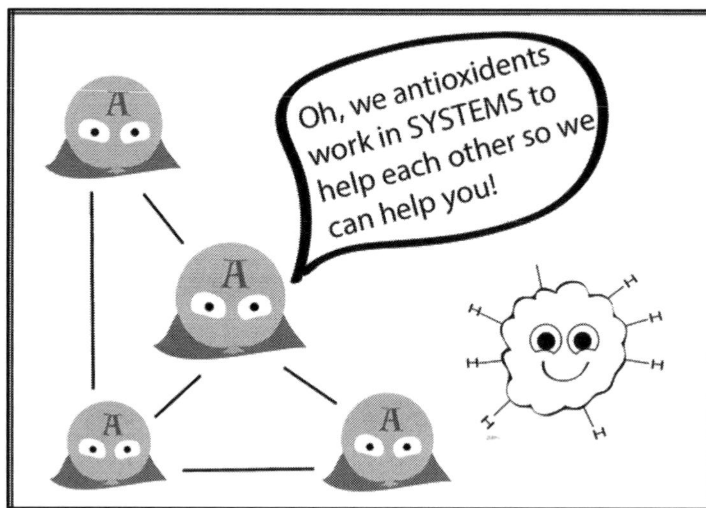

This problem is avoided by the organization of antioxidants into systems whereby the antioxidant is regenerated or recycled, preventing them from becoming reactive.

Protecting against Oxidative Stress: Nrf2 and the Antioxidant Response

Like NFkB, which activates inflammatory responses, *Nrf2* is a transcription factor. Transcription factors control the expression of many different genes. But where NFkB acts to induce and amplify inflammation, Nrf2 acts to reduce inflammation and activate the body's *endogenous antioxidant systems* (Bellezza 2018, Tu 2019). The more prominent of these are described below. When it is time for inflammation to be resolved and the healing phase to begin, Nrf2 coordinates the *antioxidant response* that protects against oxidative stress. *Endogenous antioxidants* are substances that scavenge free radicals and help prevent against oxidative stress. The liver is the main source of endogenous antioxidants, but some are made by individual cells. Even some of our gut microbes make endogenous antioxidants. Interestingly, and importantly, one of the ways that plant-based antioxidants in the diet can protect against oxidative stress is by activating Nrf2 and the antioxidant response (Stefanson 2014).

One of the most important endogenous antioxidant systems is the *glutathione system.* This system includes glutathione, which is a small peptide, plus enzymes that restore it and keep it active (Alanazi

2015). This system is enriched in the liver but is present in all cells. Glutathione is a potent antioxidant that is particularly efficient at scavenging hydrogen peroxide, a reactive oxygen species. Hydrogen peroxide can be generated during normal metabolism or produced as part of defensive responses meant to destroy pathogens. The glutathione system also acts to recycle Vitamin C, which is otherwise known as ascorbate (Linster 2007). Glutathione is made in our bodies from amino acids. Because the body can make glutathione out of simple protein building blocks, we do not need to find special dietary sources of glutathione. So long as we eat an adequate amount of protein, we can produce glutathione from amino acids in the ingested proteins. This is one reason that consuming adequate protein is important for heath. Because of its potent antioxidant capability, glutathione is potentially attractive as a supplement to ameliorate damage in conditions of oxidative stress, such as cancer chemotherapy or neurodegenerative diseases. Because it is small peptide made of three amino acids, though, it is digested before it can be absorbed. Thus, when taken in supplement form, it must be protected through encapsulation in a fatty structure called a liposome. Liposome formulations are viscous liquids. Liposomal delivery of glutathione can be absorbed into the body, where it may boost antioxidant capacity and immune function (Sinha 2018).

Superoxide dismutase (SOD) is another family of endogenous antioxidants. SOD family members are enzymes that exist in mitochondria as well as in the fluids inside cells, between cells, and in the blood (Miao 2009). As their name implies, SODs are effective at scavenging superoxide free radicals. Like hydrogen peroxide, superoxides can be generated during metabolism or in response to the presence of pathogens (Miao 2009). Both the SOD and the glutathione systems are important for limiting damage due to oxidative stress. Mutations in the SOD system have been found to be associated with diseases such as amyotrophic lateral sclerosis (ALS) (Miao 2009). Chronic hyperglycemia damages SOD proteins and may contribute to oxidative stress effects in type 2 diabetes (Reza Nazem 2019). Activity of the SOD system seems to protect against diet-induced metabolic disease, but supplements containing SOD have not been shown to be effective because they are degraded in the gut, and the kidney rapidly clears SOD from the circulation (Rosa 2021). However, SOD family members require the minerals zinc, copper, and manganese for their activity, and a recent clinical trial found that zinc supplements administered to people with type 2 diabetes boosted SOD activity and improved metabolic markers (Nazem 2019). The findings underscore the importance of adequate intake of these minerals in the diet.

Melatonin: Most people have heard of melatonin in its role as a hormone regulating circadian and reproductive cycles. The pineal gland releases large quantities of melatonin to act throughout the body as a signaling molecule. Separately, most other cells make melatonin as well because it is a very potent antioxidant (Zhang 2014). Melatonin is made in the mitochondria, the "powerhouses" of the cell. Mitochondria are in constant risk of oxidative stress due to the complex metabolism they manage. Plants also make melatonin because their powerhouses, the chloroplasts, face the same risks as our mitochondria. They differ in how much they make, but edible plants and fungi high in melatonin, such as mushrooms and nuts, could be useful for people at risk of oxidative stress. The best animal sources of melatonin are eggs and fish (Meng 2017). Older people, who may make less melatonin but need it more, may particularly benefit from consuming melatonin in foods. Fortunately, melatonin seems to have good bioavailability, and can cross the gut barrier into our bodies.

Uric Acid: In 1683, the physician Thomas Sydenham observed that "gout kills more wise men than simple" (De Giorgi 2015, Sydenham 1683). This statement perfectly describes both the benefits and risks of high *uric acid* levels. Uric acid is an antioxidant that circulates in the blood and provides more than half of the antioxidant activity there. High levels of it are associated with gout, a painful inflammatory disease of joints, as well as with increased risk of cardiovascular disease. On the other hand, high uric acid levels correlate with intelligence, and lower levels are associated with neurodegenerative diseases (De Giorgi 2015). When uric acid levels are too high, the condition called gout can occur. Historically gout has been associated with wealth, but by the 20th century, changes in diet had rendered gout rare (Kedar 2012). Sadly, the condition has made a comeback since the 1990's, coincident with increasingly available processed and high-fructose foods (Kedar 2012, Punzi 2020).

Gout is the most common type of inflammatory arthritis. It is the result of an inherited susceptibility, combined with diets high in purines, the dietary precursor of uric acid (Punzi 2020). Generally, high-purine diets result from eating lots of meats and fats, and few vegetables and other carbohydrates. High uric acid levels can become pronounced when high levels of refined sugar, especially fructose, are also a major part of the diet. In addition, alcoholic beverage intake, particularly beer and liquor, are associated with gout flare and higher uric acid levels in blood (Towiwat 2015). Interestingly, consumption of coffee and dairy products is associated with lower uric acid levels and lower risk for gout (Towiwat 2015).

Co-enzyme Q10 (CoQ10/ubiquinone/ubiquinol): Like melatonin, CoQ10 is a potent antioxidant found in mitochondria, where it helps produce energy-providing molecules, such as adenosine triphosphate (ATP), and scavenge free-radicals (Raizner 2019). It is one of the most widely used supplements because of its antioxidant properties, safety, and lack of side effects, and the fact that is absorbed into the body by the gut (Raizner 2019). Despite the popularity of CoQ10 as a supplement, there is little evidence for its efficacy as a treatment for any disease condition (Arenas-Jal 2020).

Metallothioneins and Zinc

Metallothioneins are *stress response* proteins that bind metals, especially zinc (Park 2018). They have both antioxidant and anti-inflammatory properties. They are currently being studied for the treatment of inflammatory conditions including heart disease, amyotrophic lateral sclerosis, and diabetes. One way to increase metallothionein s is through supplementation with zinc. Zinc is found in oysters, meat, dairy, hemp seed, and tofu. Zinc also has important regulatory functions of its own and is particularly important for the SOD system and immune function (Miao 2009, Jarosz 2017, Nazem 2019, Read 2019). It may also have specific anti-viral actions (Read 2019).

Dietary Antioxidants: Vitamins and Polyphenols

Many vitamins have anti-inflammatory or antioxidant properties in addition to other actions that support proper cell function. In this way, eating a diet that provides sufficient vitamins can protect health by keeping cells functioning, and by protecting against oxidative stress. Vitamins are classified into two categories: water-soluble and fat-soluble. Water-soluble vitamins are not stored in the body. They are used immediately or excreted in urine. They can be easily depleted if there are not enough in the diet, thus the risks of toxicity are low. Fat-soluble vitamins accumulate in fat and membranes, making them less vulnerable to depletion, but more apt to cause toxicity through excessive intake, and even death, in the case of vitamin A. The other best-known category of dietary antioxidants are the polyphenols, which are widely distributed in plant-based foods.

Water-Soluble Vitamins

B Vitamins are a complex of vitamins that are indispensable for the proper working of cells. Several are critical to mitochondrial function, and thus necessary for cells to generate energy to perform all their duties and stay healthy (Kennedy 2016). Some have antioxidant abilities, which may be important because of their association with energy production, as well as anti-inflammatory actions. These anti-inflammatory actions include the ability to inhibit activation of the inflammasome, a protein complex that activates pro-inflammatory cytokine molecules such as interleukins. If taken as supplements, they work best as a complex, but there are many dietary sources of B vitamins, including fish, poultry, soybeans, and mushrooms. Some B vitamins are made by our gut microbes, as well.

Our ability to absorb B vitamins, especially vitamin B-12, can be impaired as we age. B-12 deficiency causes immune and nervous system dysfunction, and can lead to cognitive impairment, mood disorders, and permanent nerve damage if not treated promptly (Kennedy 2016). Therefore, it is a good idea for older people to get their B-12 levels checked regularly.

Vitamin C, also called ascorbate or ascorbic acid, is a potent antioxidant that humans must obtain from their diet (Granger 2018). Unlike other animals, we cannot make it ourselves. It was originally famous for being discovered as the nutrient deficient responsible for scurvy, which was historically endemic among sailors. Scurvy was prevented by providing oranges for sailors to eat. Lack of vitamin C causes symptoms because of its role in collagen function. It also modulates immune function in several ways, particularly anti-viral immunity (Cerullo 2020, Halfords 2020). Vitamin C reduces oxidative stress by scavenging pro-inflammatory reactive oxygen species, and by activating endogenous antioxidant systems including the glutathione on SOD systems (Halfords 2020). Vitamin C also reduces pro-inflammatory cytokine levels, while increasing cytokines called interferons that are critical for anti-viral immunity. Vitamin C may also fight viruses directly by interfering with viral enzyme activity (Halfords 2020).

These features suggest that Vitamin C should be effective at treating or preventing viral infections. However, many studies have shown that for most people, vitamin C supplements do not prevent infection with seasonal colds and only reduce symptoms marginally (Cerullo 2020). On the other hand, vitamin C supplementation for very active people, such as marathon runners and soldiers operating in subarctic conditions, reduced the incidence of colds by half (Cerullo 2020, Halfords 2020). This suggests that intense physical exertion and thus oxidative stress may deplete Vitamin C levels. Interestingly, people with diabetes, obesity, and cardiovascular disease typically have low levels of vitamin C, which is likely linked to the chronic inflammation associated with these conditions (Cerullo 2020, Halfords 2020). At the same time, people with these conditions are at increased risk for severe COVID-19. One link may be that depletion of vitamin C during chronic inflammation leaves the lungs vulnerable to the intense oxidative stress that occurs during the immune response to COVID-19. Indeed, severe infections, such as sepsis, pneumonia, and COVID-19 are associated with dramatically depleted vitamin C levels, which is believed to due to increased use of the vitamin in the upregulated immune response (Halfords 2020). Intravenous administration of vitamin C to severely ill patients with sepsis reduces mortality and this effect seems evident for severe COVID-19 infections as well (Holford 2020).

Taken together, these observations indicate that vitamin C levels are indeed likely to be a factor in the body's response to conditions, such as infection, in which oxidative stress and inflammation can have serious consequences, including death. High-dose supplementation is indicated for people at risk for vitamin C depletion, but there does not seem to be any benefit for otherwise healthy people of daily high-dose supplements (Cerrullo 2020). Rather, a diet rich in fruits and vegetables can provide adequate vitamin C levels. Foods that are good sources of Vitamin C include citrus, berries, red peppers, and many greens, including Brussels sprouts.

Fat-Soluble Vitamins

Vitamin E refers to a group of molecules called tocopherols. Alpha-tocopherol is most prevalent in fruits, nuts, and vegetables. Vitamin E got its name, tocopherol, meaning "to carry a pregnancy" in Greek, based on studies in the 1930's showing it was a fertility factor for rats. There is no evidence that it has such actions in humans, but it has been demonstrated to be a powerful antioxidant. Because it is lipid-soluble, vitamin E may be particularly important for managing oxidation in cell membranes, which are mostly lipids. Like vitamin C, vitamin E can modulate immune functions, apparently independently from its antioxidant capability (Meydani 2018). The symptoms of vitamin E deficiency involve disturbances in membrane function, particularly in red blood cells and immune function, and sensory neuropathy (Meydani 2018). Although vitamin E deficiency is rare, there are concerns that vitamin E requirements may increase as people age, based on the observed effects of inflammaging on immune function (Meydani 2018). That is: we may require more vitamin E to protect against oxidative stress as we age. Supportive evidence for including vitamin E-rich foods in the diet is found in some small studies that show that eating whole foods containing vitamin E, such as almonds, is associated with reduced levels of inflammatory mediators (Liu 2012). Good sources of whole foods high in vitamin E include nuts, wheat germ and wheat germ oil, and most other vegetable oils including olive, canola, and avocado oil.

Vitamin A is well known for its importance for vision, but it is involved in many other functions as well, including brain development and learning (Olson 2010). It also has anti-inflammatory properties. Persons with inflammatory diseases such as Crohn's disease and Alzheimer's disease have been found to have low vitamin A levels (Zeng 2017). Vitamin A, however, is toxic at high levels, and it is safest to rely on a healthy diet to provide sufficient levels. Foods rich in vitamin A include most orange foods, such as carrots and squash.

Vitamin D, often called the "sunshine vitamin," is actually a hormone, because it is produced in the body from cholesterol with the aid of sunlight. Vitamin D can also be obtained in the diet from some mushrooms and from many fatty fish (Nair 2012). Vitamin D is most famous for its role in bone health, as it is critical for uptake of calcium (Nair 2012). But most tissues of the body contain receptors for vitamin D and thus it exerts a widespread effect on physiological function, including metabolic regulation and kidney activity. Most cells of the immune system express vitamin D receptors (Mangin 2014). Vitamin D receptors, like cortisol receptors, are located in the cell nucleus and act to coordinate gene expression, in concert with other signaling proteins such as NFkB (Mangin 2014). Thus, immune regulation is one of vitamin D's most important functions.

A perplexing current paradox is that whereas low levels of vitamin D are found in many disorders, including chronic pain, cancer, autoimmune diseases, and dementia, supplementation with vitamin D does not seem to prevent or improve any of these conditions (Chai 2019, Straub 2015, Mangin 2014, Manson 2019, Orrkaby 2019 Straube 2018). Low vitamin D levels are also seen in people who otherwise seem healthy, suggesting that low vitamin D levels in disease may be a consequence rather than cause of disease (Mangin 2014).

Normally, we can make as much vitamin D as we need by getting several minutes of sunlight exposure per day, but as we age, this ability declines (Mangin 2014, Nair 2012). Many older people have very low levels of vitamin D even if they spend a lot of time in the sun. The implications of this are yet unknown, but many practitioners recommend daily supplementation of 1000-2000 units of vitamin/day for older people with low levels of vitamin D. While Vitamin D has not been shown to increase lifespan, this dose is not toxic and may confer benefits or protection that have yet to be identified.

Vitamin K is key for the synthesis of several proteins involved in blood clotting. Blood clotting is part of the body's defense against damage and is activated as part of the inflammatory response. Vitamin K also has antioxidant capability (Samad 2021). Vitamin K is obtained from the diet from green leafy vegetables and is also found in fermented foods such as cheese. Some microbes also produce vitamin K.

Polyphenols

Polyphenols are a large class of molecules that have structural features in common. They all have phenol groups. They are found in fruits and vegetables, including whole grains. Most have antioxidant capabilities and are also anti-inflammatory (Yahfoufi 2018). Some may influence the rate at which the gut absorbs glucose, which may help glucose tolerance. These abilities are thought to contribute to the beneficial health effects of diets that are rich in fruits and vegetables.

Polyphenols are usually divided into two classes. The first class, the flavonoids, includes quercetin, catechin, and epicatechin. The second class, the non-flavonoids, includes 4 subgroups: the stilbenes, the lignans, the phenolic acids, and the anthocyanins. As an example, resveratrol, derived from grapes, is a stilbene. Brewer's yeast extract contains lignans. Caffeic acid, found in coffee, olive oil, and various fruits and vegetables, is a phenolic acid. Anthocyanins are found in fruits and beans with purple pigments, such as black beans, black rice, and some wine grapes.

Many polyphenols serve as pigments, especially in the skin of fruits. This is one reason to look for colorful food, as it is more likely to contain lots of antioxidant polyphenols. For people who like to get their fruits and vegetables by juicing, it is important to include the skins, not just the pulp, because most of the polyphenols will be in the skins. This is also one reason that red wine, which is fermented with the skins, is associated with more health benefits and higher polyphenol and other antioxidant content than white wine, which is made from just the juice.

Diet versus Supplements: What is the Best Way to Influence Oxidative Stress?

In contrast to the very encouraging results of clinical trials implementing whole-food-based dietary patterns, such as the Mediterranean Diet, for conditions such as heart disease or mood disorders, studies investigating single supplements, extracts, or single ingredients have been inconsistent and disappointing overall (Grainger 2018, Manson 2019, Zhang 2020). But supplement and "superfood" use continue to be popular in US and Europe. Is there any reason to use supplements?

The bottom line seems to be that single vitamin or mineral supplements are effective for disorders that are specifically caused by deficiencies of these vitamins or mineral, such as scurvy, pellagra, goiter, pernicious anemia, etc. but not for conditions that have a more complicated etiology (Zhang 2020).

Why don't vitamin or other supplements reliably improve disease? One source of variability can include genetic or epigenetic differences among individuals in in the uptake of vitamins (Granger 2018, Regner 2021). Aging also affects the ability of the body to absorb and use vitamins. The populations of our gut microbes also can influence uptake of vitamins and antioxidants, while whole/intact fruits, vegetables, and grains support beneficial microbes, in part by providing fiber, in ways that supplements cannot (Feng 2015).

More fundamentally, the problem may be the way we think about vitamins and other nutrients in disease. For instance, one principal rationale for supplement treatments are findings of low vitamin levels in individuals with specific diseases, and thus implying the disease is caused by the deficiency. In fact, the relationship may not be causal. For instance, some disease processes may deplete specific vitamin levels, and although supplementation might improve vitamin levels, it might not necessarily affect the disease process. Similarly, some conditions, such as cardiometabolic disorders that involve inflammation and oxidative stress, are caused by or exacerbated by a diet poor in antioxidants. Implementing healthy diet patterns does improve symptoms for such conditions.

Another concern is the tendency to think of things as either "good" or "bad". Although oxidative stress is deleterious when it is unregulated and damages cells, it can also trigger compensatory responses that are ultimately beneficial. For instance, intense exercise induces oxidative stress in muscles, which leads to growth and strengthening of the muscles. This effect is inhibited by treatment with antioxidants (Cobley 2015). There is a delicate balance between normal functions of oxidation and deleterious oxidative stress. As yet, the precise details concerning exactly when we need more antioxidant capability, which antioxidants, and how much of them are not known. Thus, evidence indicates that the safest, most effective way to prevent deleterious oxidative stress while preserving its important functions is to consume a diet that contains whole/intact plant-based antioxidants.

Bioavailability: What Gets Absorbed?

One problem with understanding the role of polyphenols involves the fact that most exhibit poor *bioavailability*. Bioavailability refers to the rate and amounts of a substance absorbed into the gut. If a substance has poor bioavailability, even eating large amounts of it may not provide benefits, because it does not get into the body. The poor bioavailability of many polyphenols has driven skepticism as to whether diets really do provide physiologically relevant antioxidant actions (Gupta 2013). Nonetheless, polyphenols may undergo biotransformation in the gut, possibly aided by gut microbes, which serve to increase their bioavailability (Feng 2015, Gupta 2013). Importantly, even polyphenols that do not get into our systemic circulation may still have important effects in our gut (Chiu 2021). For instance, they may be able to mitigate inflammation at the gut barrier. One factor that influences the ability of nutrients such as polyphenols to be absorbed into the body is cooking style. Fats, such as cooking oils, can help transport polyphenols across the gut barrier. Roasting or sautéing vegetables in oil can also improve bioavailability.

Anti-Inflammatory Dietary Ingredients

Many polyphenols have anti-inflammatory actions beyond their ability to scavenge free radicals. These agents interact with inflammatory pathways to, for example, inhibit the induction of pro-inflammatory prostaglandins, prevent the activation of NFkB and the inflammasome, or modify cytokine receptor activity. This pattern of action is essentially the same as the non-steroidal anti-inflammatory drugs (NSAIDs).

The best-studied of these ingredients is curcumin, which is found in turmeric. Curcumin can inhibit NFkB activation, which leads to reductions in levels of pro-inflammatory cytokines. Thus, curcumin may be useful for treatment or prevention of disorders related to chronic inflammation, including cardiometabolic disease, pain, and neurodegenerative diseases such as mild cognitive impairment and Alzheimer's disease (Kim 2018). Other anti-inflammatory agents found in the diet include apigenin, quercetin, and resveratrol, found in red foods such as apples, tomatoes, red peppers, red onions, chamomile, and red grapes (Bariani 2017, Bispo da Silva 2020, Li 2016, Ozdal 2019, Makanjuola 2018, Malaguarnera 2019). Like curcumin and willow bark, the original source for aspirin, these ingredients can reduce levels of inflammatory mediators, including prostaglandins, and reduce activity of NFkB (Lu, 2016, Parmu 2019). It is important to keep in mind, however, that any substance or drug that chronically suppresses inflammation can lead to side effects, such as increased susceptibility to infections.

Key Points

- Foods can have important effects on health by either increasing inflammation and oxidative stress or protecting against them.
- Antioxidants act to prevent or fix inappropriate oxidation by donating one of their own electrons or protons (hydrogen).
- The body makes antioxidants to control oxidation during normal metabolism, but during time of high demand, metabolic rate may exceed the body's stash of antioxidants. This results in oxidative stress.
- Antioxidants normally work in systems, so that they are regenerated and don't become radicalized themselves. This may explain why getting antioxidants from whole foods, which likely contain the entire system, seems to be more effective than single antioxidant supplements.
- Exogenous antioxidants can activate "anti-oxidant response" systems that are coordinated by Nrf2. In this way antioxidants can ameliorate oxidative stress both directly, and by stimulating the body's own antioxidant capability.

- Vitamins are substances that are important as either as co-factors for metabolism or as antioxidants. They provide global support for cells, preventing damage and subsequent inflammation.
- Dietary antioxidants are found in fruits, vegetables, and whole grains. They often serve as pigments, providing the color in colorful food.
- Many dietary antioxidants have poor bioavailability, meaning that they do not readily pass from the gut into the body. Even so, they make exert beneficial actions on cells of the gut lining or be metabolized by gut microbes into substances with better bioavailability. They may even help microbes in our gut stay healthy.
- Dietary antioxidants can be helpful during times of oxidative stress, such as injury, intense exercise, infection, or chronic inflammation. This is an important reason why people experiencing physical or mental stress should consume a diet rich in fresh fruits and vegetables, because such foods contain dietary antioxidants.
- Vitamin supplementation seems to be most effective in the context of treating deficiency or depletion, such as during serious infections.

References

Alanazi AM, Mostafa GAE, Al-Badr AA. Chapter Two- Glutathione. Profiles of Drug Substance, Excipients and Related Methodology, 40:43-158, 2015.

Amini L, Chekini R, Nateghi MR, Haghani H, Jamialahmadi T, Sathyapalan T, Sahebkar A. The effect of combined vitamin C and vitamin E supplementation on oxidative stress markers in women with endometriosis: A randomized, triple-blind placebo-controlled clinical trial. Pain Research and Management, 2021:5529741, 2021.

Arenas-Jul M, Sune-Negre JM, Garcia-Montoya E. Coenzyme Q10 supplementation: Efficacy, safety, and formulation challenges. Comprehensive Reviews in Food Science and Food Safety, 19:574-594, 2020.

Bariani MV, Correa F, Leishman E, Domínguez Rubio AP, Arias A, Stern A, Bradshaw HB, Franchi AM. Resveratrol protects from lipopolysaccharide-induced inflammation in the uterus and prevents experimental preterm birth. Molecular Human Reproduction, 23:571–581, 2017.

Billingsley H, Carbone S. The antioxidant potential of the Mediterranean diet in patients at high cardiovascular risk: an in-depth review of the PREDIMED. Nutrition and Diabetes, 8:8-13, 2018.

Bispo da Silva A, Cerqueira Coelho PL, das Neves Oliveira M, Luz Oliveira J, Oliveira Amparo JA, Costa da Silva K, et al. The flavonoid rutin and its aglycone quercetin modulate the microglia inflammatory profile improving antiglioma activity. Brain, Behavior, and Immunity, 85: 170-185, 2020.

Cerullo G, Negro M, Parimbelli M, Pecoraro M, Perna S, Ligouri G, et al. The long history of vitamin C: From prevention of the common cold to potential aid in the treatment of COVID-19. Frontiers in Immunology, 11:574029, 2020.

Chai B, Goa F, Wu, Dong T, Gu C, Lin Q, Zhang Y. Vitamin D deficiency as a risk factor for dementia and Alzheimer's disease: an updated meta-analysis. BMC Neurology, 19:284, 2019.

Cherian L, Wang Y, Fakuda K, Leurgans S, Aggarwal N, Morris M. Mediterranean-DASH Intervention for Neurodegenerative Delay (MIND) diet slows cognitive decline after stroke. Journal of Prevention of Alzheimer's Disease, 6:267-273, 2019.

Chiu H-F, Venkatakrishnan K, Golovinskaia O, Wanf C-K. Gastroprotective effects of polyphenols against various gastro-intestinal disorders: A mini-review with special focus on clinical evidence. Molecules, 26:2090, 2021.

Cobley JN, McHardy K, Morton JP, Nikollaidis MG, Close GL. Influence of vitamin C and vitamin E in redox signaling: Implications for exercise adaptions. Free Radical Biology and Medicine, 84:65-76, 2015.

De Giorgi A, Fabbian F, Pala M, Tiseo R, Parisi C, Misurati E, Manfredini R. Uric acid: friend or foe? Uric acid and cognitive function "Gout kills more wise men than simple". European Review for Medical and Pharmacological Sciences, 19:640-646, 2015.

Feng R, Shou J-W, Zhao Z-X, He C-Y, Ma C, Huang M et al. Transforming berberine into its intestine-absorbable form by the gut microbiota. Scientific Reports, 5:12255, 2015.

Granger M, Eck P. Dietary vitamin C in human health. Advances in Food and Nutrition Research, 83:281-310, 2018.

Gupta A, Kagliwal LD, Singhal RS. Biotransformation of polyphenols for improving bioavailability and processing stability. Advances in Food and Nutrition Research, 69:183-217, 2013.

He L, He T, Farrar S, Ji L, Liu T, Ma X. Antioxidants Maintain Cellular Redox Homeostasis by Elimination of Reactive Oxygen Species. Cellular Physiology and Biochemistry, 44:532-553, 2017.

Hemila H, Kaprio J. Modification of the effect of vitamin E supplementation on the mortality of male smokers by age and vitamin C. American Journal of Epidemiology, 169:946-953, 2009.

Halfords P, Carr AC, Jovic TH, Ali SR, Whitaker IS, Marik PE, Smith AD. Vitamin C- An adjunctive therapy for respiratory infection, sepsis and COVI19. Nutrients, 12:3760, 2020.

Huang Q, Huan Liu H, Suzuki K, Ma S, Liu C. Linking What We Eat to Our Mood: A Review of Diet, Dietary Antioxidants, and Depression. Antioxidants, 8:376, 2019.

Jacka FN, O'Neil A, Opie R, Itsiopoulos C, Cotton S, Mohebbi M, Castle D, Dash S, Mihalopoulos C, Chatterton ML, Brazionis L, Dean OM, Allison M. Hodge AM, Berk M. A randomised controlled trial of dietary improvement for adults with major depression (the 'SMILES' trial). BMC Medicine, 15:23 2017.

Jarosz M, Magdalena Olbert M, Wyszogrodzka G, Młyniec K, Librowski T. Antioxidant and anti-inflammatory effects of zinc. Zinc-dependent NF-kB signaling. Inflammopharmacology, 25:11–24, 2017.

Kedar E, and Simkin P. A perspective on diet and gout. Advances in Chronic Kidney Disease, 19:392-397, 2012.

Keewan E, Narasimhulu CA, Rohr M, Hamid S, Parthasarathy S. Are fried foods unhealthy? The dietary peroxidized fatty acid, 13-HPODE, induces intestinal inflammation in vitro and in vivo. Antioxidants, 9:926, 2020.

Kennedy DO. B vitamins and the brain: mechanisms, does and efficacy - a review. Nutrients, 8:68, 2016.

Kim Y, Clifton P. Curcumin, cardiometabolic health and dementia. International Journal of Environmental Research and Public Health, 15:2093, 2018.

Koh E, Surh J. Food types and frying frequency affect the lipid oxidation of deep frying oil for the preparation of school meals in Korea. Food Chemistry, 174:467-472, 2015.

Korkmas A, Oter S, Seyrek M, Topal T. Molecular, genetic and epigenetic pathways of peroxynitrite-induced cellular toxicity. Interdisciplinary Toxicology, 2:219–228, 2009.

Li Y, Yao J, Han C, Yang J, Tabassum Chaudhry M, Wang S, Liu H, Yin Y. Quercetin, Inflammation and Immunity. Nutrients, 8:167, 2016.

Linster CL, Van Schaftingen E. Vitamin C: Biosynthesis, recycling and degradation in mammals. FEBS Journal, 274:1-22, 2007.

Liu J-F, Liu Y-H, Chen C-M, Chang W-h, Chen O. The effects of almonds in inflammation and oxidative stress in Chinese patients with type 2 diabetes mellitus: a randomized crossover controlled feeding trial. European Journal of Nutrition, 52:927-935, 2013.

Makanjuola SBL, Ogundaini AO, Ajonuma LC, Dosunmu A. Apigenin and apigeninidin isolates from the Sorghum bicolor leaf targets inflammation via cyclo-oxygenase-2 and prostaglandin E2 blockade. International Journal of Rheumatic Diseases, 21:1487-1495, 2018.

Malaguarnera L. Influence of Resveratrol on the Immune Response. Nutrients, 11, 946; doi:10.3390/nu11050946, 2019.

Mangin M, Sinha R, Fincer K. Inflammation and vitamin D: the infection connection. Inflammation Research, 63:803-819, 2014.

Manson JE, Cook NR, Lee I-M, Christen W, Bassuck SS, Mora S, Gibson H, et al. Vitamin D supplements and prevention of cancer and cardiovascular disease. New England Journal of Medicine, 380:33-44, 2019.

Meng X, Li Y, Li S, Zhou Y, Gan R-Y, Xu D-P, Li H-B. Dietary sources and bioactivities of melatonin. Nutrients, 9:367, 2017.

Meydani N, Lewis ED, Wu D. Perspective: Should vitamin E recommendations for older adults be increased? Advances in Nutrition, 9:533-543, 2018.

Nair R, Daseeh. Vitamin D: The sunshine vitamin. Journal of Pharmacology and Pharmacotherapeutics, 3:188-126, 2012.

Nazem MR, Asadi M, Jabbari N, Allameh A. Effects of zinc supplementation on superoxide dismutase activity and gene expression, and metabolic parameters in overweight type 2 diabetes patients: A randomized, double-blind controlled trial. Clinical Biochemistry, 69:15-20, 2019.

Nellezza I, Giambanco I, Minelli A, Donato R. Nrf2-Keap1 signaling in oxidative and reductive stress. BBA-Molecular Cell Research, 1865:721-733, 2018.

Olson CR, Mello CV. Significance of vitamin A to brain function, behavior and learning. Molecular Nutrition and Food Research, 54:489-495, 2010.

Orkaby AR, Djousee L, Manson JE. Vitamin D supplements and prevention of cardiovascular disease. Current Opinion in Cardiology, 34:700-705, 2019.

Ozdal ZD, Sahmetlioglu E, Narin I, Cumaoglu A. Synthesis of gold and silver nanoparticles using flavonoid quercetin and their effects on lipopolysaccharide induced inflammatory response in microglial cells. 3 Biotech, 9:212, 2019.

Park Y, Zhang J, Cai L. Reappraisal of metallothionein: Clinical implications for patients with diabetes mellitus. Journal of Diabetes, 10:213-231, 2018.

Parmu N, Bhatnagar A. Resveratrol: from enhances biosynthesis and bioavailability to multitargeting chronic diseases. Biomedicine and Pharmacotherapy, 109:2237-2251, 2019.

Punzi L, Scanu A, Galozzi P, Luisetto R, Spinella P, Scire CA, Oliviero F. One year in review 2020: gout. Clinical and Experimental Rheumatology, 38:807-821, 2020.

Raizner AE. Coenzyme Q_{10}. Methodist DeBakey Cardiovascular Journal, 15:185-191, 2019.

Razavi Zade MR, Telkabadi MH, Bahmani F, Salehi B, Farshbaf S, Asemi Z. The effects of DASH diet on weight loss and metabolic status in adults with non-alcoholic fatty liver disease: a randomized clinical trial. Liver International, 36:563-571, 2016.

Read SA, Obeid S, Ahlenstiel C, Ahlenstiel G. The role of zinc in antiviral immunity. Advances in Nutrition, 10:696-710, 2019.

Regner-Nelke L, Nelke C, Schroeder CB, Dziewas R, Warneke T, Ruck T, Meuth SG. Enjoy carefully: The multifaceted role of vitamin E in neuro-nutrition. International Journal of Molecular Sciences, 22:100087, 2021.

Rosa AC, Brunu N, Meineri G, Corsi D, Cavi N, Gastaldi D, Dosio F. Strategies to expand the therapeutic potential of superoxide dismutase by exploiting delivery approaches. International Journal of Biological Macromolecules, 168:846-865, 2021.

Sama N, Dutta S, Sodunke TE, Fairuz A, Sapkota A, Miftah ZF, et al. Fat-soluble vitamins and the current global pandemic of COVID-19:Evidence-based efficacy from literature review. Journal of Inflammation Research, 14:2019-2110, 2021.

Schaich KM. Thinking outside the classical chain reaction box of lipid oxidation. Lipid Technology, 24:55-58, 2012.

Sinha R, Sinha I, Calcagnotto A, Trushin N, Haley JS, Schell TD, Richie JP. Oral supplementation with liposomal glutathione elevates body stores of glutathione and markers of immune function. European Journal of Clinical Nutrition, 72:105-111, 2018.

Speckmann B, Steinbrenner H, Grune T, Klotz L-O. Peroxynitrite: From interception to signaling. Archives of Biochemistry and Biophysics, 595: 153e160, 2016.

Stefanson AL, Bakovic M. Dietary regulation of Keap1/Nrf2/ARE pathway: Focus on plant-derived compounds and trace minerals. Nutrients, 6:3777-3801, 2014.

Straube S, Derry S, Straube C, Moore RA. Vitamin D for the treatment of chronic painful conditions in adults. Cochrane Database of Systematic Reviews, 5:CD007771, 2015.

Sydenham T. Tractatus de Podagra et Hydrope. London, England: G Kettilby, 1683.

Tu W, Wang H, Li S, Liu Q, Sha H. The anti-inflammatory and anti-oxidant mechanisms of the Keap1/Nerf2/ARE signaling pathway in chronic diseases. Aging and Disease, 10:637-651, 2019.

Yahfoufi N, Alsadi N, Jambi M, Matar C. The immunomodulatory and anti-inflammatory role of polyphenols. Nutrients, 10:1618, 2018.

Zeng J, Chen L, Wang Z, Chen Q, Fan Z, Jiang H, Wu Y, Ren L, Chen J, Li T, Song W. Marginal vitamin A deficiency facilitates Alzheimer's Disease pathogenesis. Acta Neuropathologica, 133:967-982, 2017.

Zhang FF, Barr SI, McNulty H, Li D, Blumberg JB. Health effects of vitamin and mineral supplements. BMJ, 369:m2511, 2020.

Zhang H-M, Zhang Y. Melatonin: a well-documented antioxidant with conditional pro-oxidant actions. Journal of Pineal Research, 57:131–146, 2014.

- WHAT ARE FATS?

- STRUCTURE DETERMINES FUNCTIONS

- FATS HAVE IMPORTANT FUNCTIONS IN THE BODY

- WHAT MAKES A FAT BAD?

- WHICH FOODS MIGHT CONTAIN OXIDIZED FATS?

- ARE SATURATED FATS REALLY BAD?

- ESSENTIAL FATTY ACIDS: OMEGA 3 AND OMEGA 6

- WHAT ABOUT HIGH FAT DIETS?

- KEY POINTS

Although high-energy, typically Western diets are associated with poor health, and oxidized lipids can drive inflammation, several clinical trials have recently reported that diets containing polyunsaturated fatty acids (PUFAs) and olive oil have health benefits. Specifically, these polyunsaturated fats may reduce inflammation, prevent blood glucose tolerance, and improve metabolic markers such as circulating low-density lipoproteins (LDL). On the other hand, saturated fats, commonly found in meat and dairy, are believed by many researchers and clinicians to cause heart disease (Wali 2020). This belief follows from epidemiological findings from the 1960s and 1970s linking high-fat diets to negative cardiovascular outcomes. However, there is still a lack of mechanistic explanation or clear evidence supporting native, non-oxidized lipids as causative agents in cardiovascular disease. More recent research has indicated that other lifestyle factors, such as physical activity levels, stress, and genetic factors play important roles in disease risk. These may interact with factors related to diet quality to predispose people to cardiovascular and metabolic diseases (Lechner 2020). Further, there are other culprits besides saturated fat in mammal products such as meat and dairy that can induce or contribute to health conditions previously attributed to saturated fat consumption (Soullilou 2020).

Nonetheless, fats still suffer from a bad reputation. Given the association of obesity with cardiometabolic disease and inflammation, it is intuitive to blame dietary fat for the relationship between diet and health outcomes (Ludwig 2018). Dietary fat has twice the calorie density of protein and carbohydrates, and thus provides more energy per unit consumed. Non-fat or low-fat versions of foods are still popular, even though studies show no benefits of these foods compared to full-fat versions (Hirahatake 2020). Unfortunately, "fat fear" may lead to unhealthy diet choices. For example, some people substitute fats with refined carbohydrates or sugars. Thus, understanding the role of fats in the body and the mechanisms by which some fats can induce inflammation can help make sense of the conflicting stories on fat.

What are Fats?

To briefly review Chapter 10, fats, or lipids, are fairly simple molecules. Fats consist of carbon chains that bind hydrogen atoms as well. Fats that consist of only 2-5 carbons are called *short-chain fatty acids* and are made by microbes in the gut (Morrison 2016). *Medium-chain fatty acids,* consisting of 6 to 12 carbons, are found in coconut milk and palm kernel oil. Carbon chains of more than 12 are termed *long-chain fatty acids;* these include the omega-3 and omega-6 polyunsaturated fatty acids.

Specific features of each kind of carbon chain affect the functioning of the fat. Carbon atoms have four valence electrons that they share with other atoms. Metaphorically, each carbon has four hands, each of which need to be holding something. Most of the carbons in a typical fatty acid are bound to other carbons to make the chain, and the other two bonds, or "hands" are holding hydrogens. Sometimes there are not enough hydrogens to go around, so the carbons make double-bonds. Within double bonds, two carbons are holding two hands, and they each also hold hands with a different carbon (on the other side to continue the chain) and in the remaining hand, or bond, they hold a hydrogen. When there are enough hydrogens to go around and there are no double bonds, the fat is said to be *saturated* with hydrogen. In other words, the hands are holding as many hydrogens as possible. Examples of saturated fats are animal fats and coconut oil. If there is only one double bond, the fat is said to be *mono-unsaturated.* Examples are olive oil and avocado oil. If there is more than one double bond, the fat is said to be *polyunsaturated.* Omega-3 and omega-6 are polyunsaturated fatty acids, or PUFA. Saturated fats tend to be more stable. They are solids at room temperature and are somewhat less vulnerable to damage by oxidation. *Trans fats* are unsaturated fats, usually made from vegetable oils that have been partially hydrogenated, meaning that hydrogens have been added so that some of the carbons no longer need to form double bonds. However, the structure of trans fat is different than that of natural fats. Trans fats are associated with health risks and inflammation. This may be caused by the shape of the fat molecule that results from the partial hydrogenation process (Qiu 2018).

Structure Determines Functions

The shape of molecules affects their functions. Among fats, the presence of double bonds influences their shape (Oteng 2020). Saturated fats are straight chains that make them "packable" and well suited for storage of energy in adipose tissue. But they are solids at room temperature, which makes them not very fluid. As such, they are not good for other functions such as forming cell membranes, where other molecules need to move around in a relatively liquid membrane environment. Unsaturated fats have "kinks" in them where they have a double bond. In most naturally occurring fats, the single hydrogens on either side of the double bond are on the same side of the molecule. This hydrogen orientation is called the *cis* structure. This makes the unsaturated fats not packable, and less suitable for storage. However, because the cis lipids are liquid, they are ideal for building cell membranes and other functions. So-called *trans* fats have hydrogens oriented such that they are on the opposite sides of the carbon-carbon double bond. This straightens out the molecule, making it more like a saturated fat (Oteng 2020). Trans fats tend to be solid at room temperature and can serve as substitutes for saturated fats, such as in margarine. Unfortunately, trans fats can incorporate into cell membranes, like unsaturated fats, and may compromise cell membrane functions (Qiu 2018). This is thought to be one reason that trans fat consumption is associated with health risks (Longhi 2017).

The dietary sources of the different fat types follow from their structure and function. Because saturated fats are suited for storage, they are found in a high-energy form in adipose tissue of most animals. Saturated fats are also found in dairy because milk is a high-energy food designed to feed growing baby mammals. The parts of animals that contain high levels of unsaturated fats, such as the brain, are not usually popular in human diets. Green leafy vegetables and fish are the best sources of unsaturated fats in most diets. With vegetables, the unsaturated fats are found in the chloroplasts, which give greens their color. Thus, the greener the vegetable the better it is as a source of unsaturated fat. Trans fats are almost exclusively found in processed foods but can occur at low levels naturally in dairy (Oteng 2020).

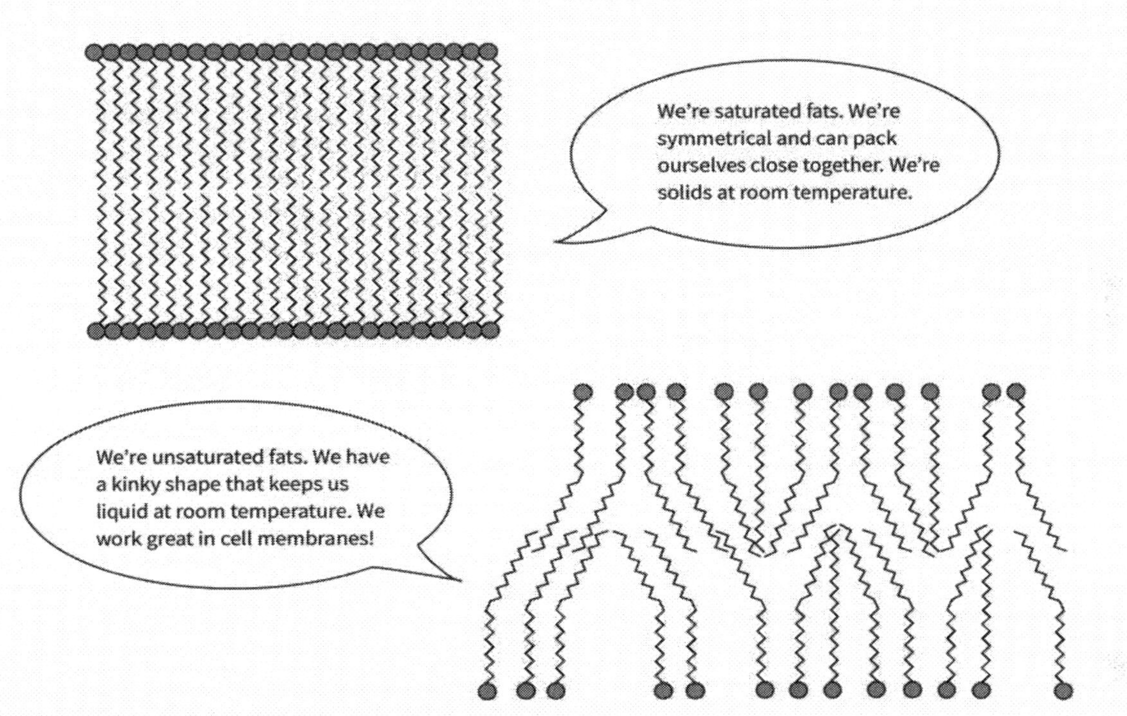

Figure Legend: The structure of fats determines their function. Saturated fats are symmetrical and create solids at room temperatures. Unsaturated fats have a bent shape that makes them harder to pack together. They are liquid oils at room temperature.

Fats have Important Functions in the Body

When we think of fat, we usually think of fats in the diet, or in our adipose tissue. Dietary fat provides more energy, described as calories, than either carbohydrate or protein, so these stable molecules are convenient and efficient for storing energy. But fats play a wide variety of roles in the body.

Cell structure and nerve insulation. Fats are not soluble in water, so they are ideal for use in cell membranes. Our cells are surrounded by fluid that might dissolve the membranes, if they were water-soluble. Many neurons, including those of peripheral nerves, have very long axons that need to be insulated to conduct the electrochemical impulses that neurons use to communicate. Fats are ideal for insulation, so the cells that insulate axons in the nervous system contain lots of fat (Poitelon 2020). This is why the brain is one of the "fattier" organs of the body.

Cell communication. In addition to their roles in cell structure, many fats also serve as communication molecules, or provide the substrate for hormones and other chemical messengers. For instance, steroid hormones such as estrogen, progesterone, testosterone, and cortisol, are derived from cholesterol, a type of fat. The *eicosanoids,* which are a big group of mediators that play critical roles in the induction and regulation of inflammation, are synthesized initially from polyunsaturated fatty acids acquired from the diet (LaGarde 2013). Prostaglandins, the targets of the non-steroidal anti-inflammatory drugs, are eicosanoids.

One of the most famous groups of fat-derived mediators are the endocannabinoids. Anandamide is an example. Endocannabinoids are synthesized from omega-6 fatty acids and are closely related to the prostaglandins (Dyall 2017). They serve as the endogenous ligands for cannabinoid receptors, which also mediate the effects of marijuana and its active ingredients (e.g., THC, CBD). Lipid mediators of the endocannabinoid system act as growth factors and neuromodulators in the brain and contribute to regulation of inflammation and appetite as well (Dyall 2017, Chiurchiu 2018, Horner 2020). There are many other lipids that also serve as signaling molecules related to control of cell growth and other critical functions.

Influencing appetite. In general, dietary fats tend to induce gut hormones associated with feelings of fullness or *satiety* (Horner 2020, Polley 2019). So far, human studies have not shown dramatic direct effects of dietary fats on appetite. Different types of fats (e.g., medium-chain versus long-chain) induce different gut hormones (e.g., GLP vs. CCK). Thus, different fats may be more appropriate for appetite control in different specific circumstances. Specifically, some fats may induce gut hormones that are effective in directly decreasing appetite, whereas others may function principally to slow down digestion, which may indirectly stimulate satiety pathways (Polley 2019). Clearly there is a need for further research addressing the effects of dietary fat on eating behavior in humans.

Interestingly, dietary fats can also be produced within our gut by microbes. These microbes make short-chain fatty acids including butyrate, acetate, propionate, and lactate, that can act in the body as substrates for metabolism or act as mediators (Morrison 2016). Short-chain fatty acids exert their effects by binding to *fatty acid receptors* that are expressed on gut endocrine cells and immune cells (Lu 2018). The actions of short-chain fatty acids seem to be to reduce appetite and regulate blood glucose (Morrison 2016).

What Makes a Fat Bad?

Studies reporting on the relationship between fats and cardiovascular disease often refer to *atherogenic* lipid particles when linking fats to disease. This term suggests that these types of lipids cause arteriosclerosis. Atherogenic lipid particles belong to the low-density lipoprotein (LDL) and very low-density lipoprotein (VLDL) categories. These particles are rich in phospholipids and PUFAs that are easily oxidized. When they are oxidized, such as in the context of inflammation or oxidative stress, they can induce or increase inflammation (Fruhwirth 2007). Thus, oxidation of lipids is the principal factor that can make a fat "bad."

When lipids are oxidized, they can form *advanced oxidized lipid end-products* (ALEs) that act as damage-associated molecular patterns (DAMPs, Chapter 7) to activate inflammation (see Chapter 10 for a description of the process). This process happens within the body during inflammatory conditions such as atherosclerosis, neurodegenerative disease, or autoimmune disease (Fruhwirth 2007, Kanner 2007). But oxidation of lipids can also happen when foods are processed for production (e.g., processed meats such hot dogs), during storage, or when heated for cooking. Oxidized fats from the diet are absorbed into the body and incorporated into VLDL molecules, which can contribute to or induce inflammation (Staprans 1996).

Which Foods Might Contain Oxidized Fats?

Because heat oxidizes lipids, especially in the presence of oxygen, fried foods often contain oxidized fats (Ho 2015, Li, 2017, Song 2017). This is particularly true of commercially fried foods, where oils are heated in open vats for hours, or even days, while cooking many batches of French fries, fried fish, and other fried foods. The longer the oils are heated, the greater the concentration of oxidized fats (Hoh 2015, Li 2017, Song 2017).

Many foods commonly eaten as part of the Western diet have been heated, fried in oils, processed, or stored for a long time, increasing the likelihood that the fats they contain will be oxidized. Many of these foods, including fish or seafood, contain easily oxidized fats, such as PUFAs, as well as substances, such as hydrogen peroxide, that oxidize fats (Legarde 2013). PUFAs are more easily oxidized than other fats because their structure makes it harder for them to hang onto their hydrogens. In other words, they are easily "mugged." Because oxidation generally increases at higher temperatures, saturated oils, which can hang onto their hydrogens longer, have been recommended for grilling or other high-temperature cooking. Coconut oil is a commonly recommended saturated oil for high-heat cooking. In addition to heat and air, light increases oxidation, so easily oxidized fats should be stored in dark-colored containers, or inside cabinets. Similarly, because metals can increase rates of oxidation, high-fat foods such as butter should not be stored in aluminum foil or other kinds of metal containers.

The saturation status of a fat is a major determinant of its vulnerability to oxidation, as well its "smoke point". The smoke point is the temperature at which an oil literally smokes, indicating that the fats are releasing carbons and are severely oxidized. It is important to note, however, that fats can be damaged at much lower temperatures.

Vegetable and nut oils contain other constituents besides fats, and many of these are antioxidants. However, many oils are refined to purify the fats, usually to make them more suitable for use in foods. Unfortunately, the refining procedures removes antioxidants, rendering the oils more easily oxidized. One vegetable oil that does not need refining is olive oil, and this may explain its well-documented health benefits, compared to other oils.

When we think of "unhealthy" fried foods, fried potatoes (e.g., French fries) often come to mind. But in fact, real-world studies assessing the levels of oxidized lipids in fried foods have found that fried vegetables and fish contain more oxidized lipids than fried potatoes do (Hoh 2015). The reason for this is that vegetables and fish contain PUFAs that become oxidized by heating, whereas potatoes are nearly all starch.

Are Saturated Fats Really Bad?

Saturated fats became controversial because diets including saturated fats, typically derived from animals, have been associated with increased risk of cardiovascular disease (Astrup 2021). But more recent studies that have focused more specifically on saturated fats have not supported this linkage (Svendsen 2017). Reducing saturated fats in the diet does not have much of an effect on cardiovascular events (Hooper 2020, Astrup 2021). Any mechanisms linking saturated fats to cardiovascular risk are as yet unknown, and it is possible that other factors that commonly co-occur with diets high in saturated fat may account for the link with cardiovascular disease. Lifestyle habits, including level of exercise, overall diet quality, and stress also contribute to cardiovascular disease and might relate to saturated fat consumption (Zhang 2021, Alstrup 2021). In addition, most studies linking fats to cardiovascular or other disease have not distinguished between the sources of saturated fats, that is, whether they come from animals (i.e. red meat), or plants (such as coconut). There is some evidence this could be an important factor (Svendsen 2017, Teng 2015, Unger 2019).

Because saturated fats are used by the body mostly for energy storage, any saturated fat intake that exceed the body's immediate needs is shipped to adipose tissue as LDL or accumulates in the liver (Luukkonen 2018). This contributes to obesity and non-alcoholic fatty liver disease, and eventually to the generation of pro-inflammatory lipid mediators and cytokines from visceral adipose tissue (Kawai 2021)). Overfeeding of saturated fat in humans also leads to gut dysbiosis and *endotoxemia*, which is a marker for gut barrier disruption and is hypothesized to drive inflammation (Luukkonen 2018). Thus, although dietary saturated fats may not contribute to cardiovascular disease, diets high in saturated fat are linked mechanistically to metabolic disease.

So how much saturated fat should be in the diet? Unfortunately, there are many likely important variables, such as total amount and quality of fats in the diet, that combined with genetic background, disease status, and lifestyle of individuals complicates making valid specific recommendations about saturated fats (Khaw 2018, Svendsen 2017). Some key questions that need to be addressed with well-designed human studies concern whether the source, such as plant versus animal or dairy versus meat makes a difference in pathophysiology of disease. In the meanwhile, the best advice would be to use saturated fats sparingly.

Because saturated fats are more resistant to chemical modifications, such as oxidation, that can generate pro-inflammatory mediators, many sources recommend using saturated fats, such as butter or coconut oil, for high-temperature cooking. This includes any cooking over 200 degrees Fahrenheit, including frying, roasting, or baking (Roldan 2014). But even saturated fats can be modified with very high temperatures or prolonged heating, such as can happen during commercial food preparation (Li 2017).

Essential Fatty Acids: Omega-3 and Omega-6

Although the body can make most of the lipids it needs, two types of polyunsaturated fatty acids (PUFA), the omega-3 and omega-6 fatty acids (alias w3 and w6, respectively), need to be obtained from the diet, and are therefore called *essential fatty acids.* These fatty acids contribute to cell structure and signaling, and they are precursors for lipid mediators that have both pro- and anti-inflammatory actions (Christie 2020). Indeed, w3 and w6-derived lipid mediators play key roles in inducing inflammation and resolving it (Christie 2020). Foods that contain these fatty acids include fatty cold-water fish (w3), vegetable and nut oils, and green leafy vegetables (both w3 and w6).

Controversy has swirled around w6, however, since w6 derivatives, including prostaglandins, can be pro-inflammatory. The assumption is that because w6 fatty acids are precursors for the synthesis of mediators, including prostaglandins and leukotrienes, which can induce and influence inflammation, dietary w6 may account for the pro-inflammatory actions of certain foods. For this to be true, synthesis of these mediators would have to be *substrate-driven*, which means that the more w6 is available, the more inflammatory mediators are produced. However, most enzyme pathways in the body are activity-dependent and tightly regulated, such that the amount of mediators synthesized is controlled by the body's perceived need for them. In this case, the quantity of mediators produced would be regulated by the need for immune system response, increasing, for example, during infection and/or inflammation. PUFA such as w3 and w6 are incorporated into cell membranes and need to be enzymatically released before they can be used as precursors for lipid mediators such as prostaglandins (Christie 2020). This occurs in response to endocrine hormones, such as epinephrine, and immune signals (Christie 2020). Further, some of the prostaglandins and eicosanoids that are derived from w6 are actually anti-inflammatory, undermining the completely "pro-inflammatory" characterization of w6 (Christie 2020, Veno 2019). It is not yet clear how synthesis of prostaglandins and eicosanoids are influenced by dietary w3 and w6.

The idea that dietary w6 fatty acids are pro-inflammatory and can increase risk of disease has been cast into serious doubt by recent large studies. An analysis of 30 large international prospective studies, with more than 68,000 participants, demonstrated that higher levels of w6 fatty acids in the body were associated with *reduced* risk of cardiovascular events (Marklund 2019). Another meta-analysis found that dietary w6 was associated with either neutral or beneficial effects on risk for cardiovascular disease (Hooper 2018).

Most foods that contain w3 and w6 fatty acids contain more w6 than w3. For many vegetable oils, the ratio of w6 to w3 is 10:1 or more. For instance, the ratio of w6 to w3 in olive oil, which is considered to be a heart-healthy oil, is an amazing 12:1 (USDA). Many processed Western diet foods contain ratios that are much higher than that. Because the Western diet is linked to increased risk for poor health outcomes, if increased w6 content is truly pro-inflammatory, this could account for these increased risks. However, it is not clear what basis is valid for recommendations for a target w6 to w3 ratio. Some claim that before the agricultural revolution 10,000 years ago, humans ate a diet that contained a 1:1 ratio of w6 to w3 and that 10,000 years is not enough to change genes in order to tolerate higher ratios of w6 to w3 (Simopoulos 2011). This is, however, both speculative and overly simplistic given the complexity of gene function. Many wellness sources recommend a ratio of 3 or 4 to 1, but because many intact, unprocessed, dietary sources of essential fatty acids contain both types, often in higher ratios, 3 or 4 to 1 may be difficult to achieve. One way to increase w3 in the diet is to eat fatty cold-water fish, such as salmon. However, this requires eating quite a lot of fish, and there are environmental risks associated with the farming of fish to meet increased demand for them.

Overall, there is no evidence base to support a "good versus bad" conceptualization of w3 and w6 essential fatty acids. The principal link of dietary w6 to health risks is their high levels in processed foods. On the one hand, these oils can be easily oxidized when heated or stored, which could link inflammation and the Western diet. On the other hand, high levels of w6 in the diet may be merely coincident to a diet high in processed foods that are deleterious for other reasons, such as containing high-energy/low-nutrient refined carbohydrates, which are also linked to health risks. The best way to avoid eating a diet with too high of an w6 to w3 ratio is to avoid processed foods.

What About High Fat Diets?

High fat diets have been linked by pre-clinical and epidemiological/observational studies to cardiometabolic diseases, which has encouraged the widespread view that dietary fats in general are deleterious to health (Wali 2020). On the other hand, ketogenic diets, which are very low in carbohydrates and high in fats, have been found to provide some benefits for treatment-resistant epilepsy. Ketogenic diets appear to result in weight loss when the diet is not high-calorie, demonstrating that a diet with a high proportion of calories from fat does not necessarily lead a person to become fat. These discrepancies imply that the effects of fat in the diet depend on factors that go beyond the overall percentage of fat in the diet.

Up until recently, the definition of a high-fat diet referred only to total amount of fat in the diet but did not distinguish between types of fats. Diets rich in saturated fats from processed meat, for instance, were not distinguished from those high in vegetable oils such as olive oil or fermented dairy products such as yogurt or cheese. Given the more recent understanding of the links between damaged fats and inflammation, the quality of fats may be more important than the percentage of them in the diet.

Although ketogenic diets have been around since the 1920's, they have surged in popularity recently. Ketogenic diets are very low carbohydrate, and the loss of calories from carbohydrate are compensated for by increased fat calories. The fuels generated from fats that can be metabolized for energy are called ketones.

One advantage of the ketogenic diet is that it is believed to preserve lean body mass or muscle while diminishing fat. In addition, ketones are "super-fuel" in that they generate more energy than glucose. This allows the body to still have adequate energy even with fewer calories. Because the ketogenic diet forces the body to use fats instead of carbohydrates, a reduced-calorie diet based on fats can be effective for weight loss, especially for people who, due to recurrent dieting, have become resistant to other low-calorie diets.

Ketogenic diets were originally developed for the treatment of severe epilepsy, and they are somewhat successful (Meira 2019). Epilepsy is a disease of neuronal hyper-excitability in the brain. Repeated seizures can damage the brain due to the oxidative stress and resultant inflammation caused by overactive neurons. Metabolism of ketones generates fewer reactive oxygen species, and thus may reduce oxidative stress and inflammation. There is some evidence that the ketogenic diet can reduce brain inflammation, which is why it may improve symptoms of epilepsy. This possible effect on neuroinflammation has also spurred clinical trials of the ketogenic diet for neurodegenerative disorders. Results are not available yet, partly because many people seem to have problems with compliance with the diet (D'Andrea Meira 2019). In people with Type 2 diabetes, the ketogenic diet may improve glucose tolerance (Gupta 2017).

One initial concern regarding the increased popularity of the ketogenic diet was risk of ketoacidosis, which can be fatal. However, when one is consuming adequate protein, ketoacidosis does not occur. As such, ketoacidosis has not been a problem as the diet has been practiced. There are other concerns about the ketogenic diet, however. Although relying on ketones for energy seems to be good for the brain, a very high-fat diet can cause problems for the gut. The most common side effect of ketogenic diets is recurrent diarrhea. This may stem from diet-induced dysbiosis, an imbalance in gut microbes that can cause inflammation, because the classic version of the diet is low in fiber and vegetables (Leeming 2019, Wisniewski 2019). In addition, high-fat diets have been consistently associated with increased incidence of disease, including cardiovascular and metabolic disease. The role of fats in this case are not established, as other lifestyle factors may be important, but currently, most physicians and dietitians recommend that if people use the ketogenic diet for weight loss, they should switch to another diet for long-term maintenance of weight. The Mediterranean diet, for which there is long-term evidence of safety, or a mixed "Med/Keto" diet that is low carbohydrate but includes and emphasizes vegetables, are commonly recommended maintenance diets.

Context may be one important predictor of whether a diet containing fats will be beneficial or not. Food constituents typically occur in the diet in a *food matrix* that contains many other things, rather than as a single nutrient (Astrup 2019). Food constituents can influence digestion, absorption, and utilization of other constituents. For instance, beans slow down the absorption of sugars, and fats slow down gut motility, possibly allowing more time for other foods to be absorbed. The food matrix in which a food constituent is consumed can alter the microbiome, as well as immune and nervous system responses to the food constituent. To illustrate, consider the general finding that high-fat diets are associated with cardiovascular risk and obesity, in the context of the effects of choices regarding whether to consume full-fat or reduced-fat dairy products. The general finding would suggest that reduced-fat dairy products would be better for minimizing risk of cardiovascular disease and obesity, but that is not what is observed. People who consume full-fat dairy products weigh less than people who eat reduced fat dairy (Alstrup 2019). This is hypothesized to be due to the effect of fats on satiety. Consumption of full-fat dairy is also associated with lower risk of cardiometabolic diseases, which may reflect the fact that dairy is a good source of calcium and proteins with antioxidant capabilities (Khan 2019). Thus, assessment of the effects of a high-fat diet on health needs to address quality of the fats and the context of the foods in which the fats occur.

Fats may be important for helping substances get across the gut barrier. Fat can help dissolve fat-soluble substances and carry them into the body for use. In other words, fats make fat-soluble substances more bioavailable. Whether this is helpful or harmful will depend on what fat-soluble substances we are consuming. If our diet contains nutrients, vitamins, and antioxidants, fat may help them get into our bodies and improve our health. But if our diet contains additives and toxins, fats can help these get across the gut barrier as well. In this case, the transported additives and toxins can induce inflammation and worsen health. Thus, eating fats along with unprocessed, fresh, nutrient-rich food may help these high-quality foods get absorbed into the body. Adding a drizzle of olive oil to a salad may make leafy greens, fruits, and nuts more nutritious, as your body absorbs their nutrients, vitamins, and antioxidants more effectively. Conversely, eating fats as part of a diet containing additives, pesticides, and pro-inflammatory foods, such as refined carbohydrates, can potentially increase the risk that these foods will induce inflammation and worsen health. For example, frying processed, refined, or pesticide-laden food may result in conveying more of these substances across the gut barrier, increasing the risk of pro-inflammatory changes. The key takeaway is that fats may amplify the benefits or harms of the matrix of foods we consume, making healthful food more nutritious and unhealthful food more damaging.

Key Points

- Fats have a variety of necessary roles in the body, and some must be obtained from the diet.
- Some fats can be easily damaged by oxidation. This damage can lead to the formation of pro-inflammatory mediators. The most vulnerable fats are polyunsaturated fatty acids (PUFA).
- Oxidized fats can be generated in the body by oxidative stress and inflammation, or they can be produced in foods during processing, cooking, or storage.
- Dietary saturated fat has been linked to disease, but the effects are likely to be secondary to overconsumption. The body does not need as many saturated fats as unsaturated fats. Extra fats are stored in adipose tissue and cause obesity and non-alcoholic fatty liver disease.
- Both omega-3 and omega-6 fatty acids have beneficial effects on health, but omega 6 is naturally present in larger amounts than omega-3 in food sources. This is the main reason most diets have a ratio of the two that favors omega-6 fats.
- The effects of high-fat diets on health depend on if the diet is also high-calorie, whether the fats in the diet are good quality (i.e., not damaged by cooking or processing), and what other food constituents are consumed with the fats.

References

Astrup A, Geiker NRW, Magkos F. Effects of full-fat and fermented dairy products on cardiometabolic disease: Food is more than the sum of its parts. Advances in Nutrition, 10:924S-930S, 2019.

Astrup A, Teicholz N, Magkos F, Bier DM, Brenna JT, King JC, et al. Dietary saturated fats and health: Are the U.S. Guidelines evidence-based? Nutrients, 13:3305, 2021.

Chiurchiu V, Leuti A, Maccarrone M. Bioactive lipids and chronic inflammation: managing the fire within. Frontiers in Immunology, 9:38, 2018.

Christie WW, Harwood JL. Oxidation of polyunsaturated fatty acids to produce lipid mediators. Essays in Biochemistry, 64:401-421, 2020.

D'Andrea I, Romao TT, Pirese do Prado HJ, Kruger LT, Tires MEP, de Conceicao PO. Ketogenic diet and epilepsy: what we know so far. Frontiers in Neuroscience, 13:5, 2019.

Dyall SC. Interplay Between n3 and n6 Long-Chain Polyunsaturated Fatty Acids and the Endocannabinoid System in Brain Protection and Repair. Lipids, 52:885-900, 2017.

Fruhwirth GO, Loidl A, Hermetter A. Oxidized phospholipids: From molecular properties to disease. Biochimica et Biophysica Acta, 1772:718-736, 2007.

Gupta L, Khandelwal D, Kalra P, Dutta D, Aggarwal S. Ketogenic diet in endocrine disorders. Current perspectives. Journal of Postgraduate Medicine, 63:242-251, 2017.

Hirahatake KM, Astrup A, Hill JO, Slavin JL, Allison DB, Maki KC. Potential cardiometabolic benefits of full-fat dairy: The evidence base. Advances in Nutrition, 11:533-547, 2020.

Hoh E, Surh J. Food types and frying frequency affect the lipid oxidation of deep frying oil for the preparation of school meals in Korea. Food Chemistry, 174:467-472, 2015.

Hooper L, Al-Khudairy L, Abdelhamid AS, Rees K, Brainard JS, Brown TJ, Ajabnoor SM, O'Brien AT, Winstanley LE, Donaldson DH, Song F, Deane KHO. Omega-6 fats for the primary and secondary prevention of cardiovascular disease. Cochrane Database of Systematic Reviews, 11: CD011094, 2018.

Horner K, Hopkins M, Finlayson G, Gibbons C, Brennan L. Biomarkers of appetite: is there a potential role for metabolomics? Nutrition Research Reviews, 33:271–286, 2020.

Kanner J. Dietary advance lipid oxidation end products are risk factors to human health. Molecular Nutrition and Food Research, 51:1094-1101, 2007.

Kawai T, Autieri MV, Scalia R. Adipose tissue inflammation and metabolic dysfunction in obesity. American Journal of Physiology Cell Physiology, 320:C375-C391, 2021.

Khan IT, Nadeem M, Imran M, Ullah R, Ajmal M, Jaspal MH. Antioxidant properties of milk and dairy products: a comprehensive review of the current knowledge. Lipids in Health and Disease, 18:41, 2019.

Khaw K-T, Sharp SJ, Finikarides L, Afzal I, Lentjes M, Luben R, Forouhi NG. Randomised trial of coconut oil, olive oil or butter on blood lipids and other cardiovascular risk factors in healthy men and women. BMJ Open, 8:e022167, 2018.

LaGarde M.,Bernoud-Habac N, Calzada C, Vericel E, Guichardant M. Lipidomics of essential fatty acids and oxygenated metabolites. Molecular Nutrition and Food Research, 57:1347-1358, 2013

Lechner K, von Schacky C, McKenzie AL, Worm N, Nixdorf U, Lechner B, et al. Lifestyle factors and high-risk atherosclerosis: Pathways and mechanisms beyond traditional risk factors. European Journal of Preventative Cardiology, 27:394-406, 2020.

Leeming ER, Johnson AJ, Spector TD, Le Roy CI. Effect of diet on the gut microbiota: Rethinking intervention duration. Nutrients, 11:2862, 2019.

Li X, Li J, Wang Y, Cao P, Liu Y. Effects of frying oil's fatty acids profile on the formation of polar lipids components and their retention in French fries over deep-frying process. Food Chemistry, 237:98-105, 2017.

Longhi R, Farina Almeida R, Machado L, Frescura Duarte MMM, Guerini Souza D, Machado P, Martimbianco de Assis A, Quincozes-Santos A, Souza DO. Effect of a trans fatty acid-enriched diet on biochemical and inflammatory parameters in Wistar rats. European Journal of Nutrition, 56:1003-1016, 2017.

Lu VB, Gribble FM, Reimann F. Free fatty acid receptors in enteroendocrine cells. Endocrinology, 159:2826-2835, 2018.

Ludwig DS, Willett WC, Volck JS, Neuhouser ML. Dietary fat: From foe to friend? Science, 362:764-779, 2018.

Luukkonen PK, Sadevirta A, Zhou T, Kayser B, Ali A, Ahonin L, et al. Saturated fat is more metabolically harmful for the human liver than unsaturated fat or simple sugars. Diabetes Care, 41:1732-1739, 2018.

Marklund M, Wu JHY, Imamura F, et al. Biomarkers of dietary omega-6 fatty acids and incident cardiovascular disease and mortality: an individual-level pooled analysis of 30 cohort studies. Circulation,139: 2422-2436, 2019.

Meira ID, Roao TT, Pires do Prado HJ, Kruger LT, Paiva Pires ME, da Conceicao PO. Ketogenic diet and epilepsy-What we know so far. Frontiers in Neuroscience, 13: Article 5, 2019.

Morrison DJ, Preston T. Formation of short chain fatty acids by the gut microbiota and their impact on human metabolism. Gut Microbes, 7:189-200, 2016.

Oteng A-B, Kersten S. Mechanisms of action of *trans* fatty acids. Advances in Nutrition, 11:697-708, 2020.

Poitelon Y, Kopec AM, Belin S. Myelin fat facts: An overview of lipids and fatty acid metabolism. Cells, 9:812, 2020.

Polley KR, Kamal F, Paton CM, Cooper JA. Appetite responses to high-fat diets rich in mono-unsaturated versus poly-unsaturated fats. Appetite, 134:172-181, 2019.

Qiu B, Wang Q, Liu W, X T-C, Lio L-N, Zong A-Z, Jia M, Li J, Du F-L. Biological effects of trans fatty acids and their possible roles in the lipid rafts in apoptosis regulation. Cell Biology International, 42:904-912, 2018.

Roldan M, Antequera T, Armenteros M, Ruiz J. Effect of different temperature-time combinations on lipid and protein oxidation in sous-vide cooked lamb loins. Food Chemistry, 149:129-135, 2014.

Simopoulos AP. Evolutionary aspects of diet: the omega-6/omega-3 ratio and the brain. Molecular Neurobiology, 44:203-215, 2011.

Song K, Kim M-J, Kim Y-J, Lee J. Monitoring changes in acid value, total polar material, and antioxidant capacity of oils used for frying chicken. Food Chemistry, 220:306-312, 2017.

Soulillou J-P, Padler-Karavani V. Editorial: Human antibodies against the dietary non-hamna Neu5Gc-carrying glycans in normal and pathological states. Fronteers in Immunology, 11:1589, 2020

Svendsen K, Arnesen E, Retterstol K. Saturated fat - a never ending story? Food and Nutrition Research, 61:1377572, 2017.

Teng K-T, Chang C-Y, Kanthimathi MS, Tan ATB, Nesaretnam K. Effects of amount and type of dietary fats on postprandial lipemia and thrombogenic markers in individuals with metabolic syndrome. Atherosclerosis, 242:281-287, 2015.

Unger AL, Torres-Gonzalez M, Kraft J. Dairy Fat Consumption and the Risk of Metabolic Syndrome: An Examination of the Saturated Fatty Acids in Dairy. Nutrients, 11:2200, 2019.

Venø SK, Schmidt EB, Bork CS. Polyunsaturated Fatty Acids and Risk of Ischemic Stroke. Nutrients,11:1467, 2019.

Wali JA, Jarzebska N, Raubenheimer D, Simpson SJ, Rodioniv RN, O'Sullivan JF. Cardio-metabolic effects of high-fat diets and their underlying mechanisms - a narrative review. Nutrients, 12:1505, 2020.

Wisniewski PJ, Dowden RA, Campbell SC. Role of dietary lipids on modulating inflammation through the gut microbiota. Nutrients, 11:117, 2019.

Zhang B-Y, Pan V-F, Chen J, Cao A, Xia L, Zhang Y, et al. Combined lifestyle factors, all-cause mortality and cardiovascular disease: a systematic review and meta-analysis of prospective cohort studies. Journal of Epidemiology and Community Health, 75:92-99, 2021.

- WHAT IS SUGAR?

- INSULIN AND INSULIN RESISTANCE

- HOW SUGAR DRIVES INFLAMMATION:

    - 1. HYPERGLYCEMIA AND ADVANCED GLYCATION END-PRODUCTS

    - 2. HYPERGLYCEMIA, MITOCHONDRIA, AND METABOLISM

    - 3. HYPERGLYCEMIA CAN DRIVE INFLAMMATION AND INSULIN RESISTANCE

    - 4. FRUCTOSE OVERDOSE

- WHY IS SUGAR SO HARD TO KICK?

- WHAT ABOUT "A SWEET TOOTH"?

- NON-NUTRITIONAL SWEETENER ISSUES: WHY WE NEED TO GET PAST NEEDING A SWEET TASTE IN EVERYTHING

- THE SPECIAL PROBLEM OF SWEETENED BEVERAGES

- KEY POINTS

A sweet taste in food is innately rewarding. Evolution has likely favored consumption of sugar because it is found in whole foods, such as fruit, that are safe to eat and nutritious. The practice of adding sweeteners such as honey, carob, or maple sugar to enhance foods has been documented since the time of the ancient Egyptians, who used honey. However, innovations in food science during the 19th century resulted in the refining of sugar from beets and cane into a pure white crystalline substance. While very sweet, table sugar differs from naturally occurring sweeteners in that it contains no other nutrients. Table sugar is more easily stored, however, and is more convenient for baking, beverages, and beyond. This has led to a dramatic increase in consumption of refined sugar since 1900, to a current average of 40 pounds per person per year worldwide (Edwards 2016). Estimates for sugar consumption in the US and UK are even higher (Johnson 2017).

Unfortunately, in addition to being a poor source of nutrients, refined sugar is pro-inflammatory. As a result, diets high in refined sugar and other refined carbohydrates are associated with obesity, type 2 diabetes, metabolic syndrome, cardiovascular disease, neurodegenerative diseases, chronic pain, mood disorders, and early all-cause mortality (Bray 2013, Johnson 2017, Malik 2019, Schultze 2015, Stanhope 2016). This association with inflammation and diverse health risks should be a strong motivator to limit the consumption of refined sugar. But the potent reward value of sugars in brain circuits may drive addictive behavior or dependence in many people (Wiss 2018). Cultural factors, convenience, and the profitability of refined sugar and sugar-containing products such as soda, also present formidable barriers to reducing the use of refined sugar in Western diets.

What is "Sugar"?

There are many kinds of sugars, but the ones most relevant to heath are glucose, fructose, and sucrose. Sucrose is also known as table sugar and is made up of equal parts glucose and fructose. These sugars are sometimes called *simple carbohydrates.* When foods containing sucrose are eaten, enzymes in the mouth and stomach break it down into glucose and fructose, and it is then absorbed into the body. The absorbed glucose and fructose travel in blood first to the liver. The liver takes of most of the fructose for its own needs, and either stores the glucose in the form of glycogen, an *animal starch*, or releases it into the general circulation. Glucose in the circulation is often called *blood sugar.*

Plants also store glucose in the form of starch. Plant starches are *complex carbohydrates* because they take longer to break down into absorbable sugars than do simple sugars/carbohydrates. Starch in plants is accompanied by fiber and other nutrients, as well, whereas simple carbohydrates only contain sugars. Some complex carbohydrates are more complex than others. This influences how quickly they are absorbed into the body.

When sugars are absorbed quickly, blood sugar levels can spike, rising rapidly and then falling dramatically as the body reacts to the peak with insulin. It is better for the body if sugars are absorbed more slowly, with a lower peak level and a more prolonged stable increase in blood sugar (Pfeiffer 2018). Eating foods that lead to blood glucose spikes may contribute to inflammation and contribute to, or worsen, metabolic diseases. But how do we know how quickly carbohydrate-containing foods are absorbed and how big of a blood glucose spike they will cause?

The *glycemic index* is a relative ranking of foods containing carbohydrates that is based on how they affect blood glucose levels (Pfeiffer 2018). Foods with a low glycemic index value contain fiber and possibly other substances that help slow down the breakdown of the starch and absorption of resulting sugars (Pfeiffer 2018). Whole grains and legumes have low glycemic index values. Foods with a high glycemic index score are typically those made from refined carbohydrates that are rapidly broken down and absorbed, leading to blood glucose spikes. Soda, fruit juices, sugary desserts, white potatoes, and white rice all have high glycemic index scores. Surprisingly *whole grain* flour that has been finely ground has the same glycemic index as refined white flour (Zafar 2020). This implies that the integrity of foods such as grains plays a crucial role in how it is absorbed into the body. This likely contributes mechanistically to the association of whole foods with better health.

Insulin and Insulin Resistance

Insulin is the hormone made in the pancreas that controls the uptake or transport of glucose and amino acids from dietary protein from the blood into cells. Insulin also spurs fat cells to take up and store lipids. The pancreas releases insulin in readiness for meals. This anticipatory insulin release can be based on the normal timing of meals or when we see, smell, or taste food. This is what is called the *cephalic phase* of insulin release (Wiedemann 2020). This anticipatory response leads to a drop in blood glucose, as the insulin triggers cells to take up glucose. This anticipatory drop in blood glucose increases the perception of hunger (Sae iab 2020). Insulin is later released in response to the absorption of sugar from the gut into our bodies. In general, the more sugar we absorb, the greater the amount of insulin released to match the levels of glucose. In this way, glucose in the blood can be efficiently absorbed by cells of the body.

In conditions in which blood glucose is persistently high, cells can become resistant to the effects of insulin. This is referred to as *insulin resistance*. When this happens, cells do not take up glucose in response to insulin and glucose continues to circulate at a high level. These high blood glucose levels are called hyperglycemia. Chronic hyperglycemia is the hallmark of type 2 diabetes and can drive inflammation in several different ways (Luc 2019). Insulin resistance raises the risk of other diseases, including cancer and Alzheimer's disease (Asimov 2016, Cehn 2013, Talbot 2012). The association of Alzheimer's disease with insulin resistance and obesity is strong enough that it is sometimes referred to as Type 3 diabetes (Nguyen 2020). In contrast, healthy centenarians tend to have good glucose tolerance, emphasizing the relationship between well-regulated glucose metabolism and successful aging (Paolisso 1996).

How Sugar Drives Inflammation

At first it seems paradoxical that molecules such as glucose and fructose, which are critical for the function of our bodies, could also be so dangerous to health. But persistent high levels of sugar in the blood, such as in the case of Type 2 diabetes, can cause blindness, neuropathy, and vascular damage. When vascular damage becomes extensive, the tissue damage can require amputation of feet or legs. We now know several mechanisms by which high blood sugar can induce inflammation and cause these serious conditions.

1. Hyperglycemia and Advanced Glycation End-Products

One of the most problematic consequences of the high-energy Western diet is the formation of advanced glycation end products (AGEs). These are formed in the blood during persistent hyperglycemia and in foods during cooking or processing, typically at high temperatures (Aragno 2017, Kellow 2015, Uribarri 2005).

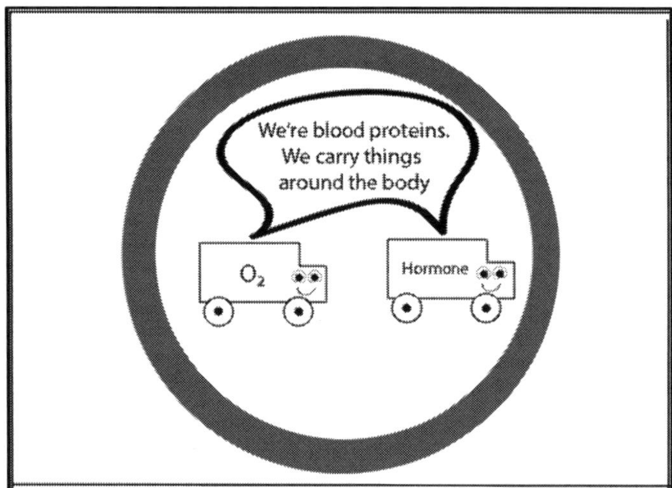

In addition to glucose and lipids, many proteins circulate in the blood. These proteins mostly carry or "chaperone" molecules such as oxygen, necessary for metabolism, or hormones. These proteins keep these molecules from being broken down on their way to their target tissues.

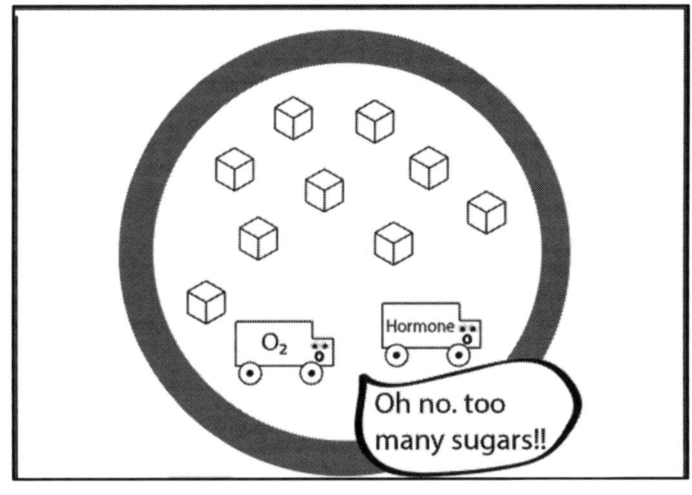

When blood sugar is high, the extra sugar binds to proteins in a process called *glycation.* This process occurs via the *Maillard reaction.* The biomarker for Type 2 diabetes, glycated hemoglobin (A1C), is an example of a protein that is glycated via this process when blood sugar is high. The amount of hemoglobin A1C that is glycated provides a record of the frequency at which blood glucose has been high in the recent past and is used as a medical indicator of persistent high blood sugar levels.

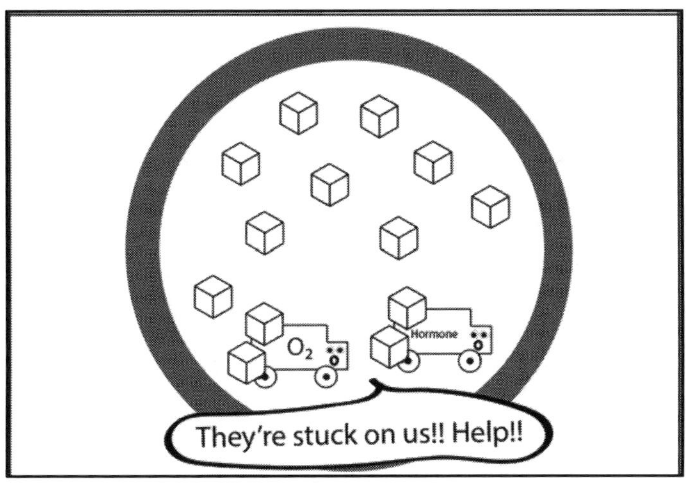

Glycation impairs the function of the proteins and triggers the formation of advanced glycation end Products (AGEs).

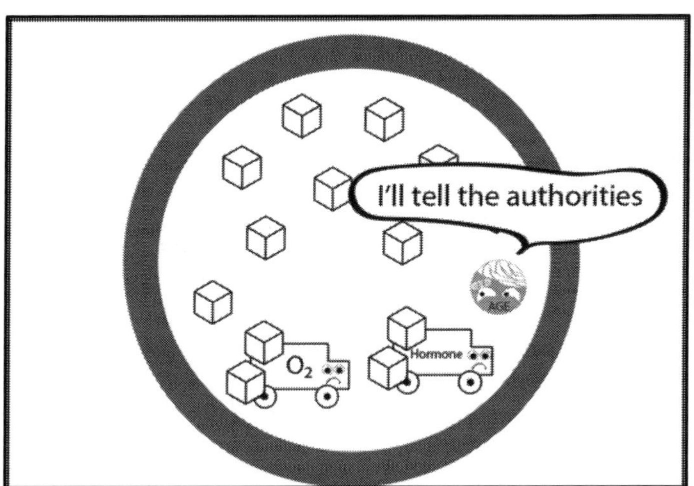

AGEs act as damage- associated molecular patterns (DAMPs, described in Chapter 7), signaling the damage to the protein.

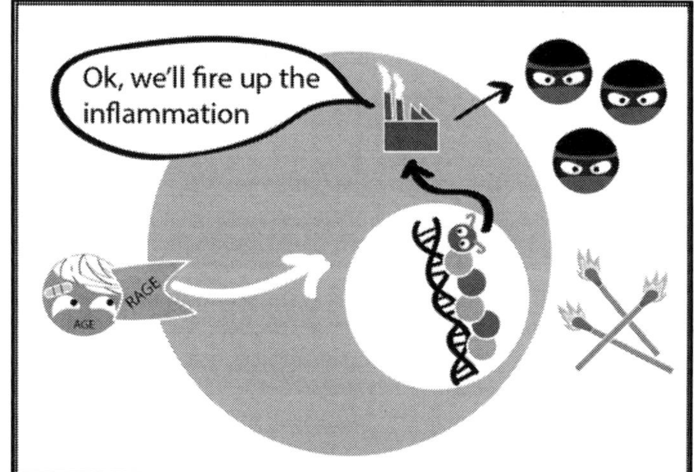

AGEs are "sensed" by the Receptor for Advanced Glycation End Products, otherwise known as the RAGE protein. Binding of AGEs to RAGE directly activates inflammatory pathways inside cells, including NFkB and inflammasomes (Kellow 2015, Kong 2017, Yeh 2017). This increases the production of cytokines and reactive oxygen species (Kong 2017).

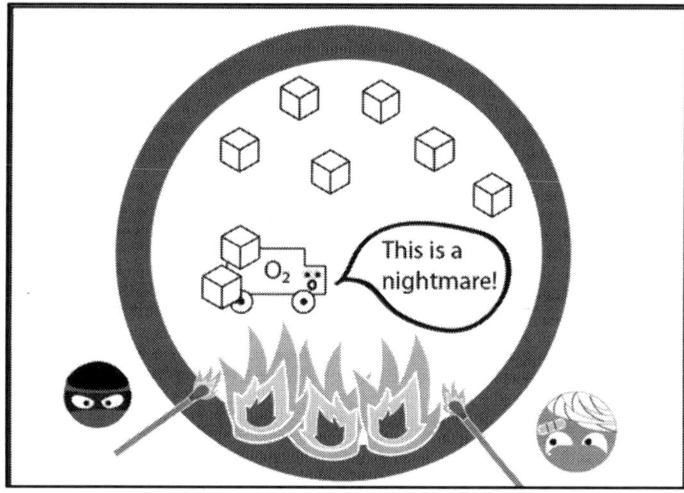

The result can be inflammation in tissues including pancreas, kidney, nervous system, and blood vessels (Kellow 2015).

The contribution of AGE formation and RAGE activation to disease cannot be overemphasized. In addition to driving pancreas, nervous system, and kidney damage associated with Type 2 Diabetes, AGE and RAGE are now linked to neurodegenerative diseases including Alzheimer's, Parkinson's, and Huntington's diseases (Kong 2017, Raichgot 2019, Yeh 2017, Butterfield 2019, Jiang 2018, Ray 2016). Further, *glycative stress* and RAGE activation contributes to the pathophysiology of cancer (Miccuci 2016, Palanissami 2018).

2. Hyperglycemia, Mitochondria, and Metabolism

To review, mitochondria act as the powerhouses of cells. Glucose is the major fuel that most cells use. Glucose circulating in the blood is transported into cells by proteins under the control of insulin. Then, enzymes in mitochondria break the chemical bonds in glucose molecules and transfer that stored energy to other molecules to use for work within the cell. This process generates reactive oxygen and nitrogen species (ROS and RNS), which at normal levels serve important functions in the cell. But if the *metabolic rate,* or the speed at which mitochondria break down glucose, is high, mitochondria can produce more ROS and RNS than the cell needs or can protect itself from. This excess of ROS and RNS constitutes oxidative stress. Oxidative stress induces inflammation and can damage the mitochondria, leading to dysfunction or even death of the cell (Sas 2007, Shah 2013).

Importantly, one of the ways metabolic rate is controlled is by the amount of glucose available in the cell (Shah 2013). During hyperglycemia, metabolic rate is increased, risking oxidative stress. In this basic way, hyperglycemia induces inflammation by increasing metabolic rate, and the overproduction of ROS and RNS which can damage mitochondria.

3. Hyperglycemia Can Drive Inflammation and Insulin Resistance

Oxidative stress can occur in the context of inflammation, due to infection, due to an injury, or following intense exercise. These conditions demand increased energy for the cells, which increases metabolic rate, leading to production of more reactive oxygen and nitrogen species. In these cases, oxidative stress is linked to metabolic rate that is increased due to needs of the body (Jimenez 2018). However, metabolic rate also increases when there is extra fuel as glucose coming into the cell (Yuan 2019). This occurs during hyperglycemia and can lead to oxidative stress. One reactive nitrogen species, *peroxynitrite*, can bind to DNA. As a consequence of oxidative stress, it induces long-lasting changes in the expression of genes related to metabolism and inflammation via the cortisol and NFkB systems (Kormaz 2008, Paixao 2012). Peroyxynitrite can also impair the function of glucose transporters (Stadler 2011, Speckmann 2016). These changes have the effect of inducing insulin resistance and inflammation, two hallmarks of Type 2 diabetes. This change in metabolic regulation, producing insulin resistance in the context of hyperglycemia, may be adaptive in the short term because it may help protect the cells from oxidative stress (Yuan 2018). Unfortunately, the side effect of this is that insulin resistance worsens hyperglycemia by preventing cells from removing glucose from the blood. What may be a beneficial protective response to brief exposures to excess sugar can become problematic when exposure to excess sugar is chronic.

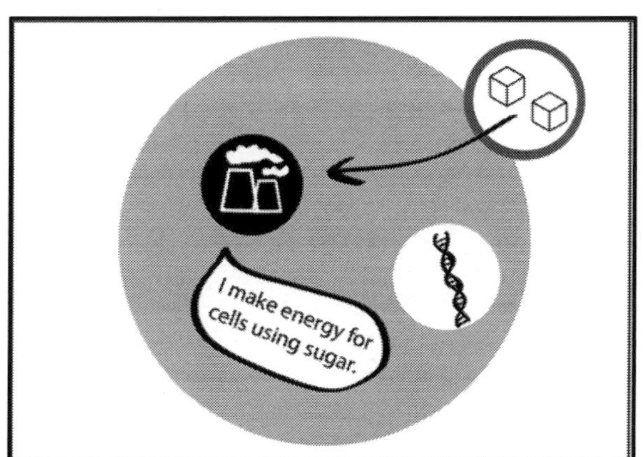

Energy needed for cell functions is mostly generated by the oxidation of glucose (in most cells).

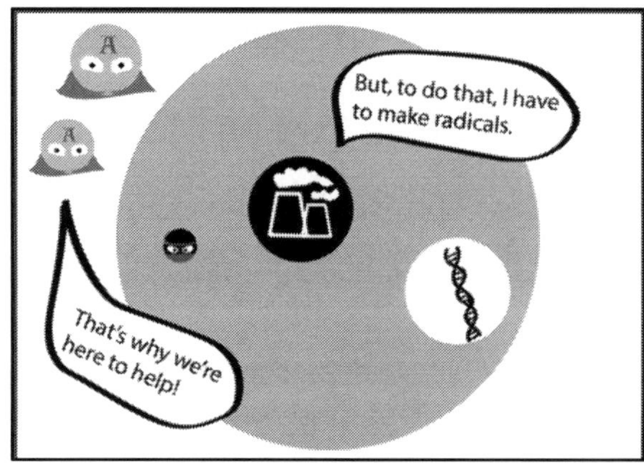

Some of the byproducts of metabolism are reactive oxygen and nitrogen species. These have important roles in the body, as long as there are not too many of them. Antioxidants manage the reactive oxygen and nitrogen species, preventing damage when metabolic rates are normal.

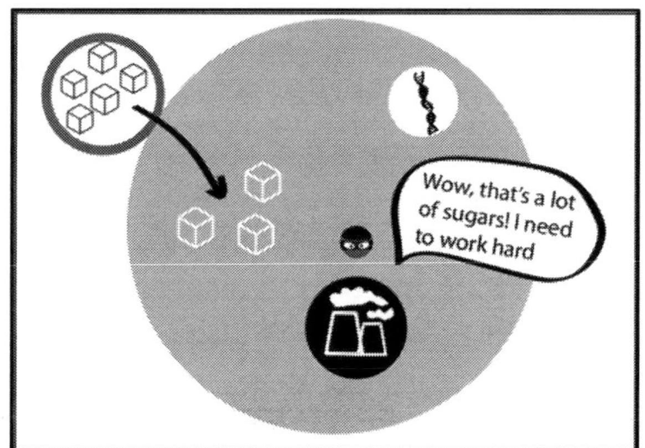

Hyperglycemia, due to diabetes or a diet high in refined carbohydrates and especially sugar, can increase metabolic rate.

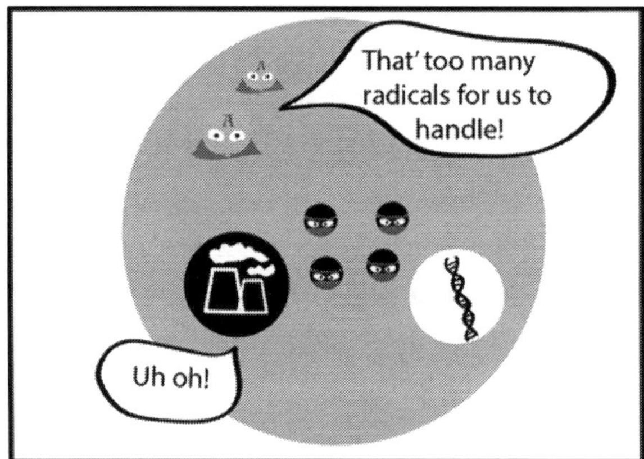

If the metabolic rate is high, it can overwhelm the cell's antioxidant capability, leading to oxidative stress.

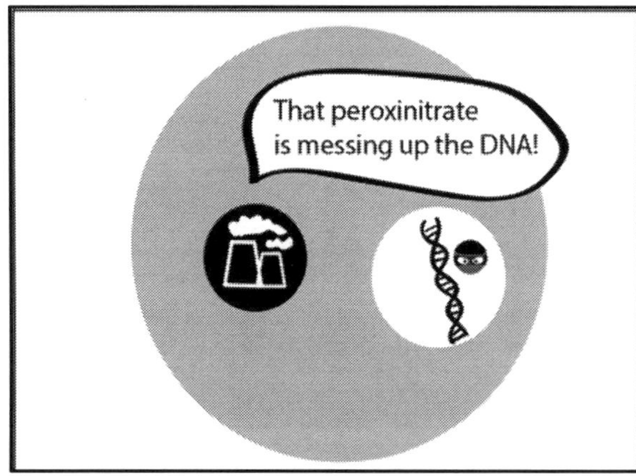

One of the normal products of metabolism, peroxynitrite, can bind DNA in cells. But high levels of peroxynitrite, such as during oxidative stress, can change gene expression, leading to serious consequences for the cell.

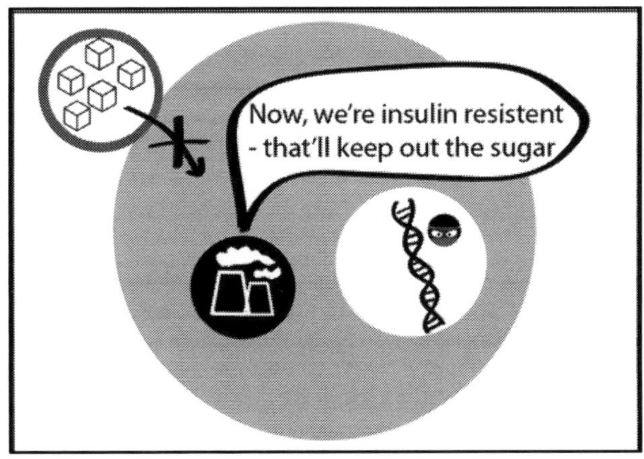

One of the consequences of gene expression changes is inflammation and insulin resistance. Insulin resistance can serve to reduce metabolic rate within the cell by keeping glucose from entering the cells and reaching mitochondria.

This will reduce the production of peroxynitrite and protect against overproduction of reactive oxygen and nitrogen species.

But the glucose that is now stuck in the blood can lead to diabetes and long-term consequences from persistent hyperglycemia. This elevated blood glucose increases the likelihood of AGE formation and RAGE activation, and thus, further inflammation.

4. Fructose Overdose

Fructose is one half of the duo, that with glucose, forms table sugar or sucrose. Of the two, fructose tastes the sweetest. Whereas glucose serves as a primary fuel of most cells of the body, fructose is only used by the liver. In the natural world, fructose is mostly found in fruit, and the amount of fructose supplied by a normal number of servings of fruit is sufficient for the liver's needs. However, in the last 30 years, food and beverage companies have been adding fructose to corn syrup as a sweetener for many foods and beverages. This, along with the concomitant increase in consumption of sweetened beverages including sodas and fruit juices, has led to a dramatic increase in the amount of fructose consumed. This provides far more fructose than the liver needs. At the same time, metabolic diseases, including Type 2 diabetes and non-alcoholic fatty liver disease, have become epidemic (Abenavoli 2019, Poluzos 2019). Fructose has been identified a major culprit (Alwafsh 2017).

When the available fructose exceeds the needs of the liver, the liver converts it into fat for storage. Some of these fats enter the circulation and are stored in adipose tissue, which contributes to obesity. But some of the fat can accumulate in liver cells and impair their functions. Non-alcoholic fatty liver (NAFL) is the name of the condition caused by fat accumulating in liver cells. Over time, a condition called non-alcoholic hepatic steatosis (NASH), in which the fatty tissue becomes inflamed, can develop. NASH can lead to liver cirrhosis, and cirrhosis can lead to liver cancer. The incidence of NAFL and NASH has been increasing since 1980, and they are now the second-leading cause for liver transplantation. The biggest risk factor for NAFL and NASH is obesity (Polyzos 2019). Fortunately, weight loss and lifestyle changes, especially diet and exercise, can halt or reverse the damage to the liver (Abenavoli 2019).

Diets that are high in fructose have been consistently associated with high incidence of insulin resistance and metabolic disease (Alwahsh 2017). Clinical and pre-clinical studies have identified several mechanisms by which fructose could induce or contribute to obesity, insulin resistance, and inflammation, the pathophysiological hallmarks of metabolic disease (Rodriguez Mortera 2019, Stanhope 2016). Thus, there are good reasons to suspect fructose is behind many of the deleterious effects of the sugary Western diet. But is this fair?

One on the main reasons fructose is blamed for increased rates of obesity is that, as just mentioned, if there is too much fructose in the diet, the liver converts the fructose to lipids for storage as fat. In addition, if there is too much glucose in the diet, the liver converts it to fructose, and then to fat via enzymatic reactions called the polyol metabolic pathway. In this way, excess calories are converted to a form appropriate for storage (Rodriguez Mortera 2019). A theme here is that problems only arise in the context of over-consumption. The idea that there may be something different about the overconsumption of fructose, however, has been supported by a meta-analysis of human studies showing that excess fructose, compared to other sugars, is associated with liver insulin resistance, a step on the road to Type 2 diabetes (ter Horst 2016). High fructose ingestion is also linked to increases in inflammatory visceral adipose tissue (Bray 2013).

Another reason fructose is suspect is that it happens to be highly reactive, and readily glycates proteins and other molecules (Rodriguez Mortera 2019). This leads to the formation of pro-inflammatory AGEs, and the activation of RAGE. Fructose, unlike glucose, has a low glycemic index (Gugliucci 2017). The gut cells responsible for absorbing nutrients transport fructose slowly, leaving it in the gut where it may glycate proteins and other molecules from food waiting to be absorbed (Gugliucci 2017). The formation of AGEs could provide a mechanism by which foods and beverages containing fructose increase inflammation.

The idea that fructose could be driving inflammation in metabolic disease is attractive, as it could explain the increase in incidence of these diseases since the low fat/high carbohydrate craze began. However, it has been difficult to show that normal levels of fructose, for example the amount found naturally in whole fruit, have adverse effects on lipid production or metabolic and inflammatory parameters (Semnani-Azad 2020). Indeed, it seems that negative effects of fructose are not seen until 75-100 grams of fructose are ingested per day (Khan 2019). But is that a lot of fructose?

Considering only sweetened beverages, where 50-65% of the sugar is fructose (Walker 2014), it would take only 3 or 4 12-ounce servings of soda or juice to provide at least 100 g of fructose (Walker 2014). Many people drink more than four 12-ounce servings of soda, energy drink, or juice per day, and may be getting even more fructose from other sweetened foods. Thus, the Western diet of sugary-refined carbohydrates is quite capable of providing enough extra fructose to drive increases in obesity and inflammation.

Why is Sugar So Hard to Kick?

Even though the dangers of sugar in the diet are becoming well-established, many people have difficulty reducing the amount that they eat. Part of the problem is that sugar, in the form of beverages, baked goods, and processed foods, is nearly ubiquitous and hard to avoid. Grocery stores typically have one or more aisles devoted to sugary snacks, candy, and soda. The little shelves or counters at the check-out areas always have sugary snacks designed to encourage impulse buying. Public health research suggests, based on the link of sugar with diabetes and other inflammatory drugs, that foods containing sugar should at least be labeled with warnings, similar to legal drugs such as nicotine and alcohol (Pomeranz 2012). However, the food and beverage industries have so far prevented any efforts that might lead to warnings, let alone reduced sugar consumption (Pomeranz 2012).

Social and cultural factors also contribute to the ubiquity of sugar. Sweet baked goods are often brought to workplaces and parties, and sweet desserts are usually offered after restaurant or dinner party meals. Anyone turning down these treats can be made to feel eccentric or unsociable. In some cultures, sweet tea or sweet coffee are parts of social rituals as well, and in other cultures, not giving candy to children is considered "mean." In this way, social pressure and temptations can seriously hamper efforts to limit sugar and other refined carbohydrates in the diet.

Perhaps one of the biggest challenges to reducing sugar in the diet involves the naturally rewarding features of sweet tastes (Ventura 2011). This may relate to the fact that sweet tastes can signal safe, nutritious food, such as fruit. In contrast, many poisons taste bitter, which may be why preferences for bitter-tasting foods usually need be to be learned. Indeed, the brain regions that respond to sweet tastes are those that control motivation and reward and are dysregulated in addiction (Wiss 2018). Chronic consumption of sugary foods can mimic some of the changes in brain reward learning circuits that are caused by addictive drugs such as heroin or cocaine (Burger 2017). Like other addictive drugs, sweet tastes have analgesic actions (Ventura 2011). Furthermore, studies with humans and animals have shown that regular consumption of sugary foods can result in symptoms of dependence and craving, similar to drug addictions (DiNicolantonio 2018).

Like other addictions, cravings for the rewarding feeling is worsened by stress (Koob 2019, Ruisoto 2019). In the case of sugar, this can lead to a vicious cycle whereby stress increases craving and dependence on sugar, but the sugar induces inflammation, worsening stress and driving further cravings for sugar. Thus, addiction or dependence on sugar is particularly a problem for people who have stress-sensitive conditions, such as chronic pain or depression, in which inflammation drives pathophysiology.

What About "A Sweet Tooth"?

Although the issue of whether sweet tastes are in fact addictive is still debated, people do differ in preferences for sweet tastes (Jayasinghe 2017). For instance, people who have a high preference for sweets are said to have a "sweet tooth". Sweet preferences seem to be determined by genetic as well as environmental factors (Ventura 2011). Among environmental factors, early life experiences strongly influence our expectations of what is a "normal" amount of sweet food in the diet, as well as the context in which sweet foods are eaten (e.g., sparingly as a treat, or daily in most meals and beverages) (Ventura 2011).

Taste, or gustation, is one of the chemical senses, which also includes smell or olfaction and the *common chemical sense*. The common chemical sense is carried by the trigeminal nerve and signals temperature as well as substances that activate these temperature sensors such as hot peppers/capsaicin, horseradish/wasabi, menthol, etc. Unlike other senses there are marked individual differences in what we can perceive and how sensitive we are to specific tastes or smells. For instance, some people, called *super tasters* have markedly greater sensitivity to tastes. They can detect tastes at a lower threshold or concentration in foods or beverages. There are genetic differences in sensitivity to certain bitter tastes, where some people are exceptionally sensitive to certain bitter tastes, while others can't taste it all. Even more strange is the fact that an odor associated with androstenone, a steroid pheromone from pigs, is experienced very differently depending on how intensely it is perceived. People with lower sensitivity report a mild pleasant scent, described as "like flowers or lotion," whereas people with higher sensitivity may respond dramatically, briefly lose their breath and report experiencing a profoundly unpleasant smell, described, for example, as a "pitted out old outhouse in the desert." Further, sensitivity of the chemical senses can change depending on experience. For instance, people who initially are unable to smell androstenone develop the ability to detect it with repeated exposure.

This malleability of perception among the chemical senses suggests that sweet taste perception and preference could be modifiable (Wise 2016), as it can be in other animals (May 2019). Preference for sweet tastes is closely linked to sensitivity to the taste, such that the more sensitive someone is to sweet tastes, the fewer sweet beverages or foods they consume (Jayasinghe 2017, Wise 2016). Interestingly, obesity is associated with lower sensitivity to sweets (Harnischfeger 2021), but sensitivity to sweet can increase with weight loss (Rohde 2020). The mechanism(s) of this change have not been established but could be related to hormonal changes associated with weight loss (Rodhe 2020), and/or may reflect changes in diet (e.g., reducing sugar) during weight loss. This suggests that "sweet tooth" preferences could change if reducing sugar in the diet increases sensitivity.

Non-Nutritional Sweetener Issues: Why We Need to Get Past Needing a Sweet Taste in Everything

Non-nutritional sweeteners are a group of substances that have been modified (e.g., sugar alcohols), synthesized (e.g., aspartame, saccharine), or extracted from plants (e.g., Stevia), and taste sweet but have few or no calories, and no nutrition (Roberts 2015). They are attractive because they allow people to still enjoy a sweet taste in foods or beverages but keep calorie consumption down. For people trying to reduce their sugar intake, either because they have diabetes or they are aware of the health risks of eating sugar, artificial sweeteners seem like a great way to still enjoy sweet tastes, without causing hyperglycemia or inflammation. But do artificial sweeteners help with weight loss, blood sugar issues, and inflammation?

So-called *diet beverages*, in fact, do not seem to help control caloric intake. It seems that drinking a beverage with artificial sweeteners (e.g., aspartame, stevia, or monk's fruit) before a meal leads to a similar number of calories consumed in the meal overall (Tey 2017). The calories "saved" by drinking a non-nutritive beverage are often gained by eating more food in the meal. This may relate to the fact that a sweet taste can lead to a cephalic phase insulin response. Here, because the brain is expecting real sugar, it triggers insulin release that leads to a drop in blood glucose and increased hunger (Wiedemann 2020). This drop in blood sugar would be compensated for when drinking a beverage containing real sugar. Thus, diet drinks, despite lacking calories, may make us hungrier. This is not helpful when trying to control appetite. Overall, studies investigating non-nutritional sweeteners to aid weight loss have not demonstrated many, if any positive effects (Edwards 2016).

Similarly, although non-nutritional beverages do not lead to acute hyperglycemia, like beverages containing sugars, longer-term assessments indicate that overall, non-nutritional sweeteners have little or no positive effect on blood glucose levels (Tey 2017, Tucker 20117). In fact, non-nutritional sweeteners seem to slightly increase the risk for Type 2 diabetes. This is true even when compensating for causality, addressing the possibility that diabetic people may consume more non-nutritional sweetener simply because they have diabetes (Fowler 2016).

Perhaps most troubling are findings indicating that cardiometabolic risks of sweeteners interact with other demographic and lifestyle factors (Fowler 2016). Notably, women, overweight/obese people, and people already at risk for diabetes may be more likely to gain weight and become insulin-resistant while consuming artificial sweeteners compared to others (Fowler 2016). The effects are more pronounced in people eating the Western diet of high-energy/low-nutrition, fatty, sugary processed foods.

The reason why non-nutritional sweeteners may increase the risk of cardiometabolic disease is not known, and indeed the findings seems counterintuitive. However, recent studies have shown that sweeteners that are non-nutritional for us may still affect certain microbes in our guts (Fowler 2016, Payne 2012, Pepino 2015). Non-nutritional sweeteners are generally not well absorbed into our bodies, and thus remain in our guts for microbes to metabolize. Not all gut microbes can metabolize these sweeteners, potentially leading to an imbalance in microbe populations called *dysbiosis*. This unbalanced microbe population can cause inflammation, which may contribute to risk of Type 2 diabetes. Other microbes that metabolize non-nutritional sweeteners are associated with obesity, possibly because they also seem to increase absorption of food (Pepino 2015). Finally, there may be a dose effect relating to safety of non-nutritional sweeteners, similar to that seen with fructose. "High" doses of aspartame, for instance seem to induce oxidative stress and inflammation, and may adversely affect protein metabolism (Choudhary 2017). Because of the increase in serving sizes of beverages, some people may be consuming "high" doses of sweeteners.

What about "natural" non-nutritive sweeteners like stevia and monk fruit? Most studies that identify potential health risks of non-nutritive sweeteners have focused on artificial sweeteners such as saccharine and aspartame. Non-nutritive "natural" sweeteners found in plants may have fewer risks for cardiometabolic disease. As yet, there is less of an evidence base for either risks or benefits of stevia or monk fruit. Natural artificial sweeteners seem to have similar effects on appetite and glycemic control (Tey 2017). Although natural sweeteners might be expected to be less toxic than artificial sweeteners, stevia is reported to have immune-modulating and bactericidal actions (Peteliuk 2021). Such action could have implications for effects of stevia-sweetened food or beverages on gut microbe populations. Although non-nutritional sweeteners are almost certainly less pro-inflammatory than sugar, risks most likely increase with dose. This implies that occasional use of non-nutritional sweeteners could be safe but that frequent use may have deleterious implications for gut microbes or the gut barrier. The bottom line is that because both sugar and non-nutritive sweeteners pose risks for cardiometabolic disease and inflammation, a healthy diet is one that contains mostly foods that don't taste sweet.

The Special Problem of Sweetened Beverages

Sweetened beverages, especially soda, seem to contribute prominently to the risks associated with excess sugar in the diet (Ahn 2021, Collin 2019, Malik 2019, Yin 2021). This may relate to the fact that beverages are often consumed with every meal, and thus contribute substantially to sugar intake. Even people who think they don't eat a lot of sweet food may get a lot of sugar in their diet from sodas or energy drinks.

In addition, artificially sweetened beverages share with nutritive-sweetened beverages such as soda, a number of other constituents, including colorings, AGEs, and bisphenol A (Fowler 2016). These additives or contaminants could have adverse effects such as increasing or inducing inflammation and impairing glucose tolerance (Fowler 2016). Although the potential risks of these constituents are recognized, there are few or no data on how they may be contributing to the health risks of sweetened beverages.

Sugar-sweetened and carbonated beverages are linked to bone problems and risk of fractures (Ahn 2021, Chen 2020). The basis for this relationship is not established but may relate to features of the beverages that are directly deleterious to bone or may simply reflect that fact that soda is being substituted for other beverages, such as milk, that are better for bone health (Tucker 2006). Although carbonation has been suggested to impair bone health, only those containing cola have been linked to low bone density (Tucker 2006). This is good news, as one alternative to sugary soda is sparkling water, which is also carbonated.

Key Points

- The amount of sugar in the typical diet has been increasing since the 1800s but has increased dramatically worldwide in the last thirty years. At the same time, the incidence of metabolic diseases, including diabetes and non-alcoholic fatty liver disease, have risen in tandem.
- The links of dietary sugar to chronic disease operate through inflammatory pathways and oxidative stress.
- Advanced glycation end-products (AGEs) are formed in the blood during persistent hyperglycemia and in foods during cooking or processing, typically at high temperatures. They are pro-inflammatory because they active RAGE, the receptor for advanced glycation end products. RAGE activates inflammatory pathways such as NFkB and is linked to cardiovascular, renal, and neurological dysfunction.
- Hyperglycemia, as can happen with a diet high in refined carbohydrates, can cause oxidative stress and inflammation, leading to insulin resistance.
- Fructose is naturally found in fruit and is a key source of energy for the liver. But if it is added to the diet, such as in table sugar or high-fructose corn syrup, this extra fructose is converted into fat. The fat can accumulate in the liver, causing non-alcoholic fatty liver disease, or be sent in the blood to visceral adipose tissue.
- Sweet tastes are naturally rewarding. This is likely because in nature they signal safe, nutritious foods such as fruit. Unfortunately, this may also make sweet tastes "addictive," especially in the context of stress.
- Non-nutritional sweeteners may seem attractive as substitutes for sugar. Although they are unlikely to contribute to oxidative stress as sugars do, they come with other risks. They may disturb gut microbial populations, and they do not seem to help curb appetite or caloric intake.

References

Abenovoli L, Boccuto L, Federico A, Dallio M, Loguercio C, Di Renzo L, De Lorenzo A. Diet and Non-Alcoholic Fatty Liver Disease: The Mediterranean Way. International Journal of Environmental Research and Public Health, 16:3011, 2019.

Ahn H, Park YK. Sugar-sweetened beverage consumption and bone health: a systematic review and meta-analysis. Nutrition Journal, 20:41, 2021.

Alwahsh SM, Gebhardt R. Dietary fructose as a risk factor for non-alcoholic fatty liver disease (NAFLD). Archives of Toxicology, 91:1545-1563, 2017.

Aragno A, Mastrocola R. Dietary Sugars and Endogenous Formation of Advanced Glycation End products: Emerging Mechanisms of Disease. Nutrients, 9:385, 2017.

Bray GA. Energy and fructose from beverages sweetened with sugar or high-fructose corn syrup pose a health risk for some people. Advances in Nutrition, 4: 220–225, 2013.

Burger, KS. Frontostriatal and behavioral adaptations to daily sugar-sweetened beverage intake: a randomized controlled trial. American Journal of Clinical Nutrition, 105:555-563, 2017.

Butterfield DA, Halliwell B. Oxidative stress, dysfunctional glucose metabolism and Alzheimer disease. Nature Reviews Neuroscience, 20:148-160, 2019.

Choudhary AK, Pretorius E. Revisiting the safety of aspartame. Nutrition Reviews, 75:718-730, 2017.

Chen L, Liu R, Zhao Y, Shi Z. High consumption of soft drinks is associated with an increased risk of fracture: A 7 year follow-up study. Nutrients, 12:530, 2020.

Chen Z, Zhong C. Decoding Alzheimer's disease from perturbed cerebral glucose metabolism: Implications for diagnostic and therapeutic strategies. Progress in Neurobiology, 108:21-43, 2013.

Collin L, Judd S, Safford M, Vaccarino V, Welsh JA. Association of sugary beverage consumption with mortality risks in US adults. A secondary analysis of data from the REGARDS Study. JAMA Network Open, 2: e193121, 2019.

DiNicolantonio JJ, O'Keefe JH, Wilson WL. Sugar addiction: Is it real? A narrative review. British Journal of Sports Medicine, 52:910-913, 2018.

Edwards CH, Rossi M, Corpe CP, Butterworth PJ, Ellis PR. The role of sugars and sweeteners in food, diet and health: Alternatives for the future. Trends in Food Science and Technology, 56:158-166, 2016.

Fowler, SPG. Low-calorie sweetener use and energy balance: Results from experimental studies in animals, and large-scale prospective studies in humans. Physiology and Behavior, 164:517-523, 2016.

Gugliucci A. Formation of fructose-mediated advanced glycation end products and their roles in metabolic and inflammatory diseases. Advances in Nutrition, 8:54-62, 2017.

Harnischfeger F, Dando R. Obesity-induced taste dysfunction, and its implications for dietary intake, International Journal of Obesity, 45:1644-1655, 2021.

Jayasinghe SN, Kruger R, Walsh DCI, Cao G, Rivers S, Richter M, Breier BH. Is Sweet Taste Perception Associated with Sweet Food Liking and Intake? Nutrients, 9:750, 2017.

Jiang X, Wang X, You M, Ma J, Xie A. RAGE and its emerging role in the pathogenesis of Parkinson's Disease. Neuroscience Letters, 672:65-69, 2018.

Jimenez AG. "The same thing that makes you live can kill you in the end": Exploring the effects of growth rates and longevity on cellular metabolic rates and oxidative stress in mammals and birds. Integrative and Comparative Biology, 58:544-558, 2018.

Johnson RJ, Sanchez-Lozada LG, Andrews P, Lanaspa MA. Perspective: A historical and scientific perspective of sugar and its relation with obesity and diabetes. Advances in Nutrition,8:412-422, 2017.

King X, Lu A-L, Yao X-M, Hua Q, Li X-Y, Qin L, et al. Activation of NLRP3 inflammasome by advanced glycation end products promotes pancreatic islet damage. Oxidative Medicine and Cellular Longevity, 2017:9692546, 2017.

Kellow NJ, Coughlan MT. Effect of diet-derived advanced glycation end products on inflammation. Nutrition Review, 73:737-759, 2015.

Khan TA, Tayyiba M, Agarwal A, Blanco Meija S, de Souza RJ, Wolever TMS, et al. Relation of total sugars, sucrose, fructose, and added sugars with the risk of cardiovascular disease: A systematic review and dose-response meta-analysis of prospective cohort studies. Mayo Clinic Proceedings, 94:2399-2414, 2019.

Kong X, Lu A-L, Yao X-M, Hua Q, Li X-Y, Qin L, Zhang H-M, Meng G-X, Su Q. Activation of NLRP3 Inflammasome by Advanced Glycation End Products Promotes Pancreatic Islet Damage. Oxidative Medicine and Cellular Longevity, 2017:9692546, 2017.

Koob G, Shulkin J. Addiction and stress: an allostatic view. Neuroscience and Biobehavioral Reviews, 106, 245-262, 2019.

Korkmaz A, Oter S, Seyrek M, Topal T. Molecular, genetic and epigenetic pathways of peroxynitrite-induced cellular toxicity. Interdisciplinary Toxicology, 2:219-228, 2009.

Luc K, Schramm-Luc A, Guzik TJ, Mikolajczyk TP. Oxidative stress and inflammatory markers in prediabetes and diabetes. Journal of Physiology and Pharmacology, 70:809-824, 2016.

Malik VS, Li Y, Pan A, De Koning L, Schernhammer E, Willett WC, Hu FB. Long-Term Consumption of Sugar-Sweetened and Artificially Sweetened Beverages and Risk of Mortality in US Adults. Circulation, 139:2113-2125, 2019.

May CE, Vaziri A, Lin YQ, Grushko O, Khabiri M, Wang Q-P, Holme KJ, Pletcher SD, Freddolino PL, Neely GG, Dus M. High Dietary Sugar Reshapes Sweet Taste to Promote Feeding Behavior in Drosophila melanogaster. Cell Reports, 27:1675-1685, 2019.

Meija E, Pearlman M. Natural alternative sweeteners and diabetes management. Current Diabetes Reports, 19:142, 2019.

Micucci C, Valli D, Matacchione G, Catalano A. Current perspectives between metabolic syndrome and cancer. Oncotarget, 7:38959-38972, 2016.

Nguyen TT, Ta QTH, Nguyen TKO, Nguyen TTD, Giau VV. Type 3 diabetes and its role implications in Alzheimer's Disease. International Journal of Molecular Sciences, 21:3165, 2020.

Paixao J, Dinis TCP, Almeida LM. Malvidin-3-glucoside protects endothelial cells up-regulating NO synthase and inhibiting peroxynitrite-induced NF-kB activation. Chemico-Biological Interactions, 199:192-200, 2012.

Palanissami G, Paul SFD. RAGE and its ligands: Molecular interplay between glycation, inflammation, and hallmarks of cancer - a review. Hormones and Cancer, 9:295-325, 2018.

Paolisso G, Gambardella A, Ammendola A, D'Amore A, Balbi V, Varricchio M, D'Onofrio F. Glucose tolerance and insulin action in healthy centenarians. American Journal of Physiology, 270: E890-4, 1996.

Payne AN, Chassard C, Lacroix C. Gut microbial adaptions to dietary consumption of fructose, artificial sweeteners and sugar alcohols: implications for host-microbe interactions contributing to obesity. Obesity Reviews, 13:799-809, 2012.

Pepino MY. Metabolic effects of non-nutritive sweeteners. Physiology and Behavior, 152:450-455, 2015.

Peteliuk V, Rybchuk L. Bayliak M, Storey KB, Lushchak O. Natural sweetener *Stevia rebaudiana*: Functionalities, health benefits and potential risks. EXCLI Journal, 20:1412-1430, 2021.

Pfeiffer AFH, Keyhani-Nejad F. High glycemic index metabolic damage - a pivotal role of PGIP and GLP-1. Trends in Endocrinology and Metabolism, 29:289-299, 2018.

Pomeranz JD. The bitter truth about sugar labeling regulations: They are achievable and overdue. American Journal of Public Health, 103: e14-e20, 2012.

Rajchgot T, Thomas SC, Wang J-C, Ahmadi M, Balood M, Crosson T, Pean Dias J, Couture R, Ciaing A, Talbot S. Neurons and microglia; a sickly-sweet duo in diabetic pain neuropathy. Frontiers in Neuroscience, 19:25, 2019.

Ray R, Juranek JK, Rai, V. RAGE axis in neuroinflammation, neurodegeneration and its emerging role in the pathogenesis of amyotrophic lateral sclerosis. Neuroscience and Biobehavioral Reviews, 62:48-55, 2016.

Roberts JR. The paradox of artificial sweeteners in managing obesity. Current Gastroenterology Reports, 17:423, 2015.

Rodriguez Mortera R, Bains Y, Gugliucci A. Fructose at the crossroads of the metabolic syndrome and obesity epidemics. Frontiers in Bioscience, 24:186-211, 2019.

Rohde K, Schamarek I, Bluher M. Consequences of obesity on taste: Taste buds as treatment targets? Diabetes and Metabolisms Journal, 44:509-524, 2020.

Ruisoto P, Contador I, The role of stress in drug addiction. An integrative review. Physiology and Behavior, 202:62-68, 2019.

Sas K, Robotka H, Toldi J, Vecsei L. Mitochondria, metabolic disturbances, oxidative stress and the kynurenine system, with focus on neurodegenerative disorders. Journal of the Neurological Sciences, 257:221-239, 2007.

Sae iab T, Dando R. Satiety, taste and the cephalic phase: A crossover designed pilot study into taste and glucose response. Foods, 9:1578, 2020.

Schultze BS, Ridner SH. Death by sugar: the impact of sugar on acutely ill patients. The Journal for Nurse Practitioners, 11:456-461, 2015.

Semniani-Azad Z, Khan TA, Blanco Meija A, de Souza RJ, Leiter LA, Kendall CWC, et al. Association of major food sources of fructose-containing sugars with incident metabolic syndrome. A systematic review and meta-analysis. JAMA Network Open, 3:e209993, 2020.

Shah GN, Morofuji Y, Banks WA, Price TO. High glucose-induced mitochondrial respiration and reactive oxygen species in mouse cerebral pericytes is reversed by pharmacological inhibition of mitochondrial carbonic anhydrases: Implications for cerebral microvascular disease in diabetes. Biochemistry and Biophysics Research Communications, 440:354-358, 2013.

Speckmann B, Seinbrenner H, Grune T, Klotz L-O. Peroxynitrite: from interception to signaling. Archives of Biochemistry and Biophysics, 595:153-160, 2016.

Stadler K. Peroxynitrite-driven mechanisms in diabetes and insulin resistance - The latest advances. Current Medical Chemistry, 18:280-290, 2011.

Stanhope KL. Sugar consumption, metabolic disease and obesity: The state of the controversy. Critical Reviews in Clinical and Laboratory Science, 53:52-67, 2016.

Talbot K, Wang H-Y, Kazi H, Han L-Y, Bakshi KP, Stuckey A, Fuino RL, Kawaguchi KR, Samoyedny AJ, Wilson RS, Arvanitakis Z, Schneider JA, Wolf BA, Bennett DA, Trojanowski JQ, Arnold SE. Demonstrated brain insulin resistance in Alzheimer's disease patients is associated with IGF-1 resistance, IRS-1 dysregulation, and cognitive decline. Journal of Clinical Investigation, 122:1316-1338, 2012.

ter Horst K, Schene MR, Holman R, Romijn JA, Serlie MJ. Effect of fructose consumption on insulin sensitivity in nondiabetic subjects: a systematic review and meta-analysis of diet-intervention trials. American Journal of Clinical Nutrition, 104:1562-76, 2016.

Tey SL, Salleh NB, Forde CG. Effects of aspartame-, monk fruit-, stevia- and sucrose-sweetened beverages on postprandial glucose, insulin and energy intake. International Journal of Obesity, 41:450-457, 2017.

Tucker KL, Morita K, Qiao N, Hannan MT, Cupples LA, Kiel DP. Colas, but not other carbonated beverages, are associated with low bone mineral density in older women: The Framingham Osteoporosis study. American Journal of Clinical Nutrition, 84:936-942, 2006.

Tucker RM, Tan S-Y. Do non-nutritive sweeteners influence acute glucose homeostasis in humans? A systematic review. Physiology and Behavior, 182:17-26, 2017.

Urribarri J, Cai W, Sandu O, Peppa M, Goldberg T, Vlassara H. Diet-derived advanced glycation end products are major contributors to the body's AGE pool and induce inflammation in healthy subjects. Annals of the New York Academy of Sciences, 1043:461-466, 2005.

Venn BJ, Mann JI. Cereal grains, legumes and diabetes. European Journal of Clinical Nutrition, 58:1443-1461, 2004.

Ventura AK, Mennella JA. Innate and learned preferences for sweet taste during childhood. Current Opinion in Clinical Nutrition and Metabolic Care, 14:379-384, 2011.

Walker RW, Dumke KA, Goran MI. Fructose content in popular beverages made with and without high-fructose corn syrup. Nutrition, 30:928-935, 2014.

Weidemann SJ, Rachild L, Illigens B, Noni-Schnetzler M, Donath MY. Evidence for cephalic phase insulin release in humans: A systematic review and meta-analysis. Appetite, 155:104792, 2020.

Wiss DA, Avena N, Rada P. Sugar addiction: From evolution to revolution. Frontiers in Psychiatry, 9:545 doi: 10.3389/fpsyt.2018.00545, 2018.

Yeh W-J, Yan H-Y, Pai M-H, Wu C-H, Chen J-R. Long-term administration of advanced glycation end product stimulates the activation of NLRP3 inflammasome and sparking the development of renal injury. Journal of Nutritional Biochemistry, 39:68-76, 2017.

Yin J, Zhu Y, Malik V, Li X, Peng X, Zhang FF, Shan Z, Liu L. Intake of sugar-sweetened and low-calorie sweetened beverages and the risk of cardiovascular disease: A meta-analysis and systematic review. Advances in Nutrition, 12:89-101, 2021.

Yuan T, Yang T, Chen H, Fu D, Hu Y, Wang J, et al. New insights into oxidative stress and inflammation during diabetes mellitus-accelerated atherosclerosis. Redox Biology, 247-260, 2019.

Zafar TA, Aldughpassi A, Al-Mussallam A, Al-Othman A. Microstructure of whole wheat versus white flour and wheat-chickpea flour blends and dough: impact on the glycemic response of pan bread. International Journal of Food Science, 2020:8834960, 2020.

CHAPTER 14: STRESS, INFLAMMATION, THE WESTERN DIET AND THE VULNERABLE BRAIN

- WESTERN DIET EFFECTS ON DIABETES AND METABOLIC SYNDROME: INSULIN RESISTANCE AND INFLAMMATION

- THE BIDIRECTIONAL INTERACTIONS BETWEEN DIABETES AND STRESS

- DEPRESSION IS A COMMON COMPANION OF DIABETES

- BRAIN INSULIN RESISTANCE: "TYPE 3 DIABETES" AND THE BRAIN

- PRE-DIABETES: IS DIABETES INEVITABLE?

- DIET STRATEGIES TO MANAGE OR PREVENT HYPERGLYCEMIA AND INFLAMMATION

- IMPLICATIONS OF THE WESTERN DIET AND LIFESTYLE FOR TYPE 2 DIABETES AND METABOLIC SYNDROME

- ADDRESSING STRESS AND DISTRESS

- KEY POINTS

The most serious consequences of the vicious cycle of stress, Western diet, and inflammation are the metabolic disorders: Type 2 diabetes, metabolic syndrome (the combination of Type 2 diabetes, obesity, and cardiovascular disease), and non-alcoholic fatty liver disease. Metabolic disorders disrupt the function of every other system in the body. The associated inflammation induces microvascular damage that affects organ functions. This results in kidney damage, heart disease, peripheral nerve damage, retinal damage leading to blindness, and circulation problems, leading to lower limb amputations and strokes (Koska 2018, Lau 2019). Further, the close relationships between metabolism, inflammation, and immunity render people with Type 2 diabetes vulnerable to infectious diseases such as SARS COVID-19 (Butler 2020, Neilsen 2017). Long-term consequences of diabetes include a dramatic increase in risk for neurodegenerative diseases, such as Alzheimer's disease (Hayden 2019). Finally, the chronic inflammation associated with diabetes and metabolic syndrome is typically associated with the sickness syndrome of fatigue, cognitive fuzziness, sleep problems, mood symptoms, and chronic pain, with important implications for quality of life. Risks of these disorders are exaggerated when the Western diet is combined with psychological and socioeconomic stress.

Globally, nearly 400 million people have Type 2 diabetes (Wang 2007), with approximately 37 million in the US alone (11% of the total US population; Centers for Disease Control and Prevention 2022). Millions more have "pre-diabetes," and about 70% of these will go on to develop Type 2 diabetes. As countries such as China begin to adopt the Western diet, the incidence of Type 2 diabetes rises dramatically there as well (Soares 2017). Worldwide, metabolic disorders and their consequences represent a tremendous burden in terms of health care costs and suffering. Fortunately, changing food habits and addressing stress can help manage the consequences of, and even prevent, metabolic disorders.

Western Diet effects on Diabetes and Metabolic Syndrome: Insulin Resistance and Inflammation

Diabetes is classified into two types: Type 1 and Type 2. Both Type 1 and Type 2 diabetes occur as a confluence of genetic and environmental factors (Petersen 2018). Type 1 diabetes is caused by autoimmune attack on pancreatic cells that make insulin, and it constitutes about 10% of diabetes cases. Type 2 diabetes is characterized by insensitivity of cells to insulin, a condition called insulin resistance, and this type constitutes about 90% of diabetes cases. The dramatic increase in incidence of both types is thought to follow from environmental factors, with global dietary changes associated with the energy-rich, but nutrition-poor, Western diet, implicated as a plausible major culprit (Soares 2017).

Diabetes mellitus means "lots of sweet urine," and historically one way it was diagnosed was by observing flies on affected individual's shoes. Thus, the most obvious commonality between the two types of diabetes is hyperglycemia. Until recently, however, it was believed that the pathophysiology of these disorders was quite different. But recent research is now pointing to commonalities in inflammation, autoimmunity, and insulin resistance associated with both types of diabetes (Brooks-Warrell 2019).

Insulin resistance is a complex phenomenon that may serve an adaptive role initially to protect cells from oxidative stress due to hyperglycemia, as noted in Chapter 13 (Peterson 2018). Insulin is released from the pancreas after a meal, and it functions to activate transport of glucose and amino acids into cells. A phenomenon called hyperinsulinemia can occur in response to diets containing high levels of carbohydrates, and especially sugars, and protein. Insulin levels must be high, initially, to remove excess glucose from the blood. High levels of insulin lead to downregulation of insulin receptors and thus less sensitivity of the cells to the insulin (i.e., insulin resistance). This has the effect of reducing glucose transport into cells. This may be a protective action because excess glucose, as a substrate for metabolism, can lead to oxidative stress (Luc 2019). However, once cells are resistant to insulin, not enough glucose can enter the cell, leading to hypometabolism and impairment of function. Thus, with insulin resistance, cells may effectively wind up starved for glucose while sitting inside a river of sugar syrup. The persistent hyperglycemia in the blood that ensues when cells don't take up glucose can drive the formation of glycated proteins, such as hemoglobin A1C. High levels of hemoglobin A1c are used clinically as an indication of chronic hyperglycemia and probable insulin resistance. At the same time, fat tissue releases hormones or adipokines that drive inflammation and further insulin resistance.

One of the main contributing factors to Type 2 diabetes is obesity. Obesity is associated with systemic inflammation, especially in the context of the high-energy Western diet (Ghanim 2004). This is suggested to, among other things, disrupt the balance between anti-inflammatory immune cells (e.g., Tregs) and pro-inflammatory immune cells (e.g., TH17) in the pancreas, contributing further inflammation and autoimmune attack on insulin-producing cells (Brooks-Warrell 2019). Although the details of autoimmunity in Type 2 diabetes are still being clarified, the mechanisms may be similar to celiac disease and inflammatory bowel disease. In these disorders, auto-reactive T cells play a prominent role in attacking and damaging one's own cells. Here, genetics and environment interact in ways that are still being understood to lead to development of these disorders. In the case of Type 2 diabetes, diet seems to be a major precipitating environmental factor.

Whereas the linkage of overweight, obesity, and insulin resistance is most obvious in Type 2 diabetes, recent studies also point to overweight and obesity contributing to Type 1 diabetes (Brooks-Warrell 2019). This is thought to follow from the increasing prevalence of weight problems, especially in children (Priya 2018). Children diagnosed with Type 1 diabetes are more likely to be overweight than other children, and this has been suggested to function as an accelerating factor for onset of the condition (Priya 2018). Insulin resistance increases demand on pancreatic cells, and this may increase antigen presentation and autoimmune damage (Brooks-Warrell 2019).

Both types of diabetes are associated with serious co-morbidities, including cardiovascular disease, retinopathy, and kidney disease. These consequences follow from an interaction of metabolic dysregulation and inflammation. To review, persistent hyperglycemia drives inflammation by several mechanisms. Glycated proteins (e.g., A1C), can be further processed into advanced glycation end products (AGEs), which can activate the receptor for advanced glycation end products (RAGE), inducing inflammation and oxidative stress (Teissier 2019). In other words, sugar modified proteins can activate receptors that turn on inflammatory immune responses. Cumulative damage from inflammation triggered by AGEs/RAGE can induce damage to arteries leading to progression of Type 2 diabetes to metabolic syndrome and increasing risk of cardiovascular events such as heart attack and stroke (Koska 2018).

The Bidirectional Interactions between Diabetes and Stress

Stress is uniquely problematic for metabolic diseases, because of the dual role that challenge or stress response systems play in regulating metabolism and inflammation (Butler 2020, Hackett 2017). Stress complicates glycemic control because a core feature of challenge responses is hyperglycemia, which occurs to ensure adequate energy is available to meet the demands of a challenge. Chronic stress also dysregulates the HPA axis, which functions to regulate metabolism, fat deposition, and appetite (Greulich 2016, Michels 2019). Both childhood stress [e.g., adverse childhood experiences (ACEs)] and adult chronic stress are associated with the development of insulin resistance (Fuller-Rowell 2019, Joseph 2017). Further, stress enhances preferences for sugary, high-energy food that can drive insulin resistance and inflammation.

Living with a chronic disease is inherently challenging. *Diabetes distress* is defined as the negative emotional impact of living with diabetes, and the difficulties, worries and frustrations of meeting the challenges associated with establishing and maintaining glycemic control. Diabetes distress is considered apart from other stress-related psychological symptoms, such as depression, and affects up to one third of people with diabetes (Owens-Gary 2018). The consequences of unaddressed diabetes distress are considerable, as it is associated with worse metabolic markers, poor glycemic control values, and increased incidence of cardiovascular disease (Winchester 2016).

The interactions of stress, diet, and diabetes result in the marked over-representation of people of color, migrants, and people with low income or low socio-economic status among the diabetic population (Sartorius 2018). People of these groups are more likely to work at stressful low wage jobs and have poor diet and sedentary and other unhealthful lifestyle habits (Nkwata 2020). At the same time, access to health care, including preventative care for those at-risk, is less available for poor rural counties. Lack of health insurance due to poor job benefits or pay can limit access to health care in some urban areas (Nkwata 2020). Further, access to affordable, highly nutritious food can be more challenging in rural and inner city "food deserts." Moreover, diabetogenic, highly processed, high-energy, Western diet junk foods are both more widely available, convenient, and likely to be consumed compulsively by people living with chronic stress. Thus, it is unsurprising that people who experience these disparities in access to health care and healthy food are at elevated risk for metabolic syndrome and the long-term consequences of hyperglycemia (Walker 2014).

Among people of color, the experience of discrimination contributes importantly to diabetes distress, which as noted, is associated with poor glycemic control. This is of serious concern, as a recent study of diabetic Latinx people reported that two thirds of participants reported experiences of discrimination, as assessed by the Everyday Unfair Treatment scale (LeBron 2019). Examples of the types of discrimination assessed by the scale include experiencing poor service or being made to feel less intelligent. The study linked discrimination with diabetes distress, implying that the stress of discrimination drives the challenges of glycemic control among people of color (Le Bron 2019). Similarly, a study of older adults diagnosed with diabetes or heart disease found that the cumulative effects of life stress, including ACEs, exert a more pronounced deleterious effect on health-related quality of life on minorities than on Caucasians (Nkwata 2020). Weight-related discrimination is often experienced by overweight/obese diabetics and is associated with higher burden of co-morbidities (Udo 2016). This adds to the burden of social stress on minorities, who are more likely to be overweight or obese (Wang 2007). Finally, a recent study comparing lifetime stress, inflammation, and insulin resistance in a large sample of middle-aged Black and White people demonstrated marked disparities (Fuller-Rowell 2019). Black adults experienced more stressful experiences both in childhood and as adults and had higher levels of inflammatory markers. Importantly, life history of stress, as well as evidence of dysregulated cortisol function, correlated with measures of insulin resistance. These findings directly link stress with risk for diabetes and underline the importance of addressing societal factors that drive risks for metabolic disease.

Depression is a Common Companion of Diabetes

The effects of diabetes distress extend beyond glycemic control. Rates of depression are more than twice as high among people with diabetes than among non-diabetics (Sartorius 2018). Nearly one third of people with diabetes experience depression or depressive symptoms, and, as in the general population, depression is more common in women (Sartorius 2018). Depressive symptoms are higher among diabetics who report symptoms of diabetic distress and experiences of discrimination (Owens-Gary 2018). Migration frequently occurs because of adverse circumstances in a person's homeland and can be associated with discrimination in both homeland and sanctuary. Like other indicators of chronic stressful life event exposure, migration has been associated with elevated rates of both depression and diabetes, again linking stress with mood and glycemic control (Sartorius 2018).

Although the pathophysiological links between diabetes and depression are not clearly established, both conditions are associated with systemic inflammation, dysregulated cortisol rhythms, and several risk factors including early childhood stress (Joseph 2017, Herder 2019). Brain insulin resistance has been reported in depression, especially in association with symptoms of anhedonia and cognitive impairment

(Hamer 2019). These symptoms are also linked to brain insulin resistance in people with diabetes, suggesting a common pathway to these symptoms, perhaps via inflammation (Herder 2019, Franklin 2018), stress-related cortisol dysregulation (Joseph 2017), or diet. Certainly, cognitive dysfunction increases risk of depression, and poor glycemic control leads to cognitive dysfunction, thus linking metabolic impairments with brain dysfunction.

Not only is diabetes a risk for depression, but depression is a risk factor for diabetes (Joseph 2017). The basis for this association is not known but may follow from lifestyle factors associated with depression, such as stress eating of high-energy foods that induce insulin resistance. Notably, depression is also a common companion to obesity, itself a major risk factor for diabetes (Milaneschi 2019). In addition, the sub-clinical hypercortisolemia that can be a feature of depression could drive hyperglycemia and insulin resistance and the development of diabetes (Joseph 2017). Unfortunately, co-morbid depression can complicate the adoption of self-care and lifestyle habits such as diet that are necessary for effective glycemic control (Sartorius 2018, Herder 2019). Thus diabetics with depression experience higher rates of complications, disability, and shorter lifespan. Notably, depression increases risk for dementia in both Type 1 and Type 2 diabetes (Gilsanz 2019).

Brain Insulin Resistance: "Type 3 Diabetes" and the Brain

Diabetes has marked consequences for the brain. The brain is the most metabolically active organ in the body. The brain uses glucose as its principal fuel and thus has high requirements for glucose. However, unlike most other tissues of the body, the brain does not need insulin to transport glucose from the blood and into cells. Rather, glucose is taken up into the brain by an insulin-dependent glucose transporter protein in a concentration-dependent manner.

Insulin is transported across the blood-brain barrier, and the brain expresses insulin receptors in a region-specific way (Banks 2012). Persistent hyperglycemia leads to persistent high levels of insulin in the brain as well. This hyperinsulinemia leads to a down-regulation of insulin receptor expression and thus fewer insulin receptors. While this is presumably an attempt to regulate the actions of insulin in the brain, it nevertheless results in *brain insulin resistance*, which is sometimes called "Type 3 diabetes".

Why does the brain transport insulin and express receptors for it if the brain does not need to insulin to take up glucose and amino acids? Clues to the function of insulin in the brain come from comparative studies that indicate that early in evolution, insulin may have had a principal role as a growth factor (Banks 2012). Over hundreds of thousands of years, the insulin gene has duplicated and mutated, leading to a whole family of insulin-related proteins. For most tissues of the body, insulin functions principally to regulate nutrient uptake and metabolism. However, other insulin protein family members retain the growth factor functions of prehistoric insulin. Studies of insulin receptor function in the brain point to it having critical roles in the regulation of behaviors such as eating behaviors, neurological influence on metabolism and peripheral insulin release, and growth factor-like support of cognition (Banks 2012). These observations imply that one possible mechanism by which brain insulin resistance contributes to depression and dementia occurs because of depriving neurons of the growth-factor abilities of insulin, leading to cognitive impairment.

People with diabetes have double the risk for late-onset Alzheimer's disease (AD), exemplifying the link between insulin resistance and cognition (Hayden 2019). Indeed, most AD patients have abnormal fasting glucose and insulin resistance, as do patients with other neurodegenerative diseases, such as fronto-temporal dementia and vascular dementia (Chen 2013). Diabetes is a common comorbidity among people with stroke, affecting about 30% of stroke patients (Lau 2019). Ischemic strokes, which result from inflammation and blockages in brain blood supply, occur in the context of chronic inflammation. This can include the activation of RAGE in brain cells which may link diabetes, neurodegenerative diseases, and depression (Matrone 2015, Franklin 2018).

Pre-Diabetes: Is Diabetes Inevitable?

Type 2 diabetes usually develops over time, passing through an intermediate stage called *pre-diabetes* where glucose tolerance and insulin sensitivity are impaired, but do not quite reach the values associated with a diagnosis of Type 2 diabetes. Nonetheless, people with pre-diabetes show similar atherosclerotic plaques in their vascular system as do people with Type 2 diabetes, indicating that they are likely to be at a similar elevated risk for cardiovascular events such as stroke and heart attack (Zand 2018). Whereas most people with pre-diabetes go on to develop full-blown Type 2 diabetes, about 30% do not, supporting the idea that interventions such as dietary change are able to prevent the progression of the disease (Roberts 2017).

To that end, pre-diabetes is usually treated with metformin, a drug that improves glucose tolerance and insulin resistance, and/or lifestyle changes including dietary improvements, weight loss, and increased exercise (Beulens 2019). Studies have indicated similar outcomes for metformin and lifestyle interventions for prevention of Type 2 diabetes, but there is an assumption that lifestyle changes have more enduring effects (Roberts 2017). Most hearteningly, a recent large study of both men and women with pre-diabetes that employed a weight loss phase, followed by an ongoing lifestyle intervention program, reported that weight loss alone was associated with marked improvements in metabolic indicators (Christensen 2019). Importantly, more than one third of the participants reverted to normal glycemic levels, indicating that it may indeed be possible to prevent the progression to Type 2 diabetes in at-risk people.

Diet Strategies to Manage or Prevent Hyperglycemia and Inflammation

Based on what we know about the effects of food on the body, and the pathophysiology of metabolic disorders, it seems intuitive that diet intervention and lifestyle approaches should be important for the prevention and management of diabetes. Indeed, studies now show that diets based on mostly plants that avoid refined carbohydrates are associated with improvements in glycemic control and other metabolic makers (Evert 2019). A recent review of studies investigating the effects of different macronutrient content (e.g., high- versus low-carbohydrate), as well as specific diet ingredients, provides guidelines for diets based on the quality of the evidence (Evert 2019). Unfortunately, most studies are targeted to Type 2 diabetes and there is comparatively little specific data regarding Type 1 diabetes.

One of the most confusing and controversial issues regarding diets targeted to diabetes and metabolic syndrome involves the benefits of high-carbohydrate versus low-carbohydrate content of the diet. Determining which is most effective is complicated by individual differences across people and the varying quality of carbohydrates (e.g., refined or whole grains, fiber, vegetables, or fruits). Evidence so far indicates that quality of the carbohydrate, defined as being high in fiber, vitamins, and minerals, is a key determinant of effects on diabetes outcomes (Evert 2019). Fiber seems to be particularly important, and beans, peas, lentils, fruits, and intact grains are recommended. Low-carbohydrate diets, defined as those with less than 45% calories from carbohydrates, can reduce A1C at least temporarily. These low-carbohydrate diets, however, can be dangerous and must be undertaken in consultation with a physician or dietician.

Another dietary approach is to substitute fats for carbohydrates. If the fats are good quality, this does seem to help glycemic control (Evert 2019). What are "good quality fats"? Good quality fats are not synthetic, meaning they have not been hydrogenated into trans fat, and are "native," meaning they are non-oxidized. Vegetable fats that are solid at room temperature are typically synthetic. Some studies have reported that saturated dairy fats, and saturated fats from vegetable sources such as coconut oil, may reduce risks for diabetes, but others have reported no association (Evert 2019). In general, clinical studies of dairy fat effects on markers associated with metabolic syndrome have shown either beneficial or neutral effects (Unger 2019). These findings indicate that diets containing full-fat dairy products are not likely to be problematic for people with diabetes or metabolic syndrome. Indeed, some dairy fats, most notably butyrate, have anti-inflammatory effects on macrophages, and might help down-regulate inflammation associated with diabetes and metabolic syndrome. Polyunsaturated fats such as omega-3s and olive oil, also seem to aid in prevention of diabetes in at-risk people and improve metabolic markers. In contrast, low-fat diets are generally not helpful unless they rely on vegetables, beans, and grains, non-fat dairy, and egg whites (e.g., Atkins Diet). Similarly, high-protein diets, providing 30% or more total calories from protein, can help with weight loss, which is an important objective. However, high-protein diets do not seem to improve glycemic control (Evert 2019).

Dysbiosis, an imbalance in gut microbes, as well as gut barrier inflammation, typically accompany metabolic diseases. These likely contribute to inflammation that drives stress and mood symptoms and may enhance insulin resistance. Thus, the idea that pro-biotic foods can improve features of diabetes is attractive. However, the evidence for a beneficial effect of probiotics is mixed (Eid 2017). A major problem for evaluating potential efficacy is that the methodology of studies varies widely. Study methods vary so much that interpretation of findings is difficult. For example, studies use different species of bacteria, each of which might be expected to have different actions. Probiotics are provided in different forms, with some consumed as pills and other as food sources, such as yogurt. The length of probiotic interventions differs substantially as well. Among the more well-designed protocols, a recent clinical study found that a probiotic formula containing microbes that produce the short-chain fatty acid butyrate improved glucose tolerance in people with Type 2 diabetes. As butyrate has immunomodulatory actions on macrophages and can downregulate inflammation, this effect supports the suspected link between gut microbes, inflammation, and diabetes (Perraudeau 2020). Thus, it seems likely that future studies that focus on specific microbes, based on their identified actions, may be able to clarify and inform approaches for ameliorating the effects of dysbiosis on features of diabetes and metabolic syndrome.

Given the clear relationship between diet and metabolic disease, what is the best diet strategy? In general, plant-based (i.e., vegetarian or vegan) diets seem to be helpful for improving glucose tolerance, and several clinical trials have shown the Mediterranean diet to be effective for improving metabolic markers associated with diabetes and metabolic syndrome (Evert 2019, Esposito 2015). Unfortunately, there is much less evidence about diet strategies for Type 1 diabetes. However, from what we know of the pathophysiology of the condition, a Mediterranean diet low in refined carbohydrates, but including plentiful vegetables and plant-based oils, might be helpful for Type 1 diabetes as well.

Implications of the Western Diet and Lifestyle for Type 2 Diabetes and Metabolic Syndrome

The Western lifestyle is characterized by sedentary activity levels and reliance on convenient high- energy, low-nutrient foods, often eaten late in the day. Indeed, many convenience food outlets offer to deliver foods, such as pizza, late at night or even 24/7. Unfortunately, the habit of consuming many calories late at night is associated with marked increases in risk for obesity, Type 2 diabetes, and metabolic syndrome (Garaulet 2014, Lopez-Minguez 2019). Alarmingly, a recent study linked night-time eating with development of severe responses leading to death from Covid-19 (Ver 2020). There are several likely mechanisms for these effects, including the disruption of circadian rhythms of cortisol and metabolism, as well as the effects of the hormone melatonin, which is released in the evening as part of preparation of the body for sleep, on glucose tolerance and metabolism. Disruption of these endocrine rhythms can dysregulate the immune and metabolic systems, enhancing the effects of Western diet foods on inflammation and insulin resistance (Focke 2020).

Normally, cortisol levels are high during the day, as cortisol contributes to control of nutrient availability, and its release is linked to meals. Cortisol release related to meals occurs in part as a consequence of gut-to-brain communication (Benedict 2005). Proper sensitivity to cortisol depends on levels declining in the evening and remaining low until right before awakening. This is aided by refraining from eating in the evening. Higher levels of cortisol at bedtime are associated with the development of insulin resistance and Type 2 diabetes, likely because cortisol regulates the sensitivity of insulin receptors (Gruelich 2016). In general, insulin sensitivity is lowest at night, meaning that glucose in the blood consequent to eating a meal at night is less likely to be absorbed by cells, resulting in persistent hyperglycemia. Indeed, among people with Type 2 diabetes, night-time eating is associated with higher A1C levels and obesity (Lopez-Minguez 2019).

Melatonin may also contribute to the relationship between night-time eating and diabetes risk. Melatonin levels begin to rise about an hour before normal bedtime. In studies where people received a 5 mg melatonin supplement at bedtime, this extra bedtime melatonin worsened glucose tolerance. Thus, if meals are eaten late, the elevated blood glucose consequent to the meal is less likely to be absorbed, leading to persistent hyperglycemia. Genetic differences may exaggerate the effects of melatonin on glucose tolerance. A version of the melatonin 1B receptor has been found to be a strong genetic risk factor associated with Type 2 diabetes (Lopez-Minguez 2019). This version of the melatonin 1B receptor is common and carried by nearly half of the Caucasian population. The effect of melatonin on glucose uptake is most pronounced among people carrying the diabetes-risk melatonin receptor gene, providing another mechanistic link of late-night eating to the development of Type 2 diabetes (Lopez-Minguez 2019).

From these observations, it seems intuitive that meals should be taken earlier during the day. Indeed, studies comparing people who eat early with those who eat later have shown that early eaters tend to be leaner and less likely to develop Type 2 diabetes (Lopez-Minguez 2019). How early is early? The answer to that question seems to depend on a person's *chronotype*, basically whether one is a morning/early person, a night/late person, or flexible. The bottom line seems to be that people who go to bed early need to eat early, and people who stay up late can eat later, but still need to have several hours awake without eating before going to bed. In this way, blood glucose and cortisol levels will have declined before melatonin levels rise.

One approach that can address the issue of eating at night is *Time-Restricted Eating* (TRF). TRF was originally developed as a weight-loss strategy because it limits the time during the day when eating can occur, usually to within a window of 6-10 hours. The idea was to also restrict caloric intake, but in addition, TRF is thought to more closely approximate historic human eating patterns. If the eating window occurs in the middle of the day, TRF prevents night-time eating and its deleterious effects on glucose tolerance and insulin sensitivity. To that end, recent studies have shown that in both healthy and pre-diabetic young men, an early TRF schedule resulted in improved insulin sensitivity, even without calorie restriction (Jamshed 2019, Jones 2020, Sutton 2018).

Addressing Stress and Distress

The entangled relationship between diabetes distress, lifetime stress, diet choices and patterns, and glycemic control give rise to several barriers that need to be addressed in order facilitate effective glycemic control (Evert 2019). These barriers include lack of education regarding the risks of certain diets, such that many diabetics don't fully understand how important their diet is in determining their disease outcomes. There may be cultural factors that affect diet choice or attitudes about health care, as well as emotional issues related to diabetes distress or lifetime stressors, especially those related to discrimination or access to health care. Given the outsized impact of stress on emotions, behavior, and physiological conditions that influence control of blood glucose levels, helping patients address and manage stress should be an important part of a treatment plan (Errisuriz 2016, Winchester 2016).

To that end, several studies from the U.S. and other countries have now reported that mindfulness-based stress reduction (MBSR) programs are able to reduce feelings of stress, ratings of diabetes distress, and mood symptoms while increasing successful coping, feelings of self-efficacy, and happiness. Moreover, these mental health improvements were linked to better glycemic control (Whitebird 2018, Zarifsanaiey 2020). Importantly, studies showing successful results from MBSR interventions have included both Type 1 and Type 2 diabetics and African-Americans in their study populations (Woods-Giscombe 2019, Guo 2019).

The success of MBSR programs in improving both stress and glycemic control suggests that such programs should be more widely implemented. To do so, it will be helpful to understand factors that influence effectiveness of the programs. To that end, a recent meta-analysis of MBSR programs for diabetes showed that group formats were more effective than one-to-one, perhaps reflecting benefits of social support within the group. The analysis also found that programs that included a home practice component were more effective than programs that did not include a home practice (Guo 2019). The studied home practice was typically 30 minutes per day and involved a "body scan," specifically a meditative sequential focus on self-awareness of specific body parts, often beginning with the feet, and moving up, sitting breathing meditations, mindful eating exercises, and routine activity with awareness. Interestingly, MBSR interventions report larger effects on reducing diabetes distress at follow-up several months after the end of the intervention, suggesting that the patients may have continued their practice beyond the study period. Taken together, studies indicate that MBSR programs can indeed provide useful "tools in the toolbox" for managing interactions between stress and glycemic control.

Key Points

- The incidence of metabolic diseases has been increasing over the years, concomitant with increases in weight and consumption of Western diet: refined carbohydrates, high-fructose corn syrup, processed meats and fats, and a food supply containing inflammation-inducing additives and pesticides.
- Hyperglycemia can cause inflammation, and inflammation causes insulin and cortisol resistance. This leads to a vicious cycle that increases hyperglycemia and inflammation, stress, and mood disorders.
- Diabetes is a highly stress-sensitive condition, and the special challenges of managing it can lead to diabetes distress. Diabetes distress impairs efforts to control blood sugar and inflammation, further driving the vicious cycle.
- Insulin resistance has serious consequences for the brain. Metabolic dysfunction impairs brain functions and contributes to inflammation, increasing risk for cognitive impairment and dementia.
- Metabolic disorders exert deleterious long-term effects on the body and on quality of life. For this reason, lifestyle factors must be addressed.
- Stress and diet are key factors in the vicious cycle that perpetuates inflammation and its consequences for metabolic disorders. Interventions addressing them, notably adopting the Mediterranean diet and mindfulness-based stress management have been shown to improve symptoms.

References

Benedict C, Hallschmid M, Scheibner J, Niemeyer D, Schultes B, Merl V, Fehm HL, Born J, Kern W. Gut Protein Uptake and Mechanisms of Meal-Induced Cortisol Release. The Journal of Clinical Endocrinology & Metabolism, 90:1692-1696, 2005.

Banks WA, Owen JB, Erickson MA. Insulin in the Brain: There and Back Again. Pharmacology and Therapeutics, 136:82-93, 2012.

Beulens JWJ, Rutters F, Ryden L, Schnell O, Mellbin L, Hart HE, Vos RC. Risk and management of pre-diabetes. European Journal of Preventive Cardiology, Vol. 26: 47-54, 2019.

Brooks-Worrell BM, Palmer JP. Setting the Stage for Islet Autoimmunity in Type 2 Diabetes: Obesity-Associated Chronic Systemic Inflammation and Endoplasmic Reticulum (ER) Stress. Diabetes Care, 42:2338-2346, 2019.

Butler MJ, Barrientos RM. The impact of nutrition on COVID-19 susceptibility and long-term consequences. Brain, Behavior, and Immunity, 87:53-54, 2020.

Centers for Disease Control and Prevention. National Diabetes Statistics Report website. Available at: https://www.cdc.gov/diabetes/data/statistics-report/index.html. Accessed February 1, 2020.

Chen Z, Zhong C. Decoding Alzheimer's disease from perturbed cerebral glucose metabolism: Implications for diagnostic and therapeutic strategies. Progress in Neurobiology, 108:21-43, 2013.

Christensen P, Meinert Larsen T, Westerterp-Plantenga M, Macdonald I, Martinez JA, Handjiev S, et al. Men and women respond differently to rapid weight loss: Metabolic outcomes of a multi-center intervention study after a low-energy diet in 2500 overweight, individuals with pre-diabetes (PREVIEW). European Journal of Preventive Cardiology, 26: 47-54, 2019.

Eid HM, Wright ML, Kumar NVA, Qawasameh A, Hassan STS, Mocan A, Nabvi SM, Rastrelli L, Atanasov A, Haddad PS. Significance of microbiota and metabolic disease and the modulatory potential by medicinal plants and food ingredients. Frontiers in Pharmacology, 8:387, 2017.

Errisuriz VL, Pasch KE, Perry CL. Perceived stress and dietary choices: The moderating role of stress management. Eating Behaviors, 22:211-216, 2016.

Esposito K, Maiorino MI, Bellastella G, Chiodini P, Panagiotakos D, Giugliano D. A journey into a Mediterranean diet and type 2 diabetes: a systematic review with meta-analysis. BMJ Open, 10: e008222, 2015.

Evert AB, Dennison M, Gardner CD, Garvey WT, Lau KHK, MacLeod J, Mitri J, Pereira RF, Rawlings K, Robinson S, Saslow L, Uelmen S, Urbanski PB, Yancy Jr YS. Nutrition Therapy for Adults with Diabetes or Prediabetes: A Consensus Report, Diabetes Care, 2019.

Focke CMB, Iremonger KJ. Rhythmicity matters: Circadian and ultradian patterns of HPA axis activity. Molecular and Cellular Endocrinology, 501:110652, 2020.

Franklin TC, Wohleb ES, Zhang Y, Fogaça M, Hare B, Duman RS. Persistent increase in microglial rage contributes to chronic stress–induced priming of depressive-like behavior. Biological Psychiatry, 83:50-60, 2018.

Fuller-Rowell TE, Homandberg LK, Curtis DS, Tsenkova VK, Williams DR, Ryff CD. Disparities in Insulin Resistance between Black and White Adults in the United States: The Role of Lifespan Stress Exposure. Psychoneuroendocrinology, 107:1-8, 2019.

Garaulet M, Gómez-Abellán P. Timing of food intake and obesity: A novel association. Physiology and Behavior, 134:44-50, 2014.

Ghanim H, Aljada A, Hofmeyer D, Syed T, Mohanty P, Dandona P. Circulating Mononuclear Cells in the Obese Are in a Proinflammatory State. Circulation, 110:1564-1571, 2004.

Gilsanz P, Schnaider Beeri M, Karter AJ, Quesenberry CP, Adams AS, Whitmer RA. Depression in Type 1 Diabetes and Risk of Dementia. Aging and Mental Health, 23:880-886, 2019.

Greulich F, Hemmer MC, Rollins DA, Rogatsky I, Uhlenhaut NH. There goes the neighborhood: Assembly of transcriptional complexes during the regulation of metabolism and inflammation by the glucocorticoid receptor. Steroids, 114:7-15, 2016.

Hackett RA, Steptoe A. Type 2 diabetes mellitus and psychological stress – a modifiable risk factor. Nature Reviews Endocrinology, 13:547-560, 2017.

Hamer JA, Testani D, Mansur RB, Lee Y, Subramaniapillai M, McIntyre RS. Brain insulin resistance: A treatment target for cognitive impairment and anhedonia in depression. Experimental Neurology, 315:1-8, 2019.

Hayden MR. Type 2 Diabetes Mellitus increases the risk of late-onset Alzheimer's disease: ultrastructural remodeling of the neurovascular unit and diabetic gliopathy. Brain Sciences, 9:262, 2019.

Herder C, Hermanns N. Subclinical inflammation and depressive symptoms in patients with type 1 and type 2 diabetes. Seminars in Immunopathology, 41:477-489, 2019.

Jamshed H, Beyl RA, Deborah L. Della Manna DL, Yang ES, Ravussin E, Peterson CM. Early time-restricted feeding improves 24-hour glucose levels and affects markers of the circadian clock, aging and autophagy. Nutrients, 11:1234, 2019.

Jones R, Pabla P, Mallinson J, Nixon A, Taylor T, Bennett A, Tsintzas K. Two weeks of early time-restricted feeding (eTRF) improves skeletal muscle insulin and anabolic sensitivity in healthy men. American Journal of Clinical Nutrition, 112:1015–102, 2020.

Joseph JJ, Golden SH. Cortisol dysregulation: the bidirectional link between stress, depression, and type 2 diabetes mellitus. Annals of the New York Academy of Sciences, 1391:20-34, 2017.

Guo J, Wang H, Luo J, et al. Factors influencing the effect of mindfulness- based interventions on diabetes distress: a meta- analysis. BMJ Open Diabetes Research and Care, 7: e000757, 2019.

Koska J, Saremi A, Howell S, Bahn G, De Courten B, Ginsberg H, Beisswenger PJ, Reaven PD. Advanced glycation end products, oxidation products, and incident cardiovascular events in patients with type 2 diabetes. Diabetes Care, 41:570-576, 2018.

Lau K-H, Lew J, Borschmann K, Thijs V, Ekinci EI. Prevalence of diabetes and its effects on stroke outcomes: A meta-analysis and literature review. Journal of Diabetes Investigation, 10:780-792, 2019.

LeBrón AMW, Spencer M, Kieffer E, Brandy Sinco B, Palmisano G. Racial/Ethnic Discrimination and Diabetes-Related Outcomes Among Latinos with Type 2 Diabetes. Journal of Immigrant and Minority Health, 21:105-114, 2019.

Lopez-Minguez J, Gómez-Abellán P, Garaulet M. Timing of Breakfast, Lunch, and Dinner. Effects on Obesity and Metabolic Risk. Nutrients, 11, 2624; doi:10.3390/nu11112624, 2019.

Luc K, Schramm-Luc A, Guzik TJ, Mikolajczyk TP. Oxidative stress and inflammatory markers in prediabetes and diabetes. Journal of Physiology and Pharmacology, 70:809-824, 2019.

Matrone C, Djelloul, Taglialatela G, Perrone L. Inflammatory risk factors and pathologies promoting Alzheimer's Disease progression: is RAGE the key? Histology and Histopathology, 30:125-139, 2015.

Michels N. Biological underpinnings from psychosocial stress towards appetite and obesity during youth: research implications towards metagenomics, epigenomics and metabolomics. Nutrition Research Reviews, 32:282-293, 2019.

Milaneschi Y, Simmons WK, van Rossum EFC, Penninx BW. Depression and obesity: evidence of shared biological mechanisms. Molecular Psychiatry, 24:18-33, 2019.

Nielsen TB, Pantapalangkoor P, Yan J, Luna BM, Dekitani K, Bruhn K, Tan B, Junus J, Bonomo RA, Schmidt AM, Everson M, Duncanson F, Doherty TM, Lin L, Spellberg B. Diabetes exacerbates infection via hyperinflammation by signaling through TLR4and RAGE. mBio 8:e00818-17, 2017.

Nkwata AK, Song X, Zhang M, Ezeamama AR. Change in quality of life over eight years in a nationally representative sample of US adults with heart disease and type 2 diabetes: minority race and toxic stress as key social determinants. BMC Public Health, 20:684, 2020.

Owens-Gary MD, Zhang X, Jawanda S, McKeever Bullard K, Allweiss P, Smith BD. The importance of addressing depression and diabetes distress in adults with type 2 diabetes. Journal of General Internal Medicine, 34:320-324, 2018.

Perraudeau F, McMurdie P, Bullard J, et al. Improvements to postprandial glucose control in subjects with type 2 diabetes: a multicenter, double blind, randomized placebo-controlled trial of a novel probiotic formulation. BMJ Open Diabetes Research and Care, 8:e001319, 2020.

Petersen MC, Shulman GI. Mechanisms of insulin action and insulin resistance. Physiological Reviews, 98:2133-2223, 2018.

Priya G, Kalra S. A review of insulin resistance in Type 1 Diabetes: Is there a place for adjunctive metformin? Diabetes Therapy, 9:349-361, 2018.

Roberts S, Barry E, Craig D, et al. Preventing type 2 diabetes: systematic review of studies of cost-effectiveness of lifestyle programmes and metformin, with and without screening, for pre-diabetes. BMJ Open, 7: e017184, 2017.

Sartorius N. Depression and diabetes. Dialogues in Clinical Neuroscience, 20:47-51, 2018.

Soares M, Muller MJ. Type 2 diabetes in Asia: where do we go from here? European Journal of Clinical Nutrition, 71:801-802, 2017.

Sutton EF, Beyl R, Early KS, Cefalu WT, Ravussin E, Peterson CM. Early time-restricted feeding improves insulin sensitivity, blood pressure, and oxidative stress even without weight loss in men with prediabetes. Cell Metabolism, 27:1212-1221, 2018.

Teissier T, Boulanger E. The receptor for advanced glycation end-products (RAGE) is an important pattern recognition receptor (PRR) for inflammaging. Biogerontology, 20:279-301, 2019.

Thivel D, Finlayson G, Miguet M, Pereira B, Duclos M, Boirie Y, Doucet E, Blundell JE, Metz L. Energy depletion by 24-h fast leads to compensatory appetite responses compared with matched energy depletion by exercise in healthy young males. British Journal of Nutrition, 120:583–592, 2018.

Thornton PL, Kumanyika SK, Gregg EW, Araneta MR, Baskin ML, Chin MH, et al. New research directions on disparities in obesity and type 2 diabetes. Annals of the New York Academy of Sciences, 1461:5-24, 2020.

Udo T, Katherine Purcell K, Grilo CM. Perceived Weight Discrimination and Chronic Medical Conditions in Adults with Overweight and Obesity. International Journal of Clinical Practice, 70:1003-1011, 2016.

Unger AL, Torres-Gonzalez M, Kraft J. Dairy Fat Consumption and the Risk of Metabolic Syndrome: An Examination of the Saturated Fatty Acids in Dairy. Nutrients, 11:2200, 2019.

Verd S, Beiro S, Fernandez-Bernaeu M, Ponce-Taylor J. Early dinner or "dinner like a pauper": Evidence, the habitual time of the largest meal of the day - dinner - is predisposing to severe COVID-19 outcome – death. Chronobiology International, 37:804-808, 2020.

Walker RJ, Gebregziabher M, Martin-Harris B, Egede LE. Independent Effects of Socioeconomic and Psychological Social Determinants of Health on Self-Care and Outcomes in Type 2 Diabetes. General Hospital Psychiatry, 36:662-668, 2014.

Wang Y, Beydoun MA. The Obesity Epidemic in the United States- Gender, Age, Socioeconomic, Racial/Ethnic, and Geographic Characteristics: A Systematic Review and Meta-Regression Analysis. Epidemiologic Reviews, 29:6-28, 2007.

Whitebird RR, Kreitzer MJ, Vasquez-Benitez G, Enstad CJ. Reducing diabetes distress and improving self-management with mindfulness. Social Work in Health Care, 57:48-65, 2018.

Winchester RJ, Williams JC, Wolfman TE, Egede LE. Depressive symptoms, serious psychological stress, diabetes distress and cardiovascular risk factor control in patients with type 2 diabetes. Journal of Diabetes Complications, 30:312-317, 2016.

Woods-Giscombe C, Gaylord SA, Li Y, Brintz CE, Bangdiwala SI, Buse JB, Mann JD, Lynch C, Phillips P, Smith S, Leniek K, Young L, Al-Barwani S, Jeena Yoo J, Faurot K. A mixed-methods, randomized clinical trial to examine feasibility of a mindfulness-based stress management and diabetes risk reduction intervention for African Americans with prediabetes. Evidence-Based Complementary and Alternative Medicine, Volume 2019, Article ID 3962623, 2019.

Zand A, Ibrahim K, Patham B. Prediabetes: Why Should We Care? Methodist Debakey Cardiovascular Journal, 14:289-297, 2018.

Zarifsanaiey N, Jamalian K, Bazrafan L, Keshavarzy, F, Shahraki HE. The effects of mindfulness training on the level of happiness and blood sugar in diabetes patients. Journal of Diabetes and Metabolic Disorders, 19:311-317, 2020.

- WHAT IS IN THE GUT?

- THE "BRAIN IN THE GUT"

- WHAT HAPPENS IN THE GUT DOES NOT STAY IN THE GUT:

    - PART 1: THE GUT IMMUNE SYSTEM

    - PART 2: THE GUT IS THE LARGEST ENDOCRINE ORGAN IN THE BODY

    - PART 3: NEURAL PATHWAYS FOR GUT-RELATED SIGNALS

- BRAIN INFLUENCES ON GUT FUNCTIONS

- KEY POINTS

Most people don't think very much about their guts. We just shovel our food down and hope for the best. Moreover, most people really don't want to think about other people's guts. Unfortunately, this aversion to thinking about guts adds something of a stigma to gut disorders, such as irritable bowel syndrome (IBS), inflammatory bowel disorder (IBD), and severe food allergies. These disorders can have immense effects on quality of life, and a lack of social support from family or co-workers can increase the stress associated with the conditions. However, gastrointestinal (GI) disorders are common, and becoming more so (Warren 2020). At least 30 million people in the U.S. have IBS, and the incidence of food allergy and celiac disease is on the rise (Warren 2020). The consequences of these GI disorders can include pain and suffering, mood and cognitive problems, loss of work, and often lack of sympathy from family, co-workers, or even health care professionals. To understand the wide-ranging effects of what goes on in the gut, it is necessary to appreciate the many functions of the gut, and the mechanisms by which "what happens in the gut does not stay in the gut." It is also useful to note that problems in the gut contribute to many pathologies outside the gut, including heart, lung, liver, kidney, pancreas, skin, and brain (Bingula 2017, Chen 2021, Forkosh 2019, Kosiewicz 2014, Lee 2021).

Because the principal function of the gut is to absorb nutrients, what we eat, and how we eat it, has huge effects on the health of the gut and therefore the rest of the body.

What is in the Gut?

The gut is basically a hollow tube that runs from the mouth to the anus. My graduate advisor, Dr. Don Novin, used to say that "we are all donuts." What he meant is that like donuts, we have an outside (skin) and an inside (bodily tissues), and like a donut hole, an outside-inside (the gut). The hollow, outside-inside part is called the lumen. The lumen contains food that is being ingested but not yet absorbed into our bodies, plus trillions of microbes. The microbes will be discussed in Chapter 17, but for now, suffice to say that having bacteria, fungi, and viruses in our outside-inside is both highly beneficial and potentially dangerous.

When we eat, food enters the gut at the mouth, where taste receptors decide whether it is something we should swallow. If so, the food is chewed up to facilitate swallowing and digestion. If not, it is spit out, and often we experience the emotion of disgust or sensation of nausea. The signals from taste receptors therefore directly influence the *hedonics* or pleasurableness of food. The taste of food is actually a combination of the odor of foods plus activation of taste receptors. Food odors travel up the back of the mouth into the sinuses to activate olfactory receptors. Taste receptors on the tongue activate in response to combinations of the five tastes: sweet, sour, bitter, salty, and umami/protein. These smell and taste signals also activate the *cephalic phase* of digestion and insulin release (Veedfald 2016). The cephalic phase serves to prepare the gut and rest of the body for digesting and absorbing food. In this way, what happens in the gut serves to influence behavior, emotions, and gut function.

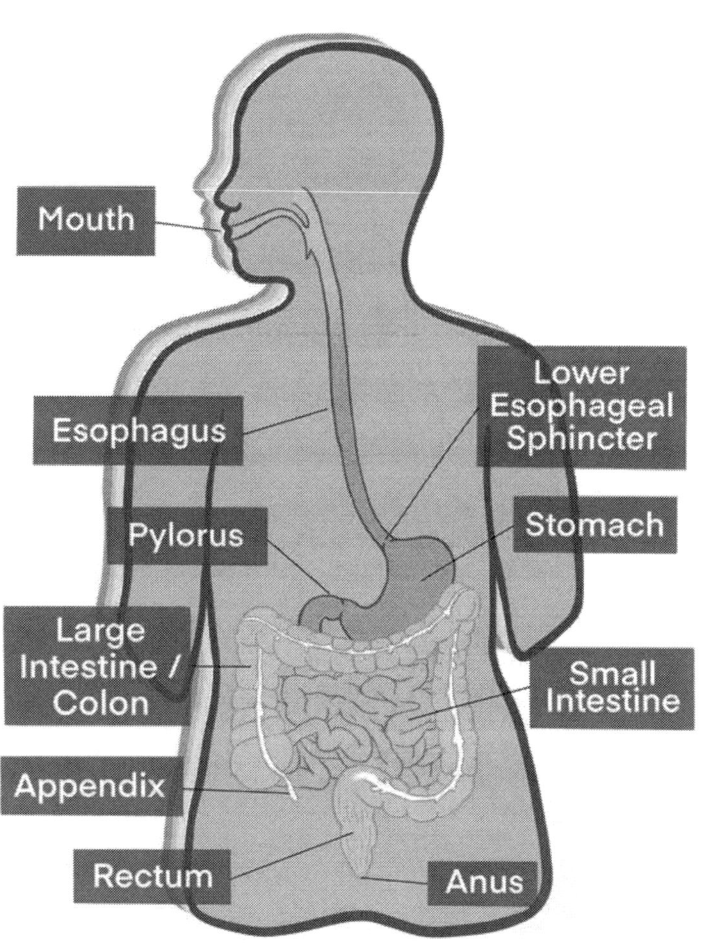

When food is swallowed it travels down the *esophagus* to the stomach. At the bottom of the esophagus is the lower esophageal sphincter, which serves as a valve to prevent food from going backwards into the esophagus. Food is supposed to move one way in the gut, but in some people, the sphincter is weak, allowing food to *reflux* back into the esophagus. Reflux can cause acid from the stomach to damage the lining of the esophagus, and may ultimately contribute to esophageal cancer (Brusselaers 2018). For this reason, *proton pump inhibitors* (PPIs) are prescribed for gastro-esophageal reflux disease (GERD), because they reduce the amount of acid the stomach can produce. Unfortunately, although PPIs can reduce pain associated with reflux, the reduction in gastric acid can cause problems with stomach function (Jaynes 2019). For instance, digestion can slow down because there is not enough acid to break down the food, causing *gastoparesis*. In gastroparesis, food empties from the stomach very slowly (Grover 2019). This can increase gastric pressure, which can increase reflux.

What happens in the *stomach*? Digestive enzymes and acids secreted in the stomach break the food into small particles and molecules to enable the food to be absorbed into the body. Although this is the stomach's principal job, it can directly absorb water, alcohol, and minerals such as calcium and iron (Sipponen 2015). Some B vitamins need to be transformed in the acid environment of the stomach to be made bioavailable. For this reason, people who have undergone gastric bypass or gastric sleeve surgery must be careful to ensure that they are consuming sufficient vitamins. The loss of vitamin availability subsequent to these stomach surgeries increases risk of deficiency diseases such as Wernicke's encephalopathy, which can lead to permanent brain damage in cognitive problems (Oudman 2018).

When food has been broken down sufficiently to be absorbed, it travels through the pylorus to the *small intestine*. Here most of our food is absorbed into the body. Food in the small intestine is basically a slurry of fluids and small suspended particles that moves slowly down the extent of the small intestine. The fluids in this mix come both from liquids we ingested, and from the body, Fluid from the body is moved into the lumen under the control of enteric *secretomotor* neurons in a carefully regulated way (Furness 2012). The fluid is necessary to absorb nutrients, but if too much is transferred into the lumen we can become dehydrated. In certain gut infections, such as food poisoning, the secretomotor neurons cause extra fluid to move into the lumen. With increased motility, this produces diarrhea, which can help expel pathogens. But if fluid is not replaced, dehydration can be fatal. An example is cholera infection. For this reason, it really is important to drink as many fluids as possible when experiencing diarrhea.

Between the small and large intestine lives the *cecum and appendix*. The appendix is a small hollow finger whose main function seems to be to serve as a reservoir for gut microbial communities (Cai 2021). This is important after we have had diarrhea or have had to clean out the intestine in preparation for colonoscopy, because microbes are washed out along with the liquid.

Because we are land animals and tend to dry out if we are not careful, it is important for the body to replace the fluids that are used to aid in digestion. As the last major part of the gut, the principal role of the *large intestine* or *colon* is to get that water back by reabsorbing it. Fecal material can become dry if the colon extracts too much water, making it hard and difficult to pass and causing constipation. This is the main reason that people who suffer from constipation need to be sure to drink lots of fluids. The colon's other major role is serving as a home for most of our gut microbes, who cheerfully feast on what's left of the food in our gut. From the colon, this residue moves on as feces into the rectum and out the anus. In this way, our "inner tube of life" manages everything we need related to absorbing food.

The "Brain in the Gut"

One important reason we don't usually have to think about our gut and what it is doing is that our gut contains its own nervous system (Spencer 2020). The gut's nervous system is able to sense conditions in the gut, such as of types of food or microbes, or presence of inflammation, and activate the appropriate responses. This nervous system is called the *enteric nervous system*, or "the brain in the gut." Like any basic nervous system, it contains sensory neurons and motor neurons, as well as interneurons that help integrate the sensory signals and determine appropriate motor responses. For example, if the sensory neurons detect the presence of pathogenic microbes or their toxins, the motor response is often vomiting and/or diarrhea, which is the gut's way of cleaning itself out.

The enteric nervous system is a complex and well-organized population of neurons (Furness 2012, Spencer 2020). There are a lot of them, extending from the esophagus to the anus. The number of neurons in the gut is about the same as in the spinal cord, and the neurons are organized into two *plexuses*. A plexus is a collection of nerve cells and their axons and dendrites, along with support cells such as glia, and immune cells.

One plexus lives in the submucosa, behind the epithelial cells, and serves a mostly sensory function (Spencer 2020). This plexus monitors the type of food in the gut, including its constituent components of fats, carbohydrates, and proteins, to help fine-tune digestion. It also monitors other factors related to conditions in the gut, such as infection or inflammation. This sensory information informs the secretomotor neurons that control fluid movement into the lumen. These neurons also live in the submucosal plexus.

The other plexus, called the myenteric plexus, lives in the muscle layer of the gut and serves a mostly motor function. The myenteric plexus serves to move food along the gut, controlling *motility*. It also regulates secretion of bile and enzymes that break food down into absorbable particles. Functional bowel disorders, such as gastroparesis and irritable bowel syndrome, are associated with dysfunction in coordination of motility (Ford 2020, Furness 2012, Grover 2019, Tack 2017).

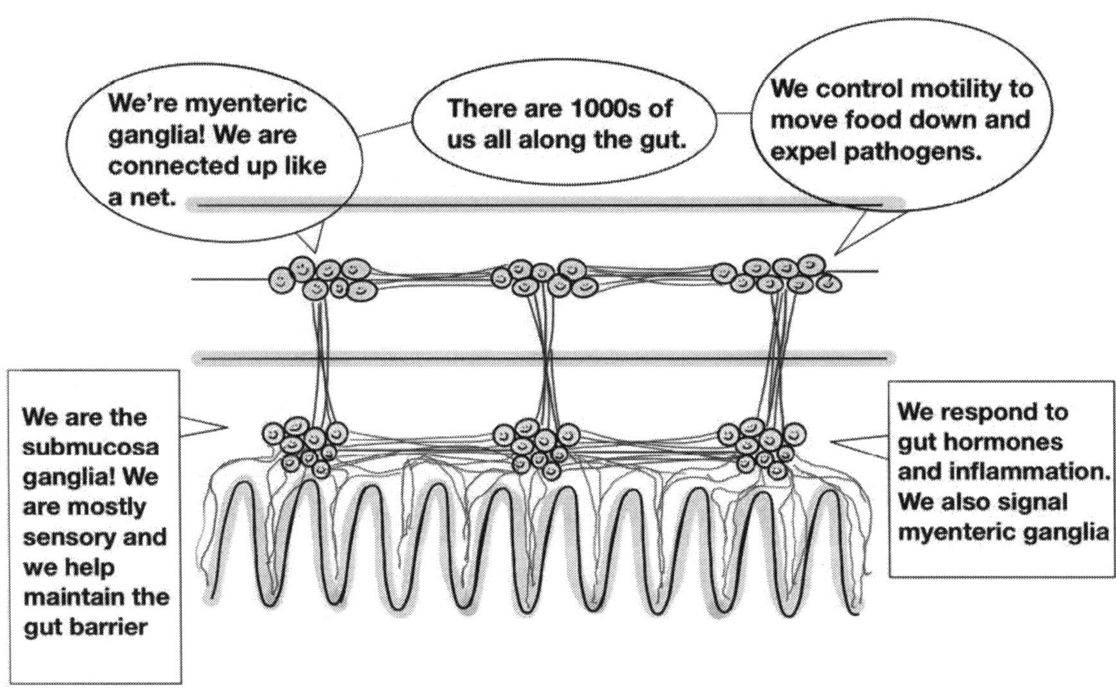

Figure Legend: The submucosa ganglia acts as the sensory nervous system for the gut. The myenteric ganglia acts as the motor nervous system for the gut.

The two plexuses have extensive connections with each other, and with the nerves that connect the gut with the brain (Spencer 2020). In this way, the "brain in the gut" coordinates digestion, and helps keep the brain informed about what is going on.

What Happens in the Gut Does Not Stay in the Gut

Many chronic conditions including neurodegenerative diseases, mood disorders, autoimmune disorders, liver disorders, asthma, autism, schizophrenia, and diabetes, are also associated with gut problems (Bingula 2017, Forkosh 2019, Kosiewicz 2014, Lee 2021). For example, Parkinson's disease, multiple sclerosis, and rheumatoid arthritis all may include gut symptoms. It has only recently been recognized that the association may be more than coincidental, and that gut problems may predispose people to these conditions or may directly be part of the pathophysiology (van Ijzendoorn 2019). Certainly, the rest of the body is dependent upon the gut to absorb nutrients, and malabsorption syndromes lead to widespread physiological dysfunction, but the gut can exert more specific actions on other tissues, especially the brain. Indeed, by "programming" immune cells, releasing hormones into the blood, and/or communicating directly with the nervous system, the gut is quite capable of exerting wide-ranging effects on most other organ systems.

What Happens in the Gut Does Not Stay in the Gut Part I: The Gut Immune System

Because the regulation of gut function is so critical to the health status of the entire body, the immune system is very interested in what is happening there. The gut provides an extensive interface with the outside world, with the human gut extending roughly 30 feet long. To patrol that length, approximately 70% of all the immune cells in the body live in the gut (Yoo 2017). The gut immune system involves collections of well-organized immune tissue that occupy the epithelium of the entire extent of the gut. These are somewhat similar to lymph nodes and are called Peyer's patches and gut-associated lymphoid tissue (GALT). Macrophages, mast cells, and the sentinel immune cells, called dendritic cells, richly populate the gut, mostly in the areas just below the epithelium and in the submucosa. Here, they are well situated to intercept any aggressive pathogen, or to identify toxins that may have slipped through the gut barrier. Even the gut barrier epithelial cells express substances called *defensins* that contribute to protecting the body from infection. Finally, the gut contains T cells and B cells that are capable of organizing both local and systemic immune responses. For instance, when B cells are activated by antigen, which can be derived from microbes, toxins, or food, they mature into *plasma cells* and produce Immunoglobulin A (IgA). IgA activates allergic responses.

The key requirement for immune cells in the gut is to respond promptly to threats such as pathogens and toxins, but to be *tolerant* of food antigens and beneficial microbes. Defense responses in the gut against pathogens such as aggressive bacteria are initiated by immune sentinels called dendritic cells, which detect potential pathogens and then activate T cells, including the pro-inflammatory TH17 *phenotype*. A phenotype is a kind of functional identity. Macrophages are related to dendritic cells and they contribute to inflammation by releasing pro-inflammatory cytokines. Tolerance is induced and maintained by the same kinds of cells, but these have a *regulatory* phenotype. In this phenotype they prevent inflammation, and are called regulatory dendritic cells (DCreg), type 2 macrophages, and regulatory T cells (Treg), which release the powerfully anti-inflammatory cytokine interleukin 10 (IL10).

Importantly, these cells exhibit *plasticity*, meaning that they may switch back and forth between phenotypes depending on the conditions in the gut (Sica 2012, Wang 2020). Although all of the mechanisms they use have not been identified, it seems that ultimately whether the gut is tolerating food antigens, or is intolerant and inflamed, depends on the balance of activity of anti-inflammatory Treg and pro-inflammatory TH17 cells (Omenettt 2015, De Martinis 2020),

How does immune function in the gut influence other tissues, such as the lung or brain? A key factor determining the phenotypes of immune cells in the gut is their interactions with microbes. Young immune cells, including some T cells and monocyte/macrophages, can be "programmed" in the gut (Bingula 2017, Kosiewicz 2014). What this means is that their interactions with other immune cells, epithelial cells, or microbes, can induce them to adopt a tolerant and anti-inflammatory phenotype or a pro-inflammatory phenotype. This process of adopting a phenotype is called *polarization* (Sica 2012). "Type 1" polarization refers to more pro-inflammatory function, where the immune cells release inflammatory mediators such as cytokines. "Type 2" polarization leads to a more tolerant state and the release of growth factors to encourage healing. Type 2 immunity is also important for managing parasites. Gut dysbiosis, which is an imbalance in microbes, can program immune cells to a pro-inflammatory phenotype. Although most of these immune cells remain in the gut, they apparently can migrate out to other tissues, such as lung, and influence immune function in these other tissues. This is suggested to contribute to the association of gut dysbiosis with conditions such as asthma and autoimmune conditions (Bingula 2017, Kosiewicz 2014, Hiltensperger 2021).

Allergic response in the gut can also exert systemic effects. Chemical mediators released consequent to IgA release from plasma cells, such as histamine or cytokines, can enter the systemic circulation and travel to distant tissues (Bingula 2017). In some circumstances, gut plasma cells can wander out of the gut to tissues such as bone marrow (Keppler 2021). These wandering cells seem to regulate systemic immune responses, but yet there is still much to learn about the details of their effects (Keppler 2021). It is likely though that factors influencing the maturation of the B cells, such as diet, will determine the whether the effects are protective or deleterious.

What Happens in the Gut Does not Stay in the Gut Part II: The Gut is the Largest Endocrine Organ in the Body

One of the ways that the gut can influence behavior, and the function of other organs, is by releasing hormones into the blood (Sternini 2008, Latorre 2016). The lining of gut contains many endocrine cells, called *enteroendocine cells*. Because the gut is so large, it contains more endocrine cells than any other organ. These cells are related to taste cells and are sometimes called the *taste cells of the gut*. Like taste cells, they detect chemical constituencies of foods, such as amino acids or fats. There are many kinds of enteroendocrine cells, and they each release a peptide or biogenic amine hormone, such as serotonin, when they are activated by food or by pressure or fullness in the gut. Peptides are small proteins and these, like biogenic amines, act as signaling molecules between cells. One example of these gut peptide hormones is ghrelin, which is secreted from the stomach early during a meal and acts as an appetite stimulant by increasing our motivation for food. In contrast, enteroendocrine cells of the small intestine release signaling molecules that serve as satiety factors. Interestingly, most of these cells are sensitive to different kinds of fats (e.g., long chain, short chain, medium chain), and this may be one reason foods containing fats tend to be more satiating than those containing simple carbohydrates, such as sugars. The amounts of fats, proteins, and carbohydrates influences features of digestion, such as enzyme or bile acid release, based on signals provided by the enteroendocrine cells. Thus, these substances serve to both coordinate digestion and to provide signals to the brain that influence eating behavior.

Gut hormones help regulate functions related to food including digestion, metabolism, and eating behavior. One substance, serotonin, also contributes to other functions. Serotonin is best known as a neurotransmitter in the brain whose signaling and regulation is a target of anxiolytic and antidepressant medications. But most of our serotonin is found in the gut. Whereas serotonin does contribute to gut-derived satiety signals, it also influences the immune system, and can signal pain, inflammation, and the feeling of nausea (Mawe 2013, O'Mahony 2015). It does this by interacting with nerves that innervate the gut, notably the vagus nerve. In this way serotonin contributes to the sensory modality of *interoception*, and may exert an influence on mood, cognition, and arousal via this pathway.

Endocrine cells are not the only source of hormones and other signaling molecules in the gut (Lyte 2013). Microbes also produce hormones and neurotransmitters such as dopamine, GABA, and serotonin. These microbial products seem to regulate gut functions and may contribute to the mechanisms by which gut microbes influence mood (Lyte 2013; and discussed further in Chapter 17).

What Happens in the Gut Does Not Stay in the Gut Part III: Neural pathways for Gut-Related Signals

What happens in the gut is relevant for every tissue of the body, but the relationship between the gut and the brain is special. The gut is a major source of signals associated with interoception, and these signals influence mood, motivation, and other brain functions. This is why gut disorders are so often accompanied by mood and other *sickness syndrome* symptoms. Interoceptive signals from the gut are carried by the vagus and the splanchnic/mesenteric sympathetic sensory nerves (Abdullah 2020, Jacobson 2021).

The vagus nerve: The vagus nerve is the major nerve of the parasympathetic system. *Vagus* means wanderer. The vagus nerve wanders all over the inside of our bodies, emerging from the brainstem to innervate the throat, the back of our ears, esophagus, heart, lungs, and everything in the abdominal cavity except the spleen (Neuhuber 2021). The vagus also innervates part of the pelvis including the uterus and possibly the urinary bladder (Neuhuber 2021). The parasympathetic system, sometimes called the cranio-sacral system, is mostly concerned with regulation of physiological systems in a way that facilitates optimal functioning or homeostasis. This involves supporting regulatory behaviors such as eating and drinking, digesting food, salivation, and returning physiology to a baseline after meeting a challenge. The wandering nature of the vagus nerve makes it well-suited to monitor and modulate most physiological systems.

Vagal sensory nerves respond to the gut hormones that signal hunger and satiety, supporting the gut factors that help control appetite and influence motivation. Vagal sensory neurons also respond to immune-related signals such as pro-inflammatory cytokines, microbe-related products, and pathogenic microbes (Dantzer 1998, Maier 1998, De La Serre 2015, Goehler 2005). For example, lipopolysaccharides (LPS) are shed by Gram-negative bacteria, and act as a PAMP, which can signal the presence of pathogens or bacterial overgrowth. Vagal transmission of these kinds of signals helps activate host-defense responses, including *sickness* behaviors. Thus, the vagus is one important pathway by which foods and inflammation can influence mood and behavior.

The sympathetic nerves: Like the vagus nerve, *sympathetic sensory* (afferent) nerves are responsive to cytokines and other immune mediators that signal inflammation. The afferent nerves of the sympathetic system are interesting, in that they can act as both sensory and motor nerves. They contain neuropeptides, such as Substance P and calcitonin gene-related peptide (CGRP). When the nerves are activated, usually because of inflammation or some foods, such as hot peppers, they send sensory signals to the spinal cord. These signals can activate brain pathways which carry information about potential threats. At the same, these nerves also release neuropeptides into the gut where they act to modulate inflammation (Populin 2021). In this way, sympathetic afferent nerve pathways both inform the brain about conditions in the gut and act to influence these same conditions.

This type of afferent nerve is found in other places in the body where it contributes to pain signaling. Indeed, these afferent nerves seem to play a critical role in the phenomenon of *visceral hypersensitivity*, which is a feature of both IBS and heartburn (Populin 2021). Both Substance P and CGRP contribute to some features of inflammation, such as swelling, but they have opposite effects on immune cells (Populin 2021). The effects of Substance P on cytokine-producing immune cells is to increase production of pro-inflammatory cytokines, but CGRP acts to down-regulate pro-inflammatory cytokines (Straub 2008, Populin 2021). The enteric nervous system also uses these and other neuropeptides (Populin 2021). This arrangement allows the nerves that innervate the gut the ability to fine-tune immune responses and inflammation.

Brain Influences on Gut Functions

Although the enteric nervous system can manage most aspects of digestion on its own, the brain influences its function based on other ongoing situations in the body, providing a direct mechanism for the effects of psychological effects of stress on the gut. The vagus and sympathetic nerves both contain motor components that regulate gut function by influencing the enteric neurons.

Vagal motor nerves play an important role in stomach emptying, and facilitate digestion and absorption, including secretions from the pancreas such as digestive enzymes and the hormone insulin. In fact, the vagus mediates the cephalic phase of digestion, in which the taste or smell of food can cause insulin and digestive enzyme release, and the perception of being hungry (Veedfald 2016). This helps prepare the gut for the arrival of food.

The most exciting recent discovery related to motor functions of the vagus is that the activation of vagal motor neurons exerts potent anti-inflammatory actions (Borovikova 2000, Populin 2021). The principal neurotransmitter used by the vagus, acetylcholine, acts directly via the ⍺-7 nicotinic cholinergic receptor on the immune cells responsible for inflammation (Populin 2021). This inhibits the activation of NFkB and the release of pro-inflammatory cytokines. Therapeutic stimulation of the vagus improves inflammatory bowel and other inflammatory disorders such as fibromyalgia and rheumatoid arthritis (Bonaz 2017, Populin 2021, Courties 2021). Mind-body modalities, such as yoga and meditation, can activate vagal motor neurons, suggesting that such practices could be helpful for reducing inflammation and managing gut disorders (Bonaz 2017).

The sympathetic motor nerves emerge from the thoraco-lumbar spinal cord and target a chain of ganglia, or collections of nerve cells, that run adjacent to the spinal column. This *sympathetic chain* interacts to co-ordinate physiological responses to challenges. The sympathetic motor nerves act broadly to ensure adequate blood supply (via effects on the cardiovascular system) and adequate metabolic fuel (e.g., via effects on the liver to release glucose into the blood) for the body to adjust to changing conditions. For the gut this means that blood flow is directed away from the gut to make it more available for the rest of the body, and digestion is slowed down. At the same time, sympathetic nerves influence secretomotor neurons to reduce the flow of fluid into the gut lumen, ensuring adequate blood volume for the rest of the body to help meet the challenge (Lomax 2010).

Bidirectional communication between the gut and brain involves both circulating mediators and neural pathways.

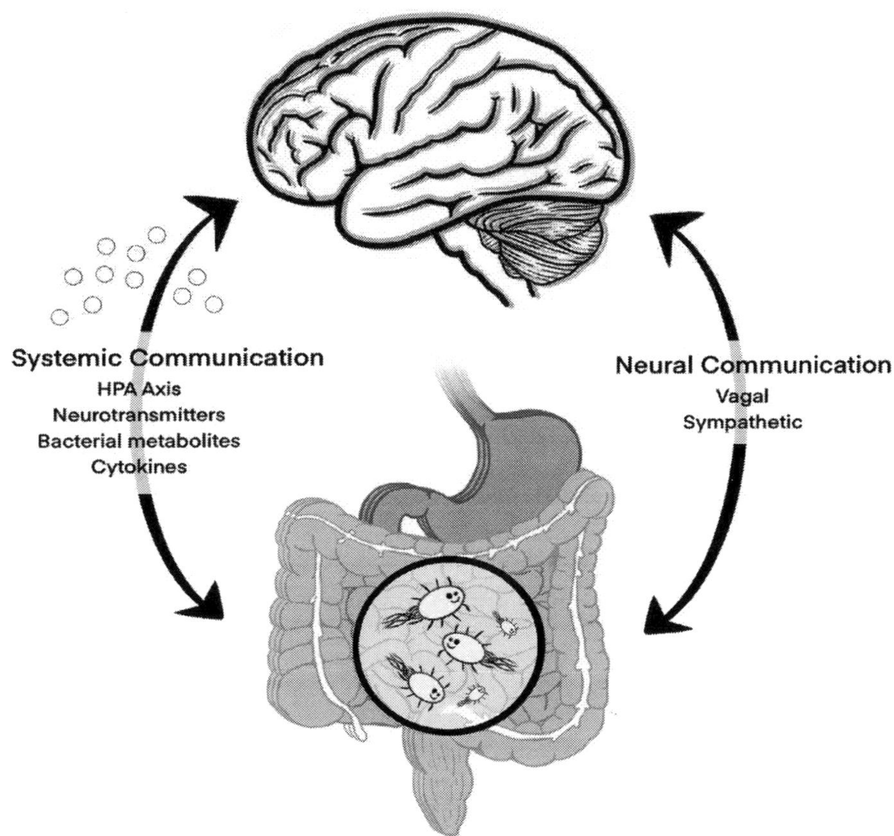

Figure legend: The brain and the gut communicate with one another in both directions. Signals can be sent from gut to brain or from brain to gut through either neuronal pathways or as chemical messengers through the blood.

Like vagal motor neurons, sympathetic motor neurons can influence immune cells in the gut. Sympathetic motor neurons release norepinephrine. When acting at beta receptors, this neurotransmitter reduces inflammation (Populin 2021). Sympathetic nerve fibers innervate Peyer's patches, and activation of beta receptors reduces the release of pro-inflammatory cytokines and polarizes macrophages to the M2 anti-inflammatory phenotype. Consistent with this, the use of beta-blocking drugs, such as for hypertension, is associated with worsening of inflammation and increased relapse in people with inflammatory bowel disorder (Populin 2021).

Together, the vagus and sympathetic nerves provide fast, bidirectional communication between the gut and the brain.

Key Points

- The gut has specialized regions along its length, including areas for chewing food, swallowing, breaking food down, absorbing it, reabsorbing water, and finally excreting. These functions are mostly coordinated by the neurons in the gut, known as the "gut brain."
- The main function of the gut is absorbing nutrients, but it also helps control eating behavior and other brain functions via the sensory modality of interoception. The gut plays an important role in immune function as well.
- What happens in the gut does not stay in the gut, because the gut communicates with the rest of the body via hormones, nervous system connections, and its influence on immune cells. Gut problems are associated with other disorders including asthma, autoimmune conditions, metabolic diseases, and neurodegenerative disorders.
- The nerves that connect the nervous system with the gut can influence inflammation, providing a pathway by which mental states can influence gut health.

References

Abdullah N, Defaye M, Altier C. Neural control of gut homeostasis. American Journal of Physiology Gastrointestinal and Liver Physiology, 319: G718-732, 2020.

Bingula R, Filaire M, Radosevic-Robin N, Bey M, Berthoud J-Y, Bernaleir-Donadille A, et al. Desired turbulence? Gut-lung axis, immunity, and lung cancer. Journal of Oncology, 2017:5035371, 2017.

Bonaz B, Sinninger V, Pellissier S. The vagus nerve in the neuro-immune axis: Implications in the pathology of the gastrointestinal tract. Frontiers in Immunology, 8:1452, 2017.

Borokovikova LV, Ivanova S, Zhang M, Yang H, Botchkina GI, Watkins LR, et al. Vagus nerve stimulation attenuates the systemic response to endotoxin. Nature, 405:458-462, 2000.

Brusselaers N, Engstrand L, Lagergren J. Maintenance proton pump inhibition and the risk of oesophageal cancer. Cancer Epidemiology, 53:172-177, 2018

Cai S, Fan Y, Zhang B, Lin J, Yang X Liu Y, et al. Appendectomy is associated with alteration of human gut bacterial and fungal communities. Frontiers in Microbiology, 12:724980, 2021.

Chen G, Chen Z-m, Fan X-y, Jin Y-l. Gut-brain-skin axis in psoriasis: a review. Dermatological Therapy, 11:25-38, 2021.

Courties A, Berenbaum F, Sellam J. Vagus nerve stimulation in musculoskeletal diseases. Joint Bone Spine, 88:105149, 2021.

Dantzer R, Bluthe RM, Laye S, Bret-Dibat JL, Parnet P, Kelly KW. Cytokines and sickness behavior. Annals of the New York Academy of Sciences, 840:289-300, 1998.

de La Serre CB, de Lartique G, Raybould HE. Chronic exposure to low dose bacterial lipopolysaccharide inhibits leptin signaling in vagal afferent neurons. Physiology and Behavior, 139:188-194, 2015.

De Martinis M, Sirufo MM, Suppa M, Ginaldi L. New perspective on food allergy. International Journal of Molecular Sciences, 21:1474, 2020.

Ford AC, Sperber AD, Corsetti M, Camilleri M. Irritable bowel syndrome. Lancet, 396:1675-1688, 2020.

Forkosh E, Ilan Y. The heart-gut axis: new target for atherosclerosis and congestive heart failure therapy. Open Heart, 2019;6: e000993, 2019.

Furness JB. The enteric nervous system and neurogastroenterology. Nature Reviews Gastroenterology and Hepatology, 9:286-294, 2012.

Goehler LE, Gaykema RP, Opitz N, Reddaway R, Badr N, Lyte M. Activation on vagal afferents and central autonomic pathways: early responses to intestinal infection with Campylobacter jejuni. Brain, Behavior, and Immunity, 19:334-344, 2005.

Grover M, Farrugia G, Stanghellini V. Gastroparesis: A turning point in understanding and treatment. Gut, 68:2238-2250, 2019.

Hiltensperger M, Beltran E, Kant R, Tyystjarvi S, Lepennetier G, Dominguez Moreno H, et al. Skin and gut imprinted T helper cell subsets exhibit distinct functional phenotypes in central nervous system autoimmunity. Nature Immunology, 22:880-892, 2021.

Jaynes M, Kumar AB. The risks of long-term use of proton pump inhibitors: a critical review. Therapeutic Advances in Drug Safety, 10:1-3, 2019.

Keppler SJ, Goess MC, Heinze JM. The wanderings of gut-derived IgA plasma cells: Impact on systemic immune responses. Frontiers in Immunology, 12:670290, 2021.

Kosiewicz MM, Dryden GW, Chhabra A, Alard P. Relationship between gut microbiota and development of T cell associated disease. FEBS letters, 588:4195-4206, 2014.

Latorre R, Sternini C, De Giorgio R, Greenwood-Van Meerveld B. Enteroendocrine cells: a review of their in brain-gut communication. Neurogastroenterology and Motility, 28:620-630, 2016.

Lee H-S, Lobbestael E, Vermeire S, Sabino J. Inflammatory bowel disease and Parkinson's disease common pathophysiological links. Gut, 70:408-417, 2021.

Lomax AR, Sharkey KA, Furness JB. The participation of the sympathetic innervation of the gastrointestinal tract in disease states. Neurogastroenterology and Motility, 22:7-18, 2010.

Lyte M. Microbial endocrinology in the microbiome-gut-brain axis: how bacterial production and utilization of neurochemicals influence behavior. PLOS Pathogens, 9:e1003726, 2013.

Maier SF, Goehler LE, Fleshner M, Watkins LR. The role of the vagus nerve in cytokine-to-brain communication. Annals of the New York Academy of Sciences, 840:289-300, 1998.

Mawe GM, Hoffman JM. Serotonin signaling in the gastrointestinal tract: Functions, dysfunctions, and therapeutic targets. Nature Reviews Gastroenterology and Hepatology, 10:473-486, 2013.

Neuhuber WL, Berhoud H-R. The functional anatomy of the vagus nerve. Autonomic Neuroscience: Basic and Clinical, 236:102887, 2021.

O'Mahony SM, Clarke G, Borre YE, Dinan TG, Cryan JF. Serotonin, tryptophan metabolism and the brain-gut-microbiome axis. Behavioral Brain Research, 277:32-48, 2015.

Omenetti A, Pizarro TT. The Treg/Th17 axis: A dynamic balance regulated by the gut microbiome. Frontiers in Immunology, 6:639, 2015.

Oudman E, Kijnia JW, van Dam M, Ulas Biter L, Postma A. preventing Wernicke encephalopathy after bariatric surgery. Obesity Surgery, 28:2060-2068, 2018.

Populin L, Stebbing MJ, Furness JB. Neuronal regulation of the gut immune system and neuromodulation for treating inflammatory bowel disease. FASEB BioAdvances, 3:953-966, 2021.

Sica A, Mantovani A. Macrophage plasticity and polarization: in vivo veritas. The Journal of Clinical Investigation, 122:787-795, 2012.

Sipponen P, Maaroos H-I. Chronic gastritis. Scandinavian Journal of Gastroenterology, 50:657-667, 2015.

Spencer NJ, Hu H. Enteric nervous system: sensory transduction, neural circuits and gastrointestinal motility. Nature Reviews Gastroenterology and Hepatology, 17:338-351, 2020.

Sternini C, Anselmi L, Rozengurt E. Enteroendocrine cells: a site of "taste" in gastrointestinal chemosensing. Current Opinion in Endocrinology, Diabetes and Obesity, 15:73-78, 2008.

Straub RH, Grum F, Strauch U, Capellino S, Bataille F, Bleich A, Falk W, Schölmerich J, Obermeier F. Anti-inflammatory role of sympathetic nerves in chronic intestinal inflammation. Gut, 57:911-921, 2008.

Tack J, Carbone F. Functional dyspepsia and gastroparesis. Current Opinion in Gastroenterology, 33:446-454, 2017.

Takiishi T, Morales Fenero CI, Olsen Saraiva Camar N. Intestinal barrier and gut microbiota: Shaping our immune responses throughout life. Tissue Barriers, 5: e1373208, 2017.

van IJzendoorn SCD, Derkinderen P. The intestinal barrier in Parkinson's disease: current state of the knowledge. Journal of Parkinson's Disease, 9: S323-S329, 2019.

Veedfald S, Plamboeck A, Deacon CF, Hartmann B, Knob FK, Vilsboll T, Holst JJ. Cephalic phase secretion of insulin and other enteropancreatic hormones in humans. American Journal of Physiology Gastrointestinal and Liver Physiology, 310: G43-G51, 2016.

Wang J, Chen W-D, Wang Y-D. The relationship between gut microbiota and inflammatory diseases: The role of macrophages. Frontiers in Microbiology, 11:1065.

Warren CM, Jiang J, Gupta R. Epidemiology and burden of food allergy. Current Allergy and Asthma Reports, 20:6, 2020.

Yoo BB, Mazmanian SK. The enteric network: Interactions between the immune and nervous systems of the gut. Immunity, 46: 910-926, 2017.

- WHAT IS THE "GUT BARRIER?"

- ORGANIZATION OF THE GUT BARRIER

- THE IMPORTANCE OF BUTYRATE

- PERMEABILITY AND "LEAKY GUT"

- GUT BARRIER INFLAMMATION: TOXINS, MICROBES, AND STRESS

- KEY POINTS

Many chronic health conditions are associated with "gut barrier" inflammation or increased permeability. This gut barrier inflammation has also been referred to as "leaky gut." Non-alcoholic fatty liver disease, Type 3 diabetes, Gulf War Syndrome, Alzheimer's disease, autism, inflammatory bowel disease, irritable bowel disease, autoimmune diseases including multiple sclerosis and rheumatoid arthritis, asthma, as well as food allergies and sensitivities have been associated with gut barrier inflammation and leaky gut (Camilleri 2019, Cui 2019, Julio-Pieper 2016, Obrenovich 2018, Sturgeon 2016, Viggiano 2015).

Most of these disorders are associated with mood and cognitive problems, and fatigue, and can seriously affect how we feel. These symptoms are characteristic of *sickness behavior*, but frequently are misidentified by clinicians and patients alike. The symptoms are mediated by the brain, and many of the disorders are not obviously associated with the gut. As such, mood and cognitive problems are often attributed to factors other than gut inflammation, for example, stress or psychosomatic illness. Often, the cause of the symptoms remains mysterious. Understanding what exactly the gut barrier is, and how problems with it can arise, can help clarify the connection between leaky gut and symptoms of chronic health conditions. This understanding can help us make dietary choices that support the gut barrier and improve the way we feel.

What is the "Gut Barrier?"

The fact that strictly speaking, the hollow part of the gut is outside the body poses serious challenges for the health of the gut. The gut barrier consists of two components: a *physical barrier* formed by a lining of epithelial cells, covered by one or two layers of protective mucus, and a *functional* barrier, formed by the activities of other cells, including immune cells, gut nervous system cells, and microbes (Hansson 2019, Cui 2019, Takiishi 2017, You 2021).

Physical barrier: The mucus or mucosa is a thinner, single-layer barrier in the stomach and small intestine, because food particles need to penetrate the mucus in order be absorbed. The mucus layer is much thicker, and double-layered in the colon (Hansson 2019). The colon contains many more microbes that might be dangerous, as well as bile acids secreted to digest fat that can damage the epithelial cells. These added threats warrant a thicker and potent layer of protection. In addition to being thick and sticky, mucus contains IgA antibodies that can bind to toxins and pathogenic microbes, neutralizing them.

The epithelium is the single layer of cells that line the hollow part, or lumen, of the gut. It contains mostly cells that absorb nutrients, as well as endocrine cells that serve as sensory detectors of the kind of nutrients released from food particles, and some specialized collections of immune cells. As the drawing below shows, the gut epithelium consists of *columnar* cells, which are lined up like columns. These columnar cells are held together by proteins, including the barrier proteins ZO-1 & gliadin among others (Camilleri 2012, Sturgeon 2016). Most nutrients are absorbed directly by the epithelial cells, but some substances enter the body between the cells.

Functional barrier: Because the gut must come into direct contact with food, the gut is inherently vulnerable to potential pathogens and toxins in that food. Protecting, supporting, and defending the gut's integrity requires a collaboration of several different cell types. These include specialized epithelial cells, immune cells, and *enteric glial cells*. These cells are even aided by certain types of bacteria.

Commensal bacteria are those that belong to our resident bacterial population. They reside on the outer, or lumenal, sides of the mucus layer. These microbes contribute to gut barrier function in a variety of ways (Hiippala 2018). They help gut barrier function by increasing the expression of the proteins that hold the epithelial cells closely together, regulating gut immune responses, and discouraging the growth of pathogens (Grainger 2013, Kumamoto 2020). The role of microbes in gut barrier health is an active area of research because management of microbial populations, for example by diet, could be an effective way to maintain healthy gut barrier function.

Organization of the Gut Barrier

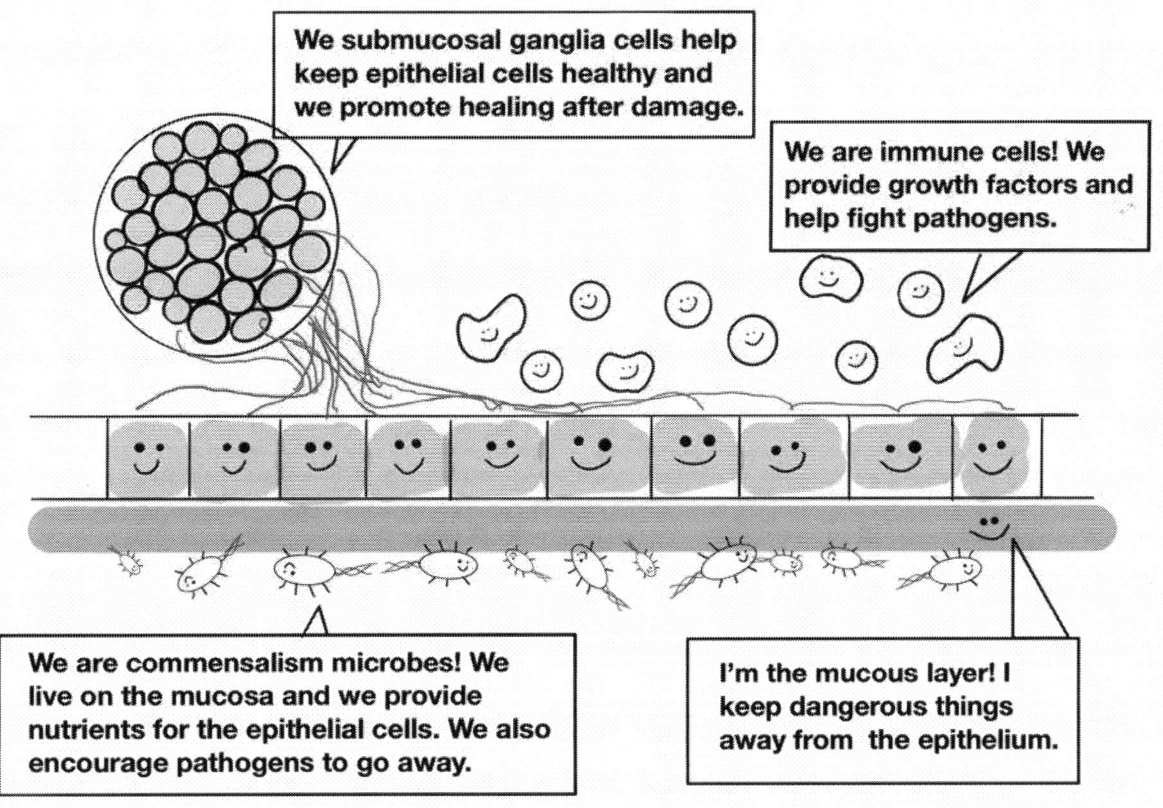

The Importance of Butyrate

One important way in which some commensal bacteria contribute to gut barrier health is by producing short-chain fatty acids (Mathewson 2016, Vital 2017). Gut epithelial cells use one of these fatty acids, butyrate, as their main source of energy. Most of the butyrate they use is provided by microbes (Bach Knudsen 2018). In addition, immune cells have receptors for butyrate, perhaps accounting for butyrate's purported anti-inflammatory effects (Bach Knudsen 2018). This is important because the gut needs to be in an anti-inflammatory state to prevent immune reactions to food. Indeed, the loss of immune cell *tolerance* to food leads to food allergies and food sensitivities that can induce and maintain inflammation at the gut barrier. Studies of microbial populations in humans have found that having fewer of the species that produce butyrate is a common feature of many diseases, including colorectal cancer (Vital 2017, Chen 2018). Thus, one way that healthy microbe populations support a healthy gut and promote health in the rest of the body is by providing butyrate.

How can we encourage the bacteria that produce butyrate? Diet is the most important factor influencing butyrate-producing bacteria (Vital 2015). The bacterial species that produce butyrate ferment fiber, especially *resistant starches* found in whole grains and legumes, and fructo-oligosaccharides, found in bananas, onions, and asparagus (Bach Knudsen 2018). Some foods also contain low levels of butyrate, including some vegetable oils, and cow's milk (Stilling 2016). The richest dietary source of butyrate is butter, and indeed the word *butyrate* is derived from the Greek word for butter. In addition, foods that contain polyphenols, such as quercetin, support the growth of gut microbes (Rodriques-Daza 2021). Fruits and vegetables including onions, red grapes, apples, cherries, green leafy vegetables, and citrus fruit help support microbes that produce butyrate.

Permeability and "Leaky Gut"

The main challenge for the gut barrier is that of determining whether a substance in the lumen is nutritious and should be absorbed, is a friendly microbe and should be tolerated, or is a toxin or unfriendly microbe that should be kept out of the body or neutralized by the immune system. This challenge of distinguishing nutritious vs. dangerous is managed by the regulation of gut *permeability*. Paracellular permeability describes how easily things are absorbed by the epithelial cells or are able to slip in between them. If the cells are too loose, toxins and aggressive microbes can get in, which is thought to account for the symptoms of leaky gut (Camilleri 2019).

A key factor driving increased permeability is inflammation (Barbara 2021). Pro-inflammatory cytokines such as TNF directly increase permeability, and inflammation can disrupt the balance of immune, neural, and microbial factors that maintain gut barrier integrity (Ahmad 2017). Increased permeability allows the translocation of pathogenic microbes and/or their pro-inflammatory products, such as lipopolysaccharides, further driving inflammation and permeability (Akdis 2021).

Symptoms of leaky gut extend far beyond the gut. Severe cases can include malnutrition because inflammation damages the cells that absorb food. But even milder cases are associated with brain-mediated symptoms. This sickness syndrome can include fatigue, mood disorders, and cognitive fuzziness (Ganda Mall 2018). These symptoms impair quality of life and can contribute to or complicate other chronic diseases. Moreover, immune dysregulation associated with increased permeability can affect skin, bone, and lungs and is suspected as a key factor in the dramatic increase in allergy and autoimmunity that is happening worldwide (Akdis 2021).

Gut Barrier Inflammation: Toxins, Microbes, and Stress

Because inflammation, including low-grade systemic inflammation, is a pathophysiological hallmark of gut barrier dysfunction, and because the gut barrier is a critical yet vulnerable interface between the inside and outside world, keeping it healthy is of utmost importance (Akdis 2021). So, to make good decisions about diet that can help maintain gut barrier health, we need to know how the gut barrier can be impaired.

Toxins and allergens: Toxins are molecules that can harm the body, or that immune cells perceive to be dangerous. Molecules that immune cells perceive as threats are called *xenobiotics.* By activating immune cells, toxins can act like the damage and danger signals DAMPS and PAMPs and directly induce inflammation at the gut barrier (Akdis 2021). Toxins include industrial by-products that find their way into food or water, or herbicides or pesticides used in the production of food (Di Tommaso 2021). For instance, glyphosate, marketed as Round-up®, is widely used in agriculture as an herbicide, and is also sprayed on grains such as wheat, to dry them just before harvest. Glyphosate residues can be detected in wheat flour, where it has been documented to induce gut barrier inflammation and leakiness (Ding 2021). It is thought that some cases of wheat or gluten sensitivity may in fact be a glyphosate reaction (Mumolo 2020). It has been hypothesized that the dramatic increase in food allergies in recent years follows from glyphosate or other toxins acting as DAMPs and sensitizing the immune system to other food constituents, such as gluten (Smith 2017). Other types of molecules used in food processing, such as dyes and preservatives, can also act as DAMPs to increase inflammation, as can advanced glycation end-products (AGEs) in processed foods (Camilleri 2019, Smith 2017). This is likely one reason highly processed foods, such as commercial baked goods, lunch meat, and hot dogs are associated with a wide variety of chronic diseases. A good way to avoid toxins and pesticides found in commercially processed food is to eat organic or homegrown foods.

Pathogenic microbes: Damage to the physical barrier can be caused by pathogenic bacteria that break down the mucin proteins that make of the mucus barrier, or by malfunction of the epithelial cells, such as goblet cells, that produce mucus (Barbara 2021, Nystrom 2021). Damage to the mucus barriers is a hallmark of the inflammatory bowel disorders Crohn's Disease and Ulcerative Colitis. Damage to the mucosa allows microbes to contact the epithelial cells, inducing an immune response, followed by inflammation that is poorly regulated due to genetic factors. On the other hand, some microbes help protect the mucus (Engevik 2019). Strategies to help maintain healthy microbes, and thus a healthy mucus barrier, will be addressed in Chapter 17.

Stress: Both physical stress and psychological stress have long been known to cause gut barrier dysfunction. Surgery and traumatic injury have particularly been associated with gut barrier dysfunction. For instance, the association of a stressful lifestyle and GI ulcers inspired decades of research into the relationships between stress pathways in the brain and increased gastric acid secretion, which was the presumed mechanism producing the ulcer. Later it was shown that an overgrowth of the bacterium,

Helicobacter pylori, was the culprit, by inducing inflammation at the gut barrier (Blosse 2018). More recent studies have shown that stress exerts a marked deleterious action on gut barrier structure and function (Hatay 2017, Keita 2010, Chen 2003, Lyte 2011, Yang 2006).

Stress can directly induce increased permeability, in association with elevated local levels of pro-inflammatory cytokines such as TNF (Barbara 2021, Hattay 2017). These cytokines act to reduce the production of the proteins that hold the epithelial cells together, directly making them leaky. Other hormones that can be associated with stress, including corticotropin-releasing hormone (CRH, produced in the gut), also lead to increased leakiness (Keita 2010). In addition, some pathogenic microbes have receptors for catecholamines such as norepinephrine, which are also elevated during stress (Lyte 2011). The activation of these receptors increases the microbes' growth and virulence. In this way stress can drive inflammation by increasing the permeability of the gut, which can allow microbes or pro-inflammatory microbe products (such as LPS, as acting as a PAMP) across the gut barrier, activating an immune response. This leads to further, often chronic inflammation, and via interoceptive gut-to-brain connections, drives feelings of fatigue, low mood, and cognitive fuzziness. This is one of the principal mechanisms by which stress in the mind can set up stress in the body, which feeds back to drive further stress in the mind.

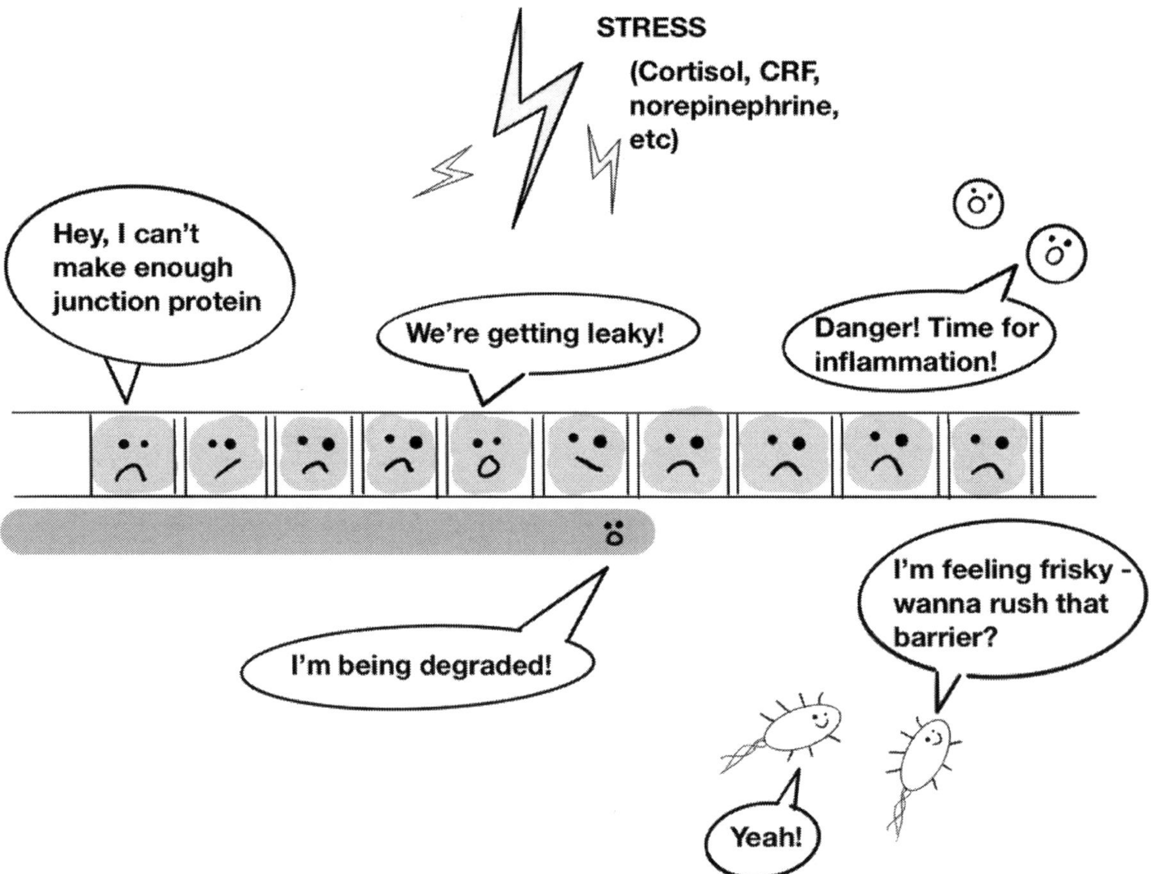

Figure legend: Stress can cause leaky gut and inflammation through multiple mechanisms. Stress may signal dangerous bacteria to grow and cause degradation of the mucous layer, and cause epithelial cells to not make enough of the proteins that hold them together.

Key Points

- The lining of the gut forms a barrier between us and the outside world.
- The gut lining is a fragile barrier and can become damaged or inflamed from toxins, pathogens, or allergens.
- When the gut barrier is inflamed, it can become more permeable, creating a "leaky gut." This can both increase inflammation in the gut and lead to many other health problems in the body including metabolic, autoimmune, respiratory, and neurological disorders.
- Stress has powerful effects on gut barrier permeability, and this is an important way that it contributes to gut disorders and brain-mediated *sickness syndrome* symptoms.

References

Ahmad R, Sorrell MF, Batra SK, Dhawan P, Singh AB. Gut permeability and mucosal inflammation: bad, good or context dependent. Mucosal Immunology, 10:307-317, 2017.

Akdis CA. Does the epithelial barrier hypothesis explain the increase in allergy, autoimmunity and other chronic conditions? Nature Reviews Immunology, 21:739-751, 2021.

Bach Knudsen KE, Lærke HN, Hedemann MS, Nielsen TS, Ingerslev AK, Gundelund Nielsen DS, et al. Impact of Diet-Modulated Butyrate Production on Intestinal Barrier Function and Inflammation. Nutrients, 10, 1499, 2018.

Barbara G, Barbaro MR, Fuscho D, Palombo M, Falagone F, Cromon C, et al. Inflammatory and microbiota-related regulation of the intestinal epithelial barrier. Frontiers in Nutrition, 8:718356, 2021.

Blosse A, Lehours P, Wilson KT, Gobert AP. Helicobacter: Inflammation, immunology, and vaccines. Helicobacter, 23: e12517, 2018.

Camilleri M. Leaky gut: mechanisms, measurement and clinical implications in humans. Gut, 68:1516-1526, 2019.

Camilleri M, Madsen K, Spiiler R, Van Meerveld BG, Verne GN. Intestinal barrier function in health and gastrointestinal disease. Neurogastroenterology and Motility, 24:503-512, 2012.

Chen C, Brown DR, Xie Y, Green BT, Lyte M. Catecholamines modulated Escherichia coli 0157:H7 adherence to murine cecal mucosa. Shock, 20:183-188, 2003.

Chen J, Vitetta L. Inflammation-Modulating Effect of Butyrate in the Prevention of Colon Cancer by Dietary Fiber. Clinical Colorectal Cancer, 17: e541-544. 2018.

Cui Y, Wang Q, Chang R, Zhou, Xu C. Intestinal barrier function- Non-alcoholic fatty liver disease interactions and possible role of gut microbiota. Journal of Agricultural and Food Chemistry, 67:2754-2762, 2019.

Ding W, Shangguan Y, Zhu Y, Sultan Y, Feng Y, Zhang B, et al. Negative impacts of microcystin-LR and glyphosate on zebrafish intestine: Linked with gut microbiota and microRNAs? Environmental Pollution, 286:117685, 2021.

Di Tommaso N, Gasbarrini A, Ponziani FR. Intestinal barrier in human health and disease. International Journal of Environmental Research and Public Health, 18:12836, 2021.

Engevik M, Luk B, Chang-Graham A, Hall A, Herrmann B, Ruan E, et al. *Bifidobacterium dentium* fortifies the intestinal mucus layer via autophagy and calcium signaling pathways. mBio, 10:01087-19, 2019.

Forkosh E, Ilan Y. The heart-gut axis: new target for atherosclerosis and congestive heart failure therapy. Open Heart, 6: e000993, 2019.

Ganda Mall, J-P, Ostlund-Lagerstrom L, Martin LindqvistC, Algilani S, Rasaol D, Repsilber D, Brummer RJ, Keita AV, Schoultz I. Are self-reported gastrointestinal symptoms among older adults associated with increased intestinal permeability and psychological distress? BMC Geriatrics, 18:75, 2018.

Grainger JR, Wohlfert EA, Fuss IJ, Bouladoux, Askenase MH, Legrand F, et al. Inflammatory monocytes regulated pathologic responses to commensals during acute gastrointestinal infection. Nature Medicine, 19:713-721, 2013.

Hansson GG. Mucus and mucins in diseases of the intestinal and respiratory tracts. Journal of Internal Medicine, 285, 479-490, 2019.

Hattay P, Prusator DK, Tran L, Greenwood-Van Meerveld B. Psychological stress-induced colonic barrier dysfunction: Role of immune-mediated mechanisms. Neurogastroenterology and Motility, 29: e13043, 2017.

Hiippala K, Jouhten H, Ronkainen A, Hartikainen A, Kainulainen V, Jalanka J, Satokari R. The Potential of Gut Commensals in Reinforcing Intestinal Barrier Function and Alleviating Inflammation. Nutrients, 10:988, 2018.

Keita AV, Soderholm JD, Ericson A-C. Stress-induced barrier disruption of rat follicle-associated epithelium involves corticotropin-releasing hormone, acetylcholine, substance P, and mast cells. Neurogastroenterology and Motility, 22:770-e222, 2010.

Julio-Pieper M, Bravo JA. Intestinal Barrier and Behavior. International Review of Neurobiology, Volume 13:127-141, 2016.

Kumamoto CA, Gresnigt, Hube B. The gut, the bad and the harmless: *Candida albicans* as a commensal and opportunistic pathogen in the intestine. Current Opinion in Microbiology, 56:7-15, 2020.

Lyte M, Vulchanova L, Brown DR. Stress at the intestinal surface: catecholamines and mucosa-bacteria interactions. Cell and Tissue Research, 343:23-32, 2011.

Mathewson ND, Jenq R, Mathew AV, Koenigsknecht M, Hanash A, Toubai T, et al. Gut microbiome-derived metabolites modulated intestinal epithelial cell damage and mitigate graft-versus-host disease. Nature Immunology, 17:505-513, 2016.

Mumolo MG, Rettura F, Melissari S, Costa F, Ricchiuti A, Ceccarelli L, et al. Is gluten the only culprit for non-celiac gluten/wheat sensitivity? Nutrients, 12:3785, 2020.

Nystrom EEL, Martinez-Abad B, Arike L, Birchenough GMH, Nonnecke EB, Castillo PA, et al. An intercrypt subpopulation of goblet cells is essential for colonic mucus barrier function. Science,372(6539), 2021.

Obrenovich MEM. Leaky gut, leaky brain? Microorganisms, 6:107, 2018.

Roager HM, Vogt JK, Kristensen M, et al. Whole grain-rich diet reduces body weight and systemic low-grade inflammation without inducing major changes of the gut microbiome: a randomised cross-over trial. Gut, 68:83-93, 2019.

Rodrigues-Daza MC, Pulido-Mateos EC, Lupien-Meilleur J, Guyonnet D, Desjardins Y, Roy D. Polyphenol-mediated gut microbiota modulation: Toward prebiotics and further. Frontiers in Nutrition, 8:689456, 2021.

Smith PJ, Masilamani M, Li X-M, Sampson HA. The false alarm hypothesis: Food allergy is associated with high dietary advanced glycation end-products and pro-glycating dietary sugars that mimic alarmins. Journal of Allergy and Clinical Immunology, 139:429-437, 2017.

Stilling RM, van de Wouw M, Clarke G, Stanton C, Dinan TG, Cryan JF. The neuropharmacology of butyrate: The bread and butter of the microbiota-gut-brain axis? Neurochemistry International, 99:111-132, 2016.

Sturgeon C, Fasano A. Zonulin, a regulator of epithelial and endothelial barrier functions, and its involvement in chronic inflammatory diseases. Tissue Barriers, 4: e1251384, 2016.

Takiishi T, Morales Fenero CI, Olsen Saraiva Camar N. Intestinal barrier and gut microbiota: Shaping our immune responses throughout life. Tissue Barriers, 5: e1373208, 2017.

Viggiano D, Ianiro G, Vanella G, Bibbo S, Bruno G, Simeone G, Mele G. Gut barrier in health and disease: Focus on childhood. European Review for Medical and Pharmacological Sciences, 19:1077-1085, 2015.

Vital M, Gao J, Rizzo M, Harrison T, Tiedje JM. Diet is a major factor governing the fecal butyrate-producing community structure across Mammalia, Aves, and Reptilia. The ISME Journal, 9:832-843, 2014.

Vital M, Karch A, Pieper DH. Colonic butyrate-producing communities in humans: an overview using omics data. mSystems, 2: e00130, 2017.

Yang P-C, Jury J, Soderholm JD, Sherman PM, McKay DM, Perdue MH. Chronic psychological stress in rats induces intestinal sensitization to luminal antigens. American Journal of Pathology, 168:104-114, 2006.

You X-y, Zhang H-y, Han X, Wang F, Zhuang P-w, Zhang Y-j. Intestinal mucosal barrier is regulated by intestinal tract neuro-immune interplay. Frontiers in Pharmacology, 12:659726, 2021.

- OUR GUT MICROBES ARE FUNCTIONALLY PART OF "US"

- IMBALANCED MICROBES: LOSS OF MICROBIAL DIVERSITY LEADS TO DYSBIOSIS

- "OLD FRIENDS" REGULATE INFLAMMATION AND HELP MAINTAIN TOLERANCE TO FOODS

- BIDIRECTIONAL RELATIONSHIP OF MICROBES AND STRESS

- "OLD FRIENDS" HELP THE GUT BARRIER

- MICROBES AND MATERNITY

- FERMENTED FOODS: ANCIENT PROBIOTICS

- MICROBES DEPEND ON OUR DIET: ALL FOOD IS "PRE-BIOTIC"

- FURTHER CONSIDERATIONS

- KEY POINTS

Like most people in 1999, I was not giving much thought to the microbes in my gut. I had no idea of the important influence that microbes have on how I feel, until a colleague in the Psychoneuroimmunology Research Society, Dr. Mark Lyte, reported that inducing dysbiosis in the gut seemed to cause anxiety-like behavior in mice (Lyte 1998). This idea was met with skepticism. How could microbes in the gut influence the brain? Working together, we were able to show that the vagus nerve was rapidly activated by feeding the mice a load of bacteria. The dose of bacteria disrupted the balance of microbes in the gut. Then the vagus nerve activation transmitted a signal to the brain through this major interoceptive gut-brain communication pathway. We showed that vagus nerve activity changes the activity of neuronal networks in the brain known to be involved in the experience of anxiety (Goehler 2007).

We have known for centuries that we share our bodies with microbes, and that our resident or commensal microbes may be beneficial to our health. However, until we were able to show that bacteria can affect behavior, the relationships between us and our bacteria were assumed to be entirely local. We had no idea the extent that microbes can influence things likes mood, cognition, and even brain development that are fundamental to our sense of self (Bastiaanssen 2019, Dickerson 2017, Dinan 2015, Gonzalez-Aranciba 2019, Kelly 2015, Koopman 2017, Nguyen 2018, Rees 2018, Yang 2019).

Studies of human tissues have revealed that there are thousands of different species of microbes that include bacteria, viruses, and fungi/yeast, which inhabit our bodies (Martinez-Guryn 2019, Musumeci 2022). Most of these microbes live in our guts, with the largest population living in our colons. But we also have microbes on our skin, and in our lungs and other internal structures. There is even evidence we may have a few microbes in our brains. Many different laboratories have now reported physiological effects of microbes in the gut that go beyond brain effects, demonstrating that when microbial populations are disordered there are broad health consequences (de Morales 2017, McCoy 2018, Weiss 2017). It is becoming increasingly clear that the condition of our associated microbe communities markedly influences how we feel. The effect of diet on our microbes may be a major reason for the interrelationship between diet, and mental and physical health.

What do we know about a "healthy" microbial population?

Our Gut Microbes are Functionally Part of "Us"

We and our microbes exist in a symbiotic relationship, providing mutual benefit. We provide food and housing for them, and they, for example, provide us with beneficial nutrients, such as vitamin K and short-chain fatty acids like butyrate. This relationship is an active one, in that we communicate with them using the same hormone and neurotransmitter signals that our cells and tissues use to communicate within our bodies. For instance, bacteria respond to challenge/stress hormones such as norepinephrine, cortisol, corticotropin-releasing hormone (CRH), and gonadal steroid hormones including estrogens (Lyte 1992, Lyte 2014, Sarkodie 2019 Vom Steeg 2017). These substances influence bacterial behavior and growth (Lyte 1992, Moriera 2016). For instance, both norepinephrine and cortisol, which are part of the challenge/stress response, increase growth of microbial colonies and increase virulence of the microbes, making them behave in aggressive ways that may be damaging to our health. This hormonal influence on our microbes could be one way that stress increases susceptibility to diseases such as gastrointestinal infections or inflammation and dental diseases.

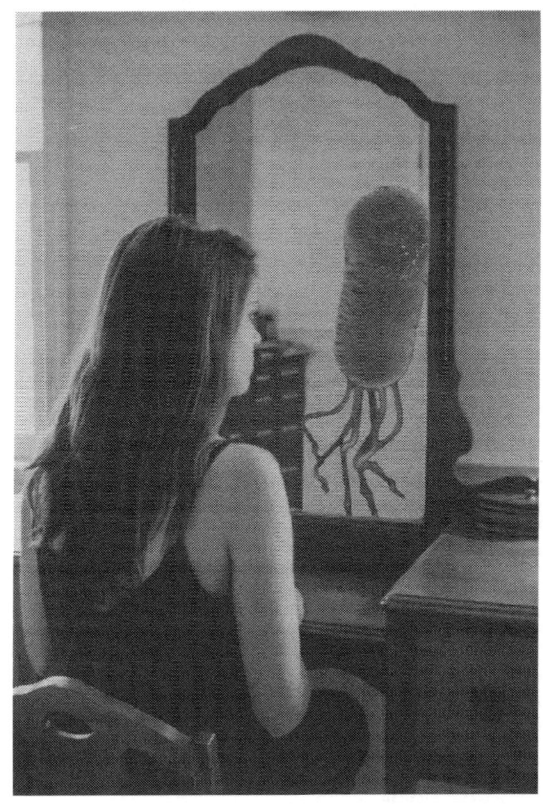

Similarly, studies have shown that gut bacteria produce many of the same signaling and metabolic substances that we do, including neurotransmitters such as serotonin, GABA, acetylcholine, and dopamine, as well as short-chain fatty acids and amino acid metabolites (Margolis 2021, Roschina 2016). These substances are known to exert biological effects on cells of our bodies, including neurons (Margolis 2021). For this reason, gut microbes can be thought as a "microbial endocrine organ" (Lyte 2016). In this way, microbes have a close and bidirectional relationship with our own cells, including brain cells.

Microbes may provide missing pieces of the puzzle of psychiatric and neurological diseases (Dickerson 2017, Firth 2019, Fitzgerald 2019, Margolis 2021, Nguyen 2018). Although the symptoms and correlates of brain-related diseases, such as Alzheimer's disease, schizophrenia spectrum disorders , autism spectrum disorders, and mood disorders, have been recognized for many years, we are still frustratingly far away from understanding just what causes them and how to reliably treat or cure them. Many different factors such as genetics, life history, and acute stress somehow interact to contribute to the causes and persistence of these conditions, resulting in rather individual experiences and etiology. It seems that some pieces of the brain disorder puzzle are missing, and decades of research have failed to close the gaps in treatment for many psychiatric disorders.

More recently, it has emerged that a hallmark of all these disorders is either systemic inflammation or neuroinflammation, raising the question of what drives persistent inflammation (Firth 2019, Maes 1995). Several lines of evidence now support a role for gut microbes. As described in Chapter 16, gut barrier dysfunction can drive inflammation, and gut microbes play key roles in keeping the gut barrier healthy. The condition called *dysbiosis* contributes to gut barrier impairment and low-grade inflammation. Dysbiosis describes the situation in which microbial populations are unbalanced and in which some microbes become aggressive. Indeed, gut dysbiosis is consistently associated with brain disorders, including Alzheimer's and Parkinson's disease, schizophrenia, autism, and mood disorders (Firth 2019, Kelly 2015, Koopman 2017, Li 2017, Rea 2016). Some studies have reported that probiotics can reduce depressive symptoms, promote resilience, and mitigate elevated cortisol during chronic stress (Park 2018). Taken together these observations support the idea that gut microbes are important factors in brain-related conditions. Indeed, perhaps the most surprising thing about our relationships with our microbes involves the influence they seem to exert on our minds.

Imbalanced Microbes: Loss of Microbial Diversity Leads to Dysbiosis

One of the main objectives driving research characterizing the patterns of microbes in the gut is to determine whether certain microbes or populations contribute to gut health, or to certain disease conditions. As yet, no pattern has been linked definitively to health or disease. Rather, having a larger number of different species, in other words having high *microbial diversity,* seems to be the most important single indicator of a healthy microbial population. Further, balance in the main groups, *Firmicutes* (mostly Gram-positive) and *Bacteroides* (Gram-negative) may be a key factor in a healthy bacterial population. Both groups contain *pathobionts,* as well as other species that are clearly beneficial. Pathobionts are resident microbes that can contribute to disease under some circumstances, but are not harmful under normal growth conditions.

Although there is still much to learn about the specific ways that microbes contribute to both health and disease, some themes are emerging from studies of people living in regions where many people live long, healthy lives. These regions have been dubbed "Blue Zones," and studies have examined the microbial populations in long-lived centenarians, or people who live beyond age 100, from these Blue Zones (Sato 2021, Tuikhar 2019). These studies provide important clues about what it takes to establish and maintain a healthy gut and microbial populations. The patterns of microbe populations in centenarians are similar across different geographical areas (Tuikhar 2019). One of the themes is that Blue Zone centenarians have microbe populations that are enriched in butyrate-producing bacteria that provide energy for the gut lining cells, as well as bacteria that are believed to help protect the mucin layer of the gut barrier (Tuikhar 2019). Similarly, Blue Zone centenarians have higher levels of the anti-inflammatory neurotransmitter GABA and the presence of GABA-producing bacteria, suggesting that microbial-produced GABA may be helping to maintain the gut barrier and the immune system in a tolerant, uninflamed state (Tuikhar 2019).

Although there are thousands of different microbial species that can inhabit humans, most healthy people living in "Westernized" countries have fewer different species than those living in non-industrialized regions. Many people, due to antibiotic use, food additives, pesticides, food choices or options, and generally poor nutrition, have low microbial diversity (Murdaca 2021). The urbanized Western lifestyle includes much more "hygienic" living conditions than the rural lifestyles typical of developing non-Westernized countries, with fewer opportunities for human interaction with microbes.

This, along with vaccination, has dramatically reduced the load of infectious diseases on human populations. These comparatively hygienic conditions are unfortunately associated with a rather dramatic increase in allergies, autoimmune diseases, and inflammatory bowel disease (IBD) (Murdaca 2021). In support of this idea, Blue Zone communities are typically rural, and people eat a traditional, diverse diet. Studies of centenarians from several different countries, including India, China, Japan, and Italy have demonstrated that unlike elderly people in Westernized cultures, who usually have less diversity in their microbial populations compared to younger people, these healthy, very elderly people have greater diversity (Tuikhara 2019).

Low microbial diversity is deleterious because it predisposes to dysbiosis, leading to overgrowth of some species, and too few of others. Symptoms of dysbiosis can include bloating, because of the excess gases produced by the overgrown bacteria, and pain. Because dysbiosis disrupts the gut barrier, leading to increased permeability or "leaky gut," it can cause neurological symptoms associated with *sickness syndrome* (Chapter 8) including mood disorders, fatigue, and cognitive "fuzziness." Food, skin, and respiratory allergies are also linked to dysbiosis. Together these may contribute to a poor quality of life and increased risk of serious illnesses such as diabetes, inflammatory bowel diseases, cardiovascular disease, and even neurological disorders (Rinninella 2019, Weiss 2017).

One well-characterized example of severe dysbiosis is infection/overgrowth with *Clostridioides difficile* (*C. difficile*). The condition is usually treated with powerful antibiotics because *C. difficile* tends to be resistant to many other antibiotics. Unfortunately, people who have antibiotic-resistant *C. difficile* overgrowth have often been treated with so many powerful antibiotics that nearly the only remaining species is *C. difficile*. This situation is life-threatening because it can lead to severe colitis. Up until a few years ago, there was no reliably effective treatment. But there is now a revolutionary treatment that is saving the lives of people hospitalized with *C. difficile*. It is called "fecal transplant" and involves giving people with overgrowth of *C. difficile* feces from a healthy person either via enema or pills. This typically leads to a cure within a few days, underlining the critical role of balanced microbial communities in maintaining gastrointestinal health.

Although most research on microbes and health has focused on the types of bacteria in our guts, recent work indicates that species of fungi also contribute benefits for gut health. This "mycobiome" seems to exist in a balance with bacteria (Jiang 2017, Patterson 2017). For instance, overgrowth of fungi, causing the condition called *thrush*, is common with antibiotic use. Probiotic yogurts can help treat thrush (Kumamoto 2021). Conversely, fungi can compensate for some of the side effects of antibiotic use that are secondary to the loss of specific bacteria (Jiang 2017). Thus, the different kinds of microbes, when in balance and not overgrown, appear to work in concert to help maintain gut health. This is a developing area of research that promises to provide important practical information relevant to keeping a healthy balance of microbes.

The correlation of low microbial diversity and dysbiosis with a wide variety of disease conditions has inspired research into the questions of what exactly microbes are doing to support health, and how having too few microbial species can drive disease. Already it is clear that microbes play critical roles in regulating inflammation and tolerance to foods, responses to stress, and maintaining gut barrier integrity.

"Old Friends" Regulate Inflammation and Help Maintain Tolerance to Foods.

This association of low microbial diversity with poor health outcomes suggest that some missing microbes may be playing critical roles in our health. The association between the "cleanliness" of the urbanized Western lifestyle with allergy and autoimmune disease has given rise to the "hygiene hypothesis," which has been refined into the "Old Friends" hypothesis (Rook 2014). The idea is that urbanized lifestyles lead to reduced microbial diversity. Urbanized lifestyles cause a loss of specific microbes, including bacteria (*Lactobacillus*, *Bifidobacteria*, *Bacteroides*, *Clostridia* species and others), yeast (*Saccharomyces* species, aka brewer's yeast) and helminths (worms) that co-evolved with humans and perform important immunoregulatory functions (Murdaca 2021). These microbes comprise the group of "Old Friends." When children are raised in "hygienic" environments with low exposure to these microbes, their immune systems do not develop in a way that supports a balance between inflammation/defense against pathogens and tolerance to food antigens or commensal microbes. This effect may be exaggerated in the context of the Western diet, which doesn't support microbial diversity and the presence of Old Friends (Murdaca 2021).

The key requirement for immune cells in the gut is to respond promptly to threats such as pathogens and toxins, but to be "tolerant" of food antigens and beneficial microbes. Commensal microbes help maintain this balance, and the principal ways they do that is by influencing *phenotypes* or activity of T cells and dendritic cells/macrophages (McCoy 2018). In short, they affect whether our immune cells behave in a pro-inflammatory or regulatory and anti-inflammatory manner, and when our immune cells are active versus inhibited.

Importantly, these immune cell populations exhibit *plasticity,* meaning that they can switch back and forth between phenotypes depending on the conditions in the gut (Sica 2012, Wang 2020). Influencing this plasticity is an important way that microbes control gut inflammation and tolerance to foods. Although all mechanisms have not been identified, it seems that whatever determines how the gut is tolerating food antigens, or whether the gut is intolerant and inflamed, depends on the balance of Treg and TH17 cell activity. This activity is controlled in large part by the signals the T cells receive from microbes (Omenetti 2015). This implies that the pro-inflammatory effects of stress and/or a poor diet can be ameliorated by changing to diets that support beneficial Old Friends.

How might Old Friends help maintain tolerance and constrain inflammation? Old Friend bacteria tend to be GABA- and butyrate-producers. Immune cells, including Tregs, TH17, and macrophages, express GABA receptors, and the effects of GABA are anti-inflammatory (Prud'homme 2015). Butyrate, produced by "Old Friends" such as bifidobacterial and certain *Clostridia* species, seems to be an important signal to induce Treg cells, and inhibit pro-inflammatory TH17 cells (Chen 2018). Tryptophan metabolites generated by microbes can also induce Tregs (Langgartner 2019). The ways that "Old Friend" helminths (such as *Heligmosomoides polygyrus*) are able to induce tolerance are less clear, but seem to involve programming macrophages, dendritic cells, T cells, and B cells to a regulatory phenotype (Rook 2014). Pre-clinical studies investigating the effects of probiotic bacteria (e.g., *lactobacillus* species and the VSL3 combination of five Old Friends) support the idea that these Old Friends do indeed program gut immune cells (Rook 2014).

Bidirectional Relationship of Microbes and Stress

Thanks to the close connections of the gut and the brain, the effects of psychological stress are very often felt in the gut. Microbes modulate stress responses in the gut by influencing the balance of tolerance versus immunity, by their influence on the gut barrier, and by their interactions with interoceptive nerves that influence mood states, activity, emotion, and cognition (Langgartner 2019). The actions of some microbes, typically pathobionts, can contribute to or exacerbate stress, whereas other microbes seem to confer resilience (Langgartner 2019). The resilience-promoting microbes are typically the Old Friends that rely on a varied diet of fiber-containing foods. One of the deleterious effects of stress is that it causes the brain to favor food choices that include fatty, sugary, low-fiber processed foods. These foods do not support the bacteria that mitigate stress responses.

Stress is associated with reorganization of microbial populations and the loss of Old Friends such as *Lactobacillus* species (Langgartner 2019, Rook 2014). Stress-related hormones can directly influence pathobiont bacteria via the hormone receptors they possess (Lyte 1992, Moriera 2016). Hormonal activation of pathobionts leads to increased growth in numbers of these bacteria, disruption of the balance with other species (dysbiosis), and increased virulence (the ability of a microbe to cause disease). Increased virulence means increased release of toxins and increased *adherence*, or the tendency to stick to the mucus or epithelial cell layer. This adherence can induce or enhance inflammation and disturb gut barrier function. Together these conditions induce inflammation and disruption of the balance between Treg and TH17 cells, which can reduce tolerance to food antigens. In this way, the "top-down" effects of stress can predispose to food allergies, insensitivities, and other bowel disorders that are associated with gut barrier dysfunction and inflammation. In addition, pro-inflammatory cytokines generated during gut inflammation can activate the interoceptive vagus nerve pathway, contributing to mood disorders, pain and the negative emotions associated with stress.

"Old Friends" Help the Gut Barrier

One of the most deleterious consequences of stress for the gut is increased gut barrier permeability. Gut barrier permeability, or "leaky gut" is a consistent pathological feature associated with dysbiosis. This implies that some of the "missing microbes" are normally helping to maintain gut barrier integrity. This is likely a principal mechanism by which microbial populations containing Old Friends can support resilience to stress. This reinforces the importance of a diet that supports these Old Friends.

Because many Old Friend bacteria, including *Bifidobacteria*, *Clostridium* clusters IV and XIVa, and others, produce butyrate, they play a pivotal function in gut barrier health. This is because butyrate serves as the principal source of energy of the gut epithelial cells. Indeed, these bacteria provide approximately 80% of the energy needs for the epithelial cells. Thus, butyrate-producing Old Friend bacteria may prevent or help heal damage to the gut barrier by ensuring cells have adequate energy to perform their functions.

In addition, butyrate can influence the expression of the junction proteins that bind the epithelial cells and act to reduce permeability. Support for the idea that butyrate-producing bacteria can help heal the gut comes from studies of fecal transplant donors. Some donors, called "super-donors," provide material that is significantly more effective for curing *C. difficile* infections than material from other donors (Wilson 2019). Characterization of the material from super-donors has shown that this material contains more of the Old Friend *Clostridium* clusters IV and XIVa, which are good butyrate producers (Wilson 2019).

The mucin layer is a key component of the gut barrier, and degraded mucin is associated with increased permeability and inflammation (Engevik 2019, Sicard 2017). Notably, mucin degradation is a key pathophysiological feature of inflammatory bowel disease. Microbes play a role in maintaining the integrity of the mucin layer by several mechanisms, including butyrate production and influence on mucin production by the goblet cells (Engevik 2019). Mucin is made up mostly of protein that is attached to a protective carbohydrate, glycan. Microbes live on the mucin layer, and some of them form biofilms. These microbes have a symbiotic relationship with the mucin. The microbes can digest and metabolize mucin carbohydrates and glycoprotein, basically feeding on the mucus while protecting the mucus/gut barrier (Paone 2020, Sicard 2017).

One dramatic example of stress and dysbiosis is necrotizing enterocolitis (NEC), a life-threatening inflammatory condition of the gut that can develop in premature infants. This condition can be ameliorated by treatment with *bifidobacteria* (Aceti 2015). In a pre-clinical model of NEC, *bifidobacteria* down-regulated a substance called zonulin, which is associated with increased gut permeability, and reduced expression of pro-inflammatory cytokines (Ling 2016). *Bifidobacteria* is normally found in breast milk. These findings reinforce the importance of microbes in gut barrier health and provide further support for the importance of breast-feeding of infants.

Microbes and Maternity

Not only do gut microbes play pivotal roles in gut health, but they also contribute to healthy pregnancies (Socha-Banasiak 2021). Microbes support pregnancy by providing important nutrients that support metabolic needs and may play a role in immune tolerance (Socha-Banasiak). This is important because the immune system plays a key role in many aspects of pregnancy, including implantation of the fetus in the womb, tissue changes in the cervix, and the onset of labor (Yockey 2018). The maternal immune system must stay in a tolerant state to avoid rejecting the fetus. But the immune system must also be able to prevent infections that could damage the baby or induce pre-term labor. It is a delicate balance. The likely benefits of a healthy microbe population underline the importance of good diet during pregnancy.

We once thought that babies were sterile until they are born, but that is not the case, as a few microbes have been found to colonize babies in the womb (Gagliardi 2018). The type of delivery, Caesarian section or vaginal, determines the immediate population of bacteria that colonize babies (Mei 2019). This difference may not be important in the long term, however, because the populations of microbes change immediately when babies begin to eat and are modified continuously until they are 1-3 years old (Yatsunenko 2012). Breast milk contains beneficial microbes, notably *Bifidobacteria*, so whether babies are nursed may be more of an important factor than delivery type in determining early infancy microbe populations (Socha-Banasiak 2021).

Prenatal microbes may play a role in neurodevelopmental disorders such as autism. Both gut microbe and immune abnormalities are seen in some autistic individuals and their mothers, which is significant because the immune system plays important roles in support of developing brains (Li 2019, Mei 2019). Interestingly, studies in animals have implicated microbes in a variety of developmental functions, including "wiring" of the fetal brain, emotionality, and cognition (Dinan 2015). The precise link between microbes and brain development is not established, but some evidence suggests microbial influence on immune system function. One idea is that "disordered" microbes in the mother may program her immune system in such a way that it compromises certain features of brain development in her child (Dinan 2015).

Fermented Foods: Ancient Pro-biotics

Fermented foods, such as yogurt, kefir, cheese, sauerkraut, kombucha, beer, etc., have been a part of the human diet for thousands of years (Gasparrini 2016). It has been estimated that sheep, cattle, and goats were domesticated more than 10,000 years ago, and there are records of fermented dairy products from ancient Sumerian texts dating to 2500 BCE. In the chapter Genesis of the Hebrew Torah and Christian Bible (18:8), when the Lord visits Abraham, he is offered "curds," a type of fermented milk or cheese. These ancient books include later references to "curds" as well. Evidence of fermented beverages dating to 7000 BCE has been found in China, and in Mesopotamia, dating to 5000 BCE. There are references to health benefits of fermented dairy for gastrointestinal infections in Ayurvedic texts, and a Persian translation of Genesis is said to report that Abraham used "curds" for gastrointestinal problems. Later, Pliny the Elder, a second-century Roman, recommended thick, fermented, sour milk for gastrointestinal infections (Gasbarrini 2016).

The idea that microbes are responsible for the health benefits of fermented foods was first noted by Elie Metchnicoff, a Nobel Laureate for his work in immunology, in the late 1800s. He had become concerned with lifestyle and aging and attributed the longevity of Bulgarian country people to their prized yogurt. From this yogurt he isolated *Lactobacillus* species, including one he named *L. bulgaricus* (Gasparrini 2016). As these people often lived to be centenarians, they were perhaps the first "Blue Zone" population identified. Metchnikoff came to believe that disease and aging were caused by bacterial toxins released into the colon, and that fermented foods benefited human health by replacing toxic bacteria with beneficial ones.

The term *probiotic* was coined in the 1960s, but it was not until high-throughput gene sequencing technology was applied to the human microbiome to identify microbial genes, that the association of microbial diversity and dysbiosis with health and disease became clear. Metchnikoff's idea that certain "beneficial" microbes can prevent or mitigate the effects of dysbiosis on GI disorders and other conditions is now being tested by both basic science and clinical studies.

Currently, there is no clear consensus on the benefits of probiotics for specific conditions. Interpretation of studies is difficult because of differences in the probiotics tested and in other methodological inconsistencies. However, probiotic preparations that contain strains of Old Friends such as *Lactobacillus*, *Bifidobacteria*, and *Saccharomyces*, as well as high-fiber diets that support Old Friends (next section), have been reported fairly consistently as conferring benefits for GI problems such as traveler's diarrhea, irritable bowel syndrome, and mood in nonhuman and human animals (Dale 2019, McFarland 2019, Park 2018, Wastyk 2021). These findings emphasize the connections between microbes, gut, and brain (Bastianssen 2019, Koopman 2017, Langgartner 2019). Interestingly, and maybe importantly, the naturally occurring microbes in fermented foods such as Greek yogurt typically belong to the Old Friends group.

Microbes Depend on our Diet: All Food is "Pre-Biotic"

Our specific populations of microbes are unique to us as individuals. Although genetic factors may influence which microbes inhabit our gastrointestinal system, environmental factors seem to be the most important determinants of microbial populations in our guts. These factors include whether we have pets, with whom we end up sharing microbes, the people we live with, our history of antibiotic use, but most especially our diets (Davis 2016). The dependence of microbe populations on our diet is demonstrated by studies in laboratory animals and people showing that changes in diet can have dramatic effects on composition of microbial populations. For example, changing from a meat-based diet to a plant-based diet complexly reorganizes our microbe population, as does bariatric surgery, which also necessitates a change in diet (David 2014). What we eat provides microbes with the kinds of foods that they can metabolize, or ferment. Thus, our overall diet has *"prebiotic"* functions. Broadly speaking, "prebiotics" are any kind of nutrient that microbes can metabolize. Thus, they support the "care and feeding" of our gut microbes.

That diet plays such an outsized role in microbial diversity was a bit of a surprise. Most microbes live in the colon, and thus they ferment foods, such as fibers, that we cannot digest or absorb. Until recently, the only way to study gut microbes was to culture them in test tubes from feces, and few kinds of microbes are able to grow in this way. The ones that could be studied fermented a restricted set of nondigestible fibers, such as inulin, a commercially available fiber "prebiotic" supplement. But it is clear now that the types of food substances that can support microbes is far more diverse. In addition, we now know that there are microbe populations throughout the gut, including the mouth, esophagus, stomach, and small intestine (Martinez-Guryn 2019). They are harder to study than microbes from the colon, which can be isolated non-invasively from feces. These microbes are exposed to food before it is digested, and thus are likely fermenting pretty much whatever we eat.

Because diet is such an important factor regulating microbial growth, diversity of food is also critical for our own diets. For instance, the Western diet has been linked repeatedly to a wide variety of poor health conditions, all of which are associated with dysregulated inflammation (Christ 2019). The Western diet consists of mostly only a few types of food, such as refined carbohydrates like sugary and starchy foods. This refined carbohydrate diet can lead to overgrowth of certain yeast and bacteria that can survive on that diet and discourage growth of the many other species that prefer fiber and other components of a fresh, plant-based diet. Overgrowth of yeast and bacteria cause dysbiosis, bloating, and symptoms of irritable bowel syndrome (IBS) and small intestinal bacterial overgrowth (SIBO), such as cramping and pain (Saffouri 2019). This dysbiosis can contribute to inflammation at the gut barrier as well as leaky gut. Leaky gut can induce or exacerbate problems elsewhere in the body. The lack of Old Friends that normally regulate inflammation in the gut can further contribute to GI pathology as well as systemic conditions.

In contrast, multiple lines of evidence, including epidemiological, cross-sectional, and clinical trials indicate that diets that include plenty of fiber from whole grains, fruits, and vegetables support a diverse microbiome, lower incidence of mood disorders, and less inflammation (Wastyk 2021).

One possible mechanism by which a diverse microbial population supports health and mitigates against inflammation involves "biotransformation" of dietary antioxidants. The structure of many dietary antioxidants makes them difficult for the gut to absorb. This low bioavailability has led to skepticism regarding the true benefits of dietary antioxidants. However, gut microbes can metabolize, or "biotransform," these molecules into smaller, more easily absorbed molecules (Maria Monagas 2010).

Further Considerations

Be mindful of chemicals in foods. Antibiotic and pesticide residues in food can be metabolized by microbes (Koppel 2017). These substances can affect microbial growth, potentially contributing to dysbiosis, and some may be toxic to the microbes as well. This is one of the most compelling reasons for eating organic foods. Similarly, it's important to avoid antibiotics, including "sanitizing" cleaning or topical products unless they are truly necessary. Antibiotic overuse is an important contributor to the development of dysbiosis, with resistant *C. difficile* infections being an extreme example of what high doses of antibiotics can do.

Manage stress to control the emotional eating that is more likely to involve Western diet-type foods that encourage low microbial diversity and/or dysbiosis. Chronic stress can contribute to increased gut barrier permeability. This "leaky gut" can drive inflammation and immune responses to foods and thus food allergies or sensitivities which cause further reduction in dietary diversity, and consequently reduction in microbial diversity, contributing to dysbiosis.

Healthy aging: We are aging as soon as we are born, and our diet in youth can influence our health in old age. A healthy diet is increasingly linked to better cognitive functioning in older people (Bramorska 2021, Morris 2017). The studies of centenarians living in Blue Zones reinforce the idea that diverse populations of gut microbes are likely playing a pivotal role in the resilience of these people.

Key Points

- Our microbial populations provide important benefits for us, including making vitamins, providing fuel for gut epithelial cells, and helping us digest plants.
- A healthy population of gut microbes is one that is *diverse*, in that there are many different species. Having lots of different species in the gut seems to prevent any one of them from overgrowing.
- Low microbial diversity is associated with *dysbiosis*, which is when one or a few species of microbes overgrows. Dysbiosis can lead to symptoms such as gassiness and bloating, irritable bowel syndrome,

and gut barrier inflammation, and is associated with many chronic diseases including diabetes and other metabolic diseases, cardiovascular disease, autoimmune diseases, and neurodegenerative and neurodevelopmental disorders.
- Healthy microbial populations are also important in pregnancy and infancy.
- There is a notable connection between gut microbe populations, dysbiosis, and brain health.
- The main influence on the types of microbial species we harbor and how much they grow is what we eat. Thus, diet is key to a healthy microbial community.
- The most important way that we can maintain a diverse, balanced microbe population is by eating a varied diet of whole foods, especially whole grains and vegetables, high-fiber foods such as beans and legumes, and probiotic foods. Highly processed foods that may also contain toxins such as pesticides and additives that can disrupt our microbes should be avoided, as should other low-fiber/low-nutrition Western-diet foods.

References

Aceti A, Gori D, Barone G, Callegari ML, Di Mauro A, Fantini MP, et al. Probiotics for prevention of necrotizing enterocolitis in preterm infants: systematic review and meta-analysis. Italian Journal of Pediatrics, 41:89, 2015.

Bastiaanssen TFS, Cowan CSM, Claesson MJ, Dinan TG, Cryan JF. Making sense of … the microbiome in psychiatry. International Journal of Neuropsychopharmacology, 22:37-52, 2019.

Bramorska A, Zarzycka W, Podilecka W, Kuc K, Brzezicka A. Age-related cognitive decline may be moderated by frequency of specific food products consumption. Nutrients, 13:2504, 2021.

Chen J, Vitetta L. Inflammation-modulating effect of butyrate in the prevention of colon cancer by dietary fiber. Clinical Colorectal Cancer, 17: e54-544, 2018.

Christ A, Lauterbach M, Latz E. Western diet and the immune system: an inflammatory connection. Immunity Review, 51:794-811, 2019.

Dale HF, Rasmussen SH, Asiller OO, Lied GA. Probiotics in irritable bowel syndrome: an up-to-date systematic review. Nutrients, 11:2048, 2019.

David LA, Maurice CF, Carmody RN, Gootenberg DB, Button JE, Wolfe BE, et al. Diet rapidly and reproducibly alters the human gut microbiome. Nature, 505:559-563, 2014.

Davis S, Yadav JS, Barrow AD, Robertson BK. Gut microbiome diversity influences more by the Westernized dietary regime than the body mass index as assessed using effect size statistic. Microbiology Open, 623e:e476, 2016.

de Morales ACF, Fernandes GR, da Silva IT, Almeida-Pititto B, Gomes EP, da Costa Pereira A, Ferreira SRG. Enterotype may drive the dietary-associated cardiometabolic risk factors. Frontiers in Cellular and Infection Microbiology, 7:47, 2017.

Dickerson F, Severance E, Yolken R. The microbiome, immunity, and schizophrenia and bipolar disorder. Brain, Behavior, and Immunity, 62:46-54, 2017.

Dinan TG, Stilling RM, Stanton C, Cryan JF. Collective unconscious: How gut microbes shape behavior. Journal of Psychiatric Research, 63:1-9, 2015.

Engevik MA, Luk B, Chang-Graham AL, Hall A, Herrmann B, Ruan W, Endres BT, Shi Z, Garey KW, Hyser JM, Versalovic J. Bifidobacterium dentium fortifies the intestinal mucus layer via autophagy and calcium signaling pathways. mBio 10: e01087, 2019.

Firth J, Veronese N, Cotter J, Shivappa N, Hebert JR, Ee C, Smith L, Stubbs B, Jackson SE, Sarris J. What is the role of dietary inflammation in severe mental illness? A review of observational and experimental findings. Frontiers in Psychiatry, 10:350, 2019.

Fitzgerald E, Murphy S, Martinson HA. Alpha-synuclein and the role of the microbiota in Parkinson's disease. Frontiers in Neuroscience, 13:369, 2019.

Gasbarrini G, Bonvicini F, Gramenzi A. Probiotics History. Journal of Clinical Gastroenterology, 50, Supp. 2: S116-S119, 2016.

Gagliardi A, Totino V, Cacciotti F, Iebba V, Neron Bi, Bonfiglio G, et al. Rebuilding the gut microbiota ecosystem. International Journal of Environmental Research and Public Health, 15:1679, 2018.

Goehler LE, Lyte M, Gaykema RP. Infection-induced viscerosensory signals from the gut enhance anxiety: implications for psychoneuroimmunology. Brain, Behavior, and Immunity, 21:721-726, 2007.

Gonzalez-Aranciba C, Urrutia-Pinones J, Illanes-Gonzales J, Sotomayor-Zarate R, Julio-Pieper M. Bravo JA. Do your gut microbes affect your brain dopamine? Psychopharmacology, 236(5): 1661-1622, 2019.

Jiang TT, Shao T-Y, Ang G, Kinder JM, Turner LH, Pham G, Whitt J, Alenghat T, Way SS. Commensal fungi recapitulate the protective effects of intestinal bacteria. Cell Host & Microbe, 22:809-816, 2017.

Kelly JR, Kennedy PJ, Cryan JF, Dinan TG, Clarke G, Hyland NP. Breaking down the barriers: the gut microbiome, intestinal permeability and stress-related psychiatric disorders. Frontiers in Cellular Neuroscience, 9:392, 2015.

Kong, F, Deng F, Ying Li Y, Zhao J. Identification of gut microbiome signatures associated with longevity provides a promising modulation target for healthy aging. Gut Microbes, 10:210-215, 2019.

Koopman M, El Aidy S. Depressed gut? The microbiota-diet-inflammation trialogue in depression. Current Opinion in Psychiatry, 30:369-377, 2017.

Koppel N, Maini Rekdal V, Balskus EP. Chemical transformation of xenobiotics by the human gut microbiota. Science, 356: eaag2770, 2017.

Kumamoto CA, Gresnigt, Hube B. The gut, the bad and the harmless: Candida albicans as a commensal and opportunistic pathogen in the intestine. Current Opinion in Microbiology, 56:7-15, 2021.

Langgartner D, Lowry CA, Reber SO. Old Friends, immunoregulation, and stress resilience. Pflügers Archive - European Journal of Physiology, 471:237-269, 2019.

Li N, Yang J, Zhang J, Liang C, Wang Y, Chen B, et al. Correlation of gut microbiome between ASD children and mothers and potential biomarkers for risk assessment. Genomic Proteomics Bioinformatics, 17:26-38, 2019.

Li Y, Lu M-R, Wei Y-J, Sun L, Zhang J-X, Zhang H-G, Li B. Dietary patterns and depression risk: A meta-analysis. Psychiatry Research, 253:373-382, 2017.

Ling X, Linglong P, Weixia D, Hong W. Protective Effects of Bifidobacterium on Intestinal Barrier Function in LPS-Induced Enterocyte Barrier Injury of Caco-2 Monolayers and in a Rat NEC Model. PLoS ONE 11:e0161635, 2016.

Lyte M, Ernst S. Catecholamine-induced growth of Gram-negative bacteria. Life Sciences, 50:203-212, 1992.

Lyte M, Varcoe JJ, Bailey MT. Anxiogenic effect of sun-clinical bacterial infection in mice in the absence of overt immune activation. Physiology and Behavior, 65:63-68, 1998.

Lyte M. Microbial endocrinology and the microbiota-gut-brain axis. Advances in Experimental Medicine and Biology, 817:3-24, 2014.

Lyte M. Microbial endocrinology: and ongoing personal journey. In M Lyte (ed) Microbial Endocrinology: Interkingdom Signaling in Infectious Disease and Health, Advances in Experimental Medicine and Biology, 874:1-24, 2016.

Maes M. Evidence for an immune response in major depression: A review and hypothesis. Progress in Neuro-Psychopharmacology, 19:11-38, 1995.

Margolis KG, Cryan JF, Mayer EA. The microbiota-gut-brain axis: from motility to mood. Gastroenterology, 160:1486-1501, 2021.

Maria Monagas M, Urpi-Sarda M, Sanchez-Patan F, Llorach R, Garrido I, Gomez-Cordoves C, Andres-Lacueva C, Bartolome B. Insights into the metabolism and microbial biotransformation of dietary flavan-3-ols and the bioactivity of their metabolites. Food & Function, 1: 233-253, 2010.

Martinez-Guryn K, Leone V, Chang EB. Regional diversity of the gastrointestinal microbiome. Cell Host Microbe, 26:314-324, 2019.

McCoy KD, Ignacio A, Geuking MB. Microbiota and Type 2 immune responses. Current Opinion in Immunology, 54:20-27, 2018.

McFarland LV, Goh S. Are probiotics and prebiotics effective in the prevention of travellers' diarrhea: a systematic review and meta-analysis. Travel Medicine and Infectious Disease, 27:11-19, 2019.

Mei C, Yang W, Wei X, Wu K, Huang D. The unique microbiome and innate immunity during pregnancy. Frontiers in Immunology, 10:2886, 2019.

Moreira CG, Russell R, Mishra AA, Narayanan S, Ritchie JM, Waldor MK, Curtis MM, Winter SE, Weinshenker D, Sperandio V. Bacterial adrenergic sensors regulate virulence of enteric pathogens in the gut. mBio 7: pii:e00826-16, 2016.

Morris MC, Wang Y, Barnes LL, Bennett DA, Dawson-Hughes B, Booth SL. Nutrients and bioactives in green leafy vegetables and cognitive decline. Neurology, 90:e214-e222, 2017.

Murdaca G, Greco M, Borro M, Gangemi S. Hygiene hypothesis and autoimmune disease: A narrative review of clinical evidence and mechanisms. Autoimmunity Reviews, 20:102845, 2021.

Musumeci S, Coen M, Leidi A, Schrenzel J. The human gut mycobiome and the specific role of *Candida albicans*: where do we stand, as clinicians? Clinical Microbiology and Infection, 28:58-63, 2022.

Nguyen TT, Kosciolek T, Eyler LT, Knight R, Jeste DV. Overview and systematic review of studies of microbiome in schizophrenia and bipolar disorder. Journal of Psychiatric Research, 99:50-61, 2018.

Omenetti S, Pizarro TT. The Treg/Th17 Axis: A Dynamic Balance Regulated by the Gut Microbiome. Frontiers in Immunology, 6:639, 2015.

Paone P, Cani PD. Mucus barrier, mucins, and the gut microbiota: the expected slimy partners? Gut, 69:2232-2243, 2020.

Park C, Brietzke E, Rosenblat JD, Musial N, Zuckerman H, Ragguett R-M, et al. Probiotics for the treatment of depressive symptoms: An anti-inflammatory mechanism? Brain, Behavior, and Immunity, 73:115-124, 2019.

Patterson MJ, Oh S, Underfill DM. Host-microbe interactions: commensal fungi in the gut. Current Opinion in Microbiology, 40:131-137, 2017.

Prud'homme, GJ, Glinka Y, Wang Q. Immunological GABAergic interactions and therapeutic applications in autoimmune diseases. Autoimmunity Reviews, 14:1048-10, 2015.

Rea K, Dinan TG, Cryan JF. The microbiome: A key regulator of stress and neuroinflammation. Neurobiology of Stress, 4:23-33, 2016.

Rees T, Bosch T, Douglas AE. How the microbiome challenges our concept of self. PLoS Biology, 16:e2005358, 2018.

Rinninella E, Raoul P, Franceschi F, Miggiano GAD, Gasbarrini A, Mele MC. What is the healthy gut microbiota composition? A changing ecosystem across age, environment, diet, and disease. Microorganisms, 7:14, 2019.

Rook GAW, Raison CL, and Lowry CA. Microbiota, Immunoregulatory Old Friends and Psychiatric Disorders. In M Lyte and JF Cryan (eds), Microbial Endocrinology: The Microbiota-Gut-Brain Axis in Health and Disease. Advances in Experimental Medicine and Biology, 817, Springer New York, 2014.

Roshchina VV. New trends and perspectives in the evolution of neurotransmitters in microbial, plant and animal cells. In M Lyte (ed) Microbial Endocrinology: Interkingdom Signaling in Infectious Disease and Health, Advances in Experimental Medicine and Biology, 874:25-77, 2016.

Rothschild D, Weissbrod O, Barkan E, Kurilshikov A, Korem T, Zeevi D, Costea PI, et al. Environment dominates over host genetics in shaping human gut microbiota. Nature, 555:210-228, 2018.

Saffouri GB, Shields-Cutler RR, Chen J, Yang Y Lekatz HR, Hales VL, et al. Small intestinal microbial dysbiosis underlies symptoms associated with functional gastrointestinal disorders. Nature Communications, 10:2012, 2019.

Sarkodie EK, Zhou S, Baidoo SA, Chu W. Influences of stress hormones on microbial infections. Microbial Pathogenesis, 131:270-276, 2019.

Sato Y, Atarashi K, Plichta DR, Arai Y, Sasajima S, Kearney SM, et al. Novel bile acid biosynthetic pathways are enriched in the microbiome of centenarians. Nature, 599:458-464, 2021.

Sica A, Montovani A. Macrophage plasticity and polarization: in vivo veritas. The Journal of Clinical Investigation, 122:787-795, 2012.

Sicard J-F, Le Bihan G, Vogeleer P, Jacques M, Harel J. Interactions of Intestinal Bacteria with Components of the Intestinal Mucus. Frontiers in Cellular and Infection. Microbiology, 7:387, 2017.

Socha-Banasiak A, Pawlowska M, Czkwianianc E, Pierzynoiwska K. From intrauterine to extrauterine- the role of endogenous and exogenous factors in the regulation of the intestinal microbiota community and gut maturation in early life. Frontiers in Nutrition, 8:696966, 2021.

Stilling RM, van de Wouw M, Clarke G, Stanton C, Dinan TG, Cryan JF. The neuropharmacology of butyrate: The bread and butter of the microbiota-gut-brain axis? Neurochemistry International, 99:110-132, 2016.

Strandwitz P, Kim KH, Terekhova D, Liu JK, Sharma A, Levering J, McDonald D, Dietrich D, Ramadhar TR, Lekbua A, Mroue N, Liston C, Stewart EJ, Dubin MJ, Zengler K, Knight R, Gilbert JA, Clardy J, Lewis K. GABA Modulating Bacteria of the Human Gut Microbiota. Nature Microbiology, 4:396-403, 2019.

Subramoni S, Venturi V. LuxR-family "solos": bachelor sensors/regulators of signaling molecules. Microbiology, 155:1377-1385, 2009.

Tian J, Dang H, Wallner M, Olsen R, Kaufman DL. Homotaurine, a safe blood-brain barrier permeable GABAA-R-specific agonist, ameliorates disease in mouse models of multiple sclerosis. Scientific Reports, 8:16555, 2018.

Tuikhara N, Keisam S, Labala RK, Imrata L, Ramakrishnand P, Cha Arunkumar M, Ahmed G, Biagi E, Jeyaram K. Comparative analysis of the gut microbiota in centenarians and young adults shows a common signature across genotypically non-related populations. Mechanisms of Aging and Development, 179:23-35, 2019.

Vitetta L, Vitetta G and Hall S. Immunological Tolerance and Function: Associations Between Intestinal Bacteria, Probiotics, Prebiotics, and Phages. Frontiers in Immunology, 9:2240, 2018.

vom Steeg LG, Lein SL. Sex steroids mediate bidirectional interactions between hosts and microbes. Hormones and Behavior, 88:45-51, 2017.

Wang J, Chen W-D, Wang Y-D. The relationship between gut microbiota and inflammatory diseases: The role of macrophages. Frontiers in Microbiology, 11:1065, 2020.

Wastyk HC, Fragiadakis GK, Perelman D, Dahan D, Merrill BD, Yu FB, et al. Gut-microbiota-targeted diets modulate human immune status. Cell, 184:4137-4153, 2021.

Weiss GA, Hennet T. Mechanisms and consequences of intestinal dysbiosis. Cellular and Molecular Life Sciences, 74:2959-2977, 2017.

Wilson BC, Vatanen T, Cutfield WS, O'Sullivan JM. The super-donor phenomenon in fecal microbiota transplantation. Frontiers in Cellular and Infection Microbiology, 9:2, 2019.

Wu L, Zeng T, Zinellu A, Rubino S, Kelvin DJ, Carru C. A cross-sectional study of compositional and functional profiles of gut microbiota in Sardinia centenarians. mSystems, 4:e00325-19, 2019.

Xu Z, Knight R. Dietary effects on human gut microbiome diversity. British Journal of Nutrition, 113:S1-S5, 2015.

Yang B, Wei J, Ju P, Chen J. Effects of regulating intestinal microbiota on anxiety symptoms: A systematic review. General Psychiatry, 32:e100056, 2019.

Yatsunenko T, Rey FE, Manary MJ, Trehan I, Dominguez-Bello MG, Contreras M, et al. Human gut microbiome viewed across age and geography. Nature, 486:222-227, 2012.

Yocker LJ, Iwasaki A. Role of interferons and cytokines in pregnancy and fetal development. Immunity, 49:397-412, 2018.

CHAPTER 18: GUT PROBLEMS: WHY SOME FOODS ARE THE PROBLEM AND OTHER FOODS ARE THE SOLUTION

- WHY ARE GUT PROBLEMS SO COMMON? DYSBIOSIS AND THE WESTERN DIET
- STRESS, EMOTION, AND THE GUT
- FOOD ALLERGIES
- NON-IGE-MEDIATED ALLERGIES AND SENSITIVITIES
- DISORDERS OF BRAIN GUT INTERACTION
- GASTRO-ESOPHAGEAL REFLUX DISEASE (GERD)
- INFLAMMATORY BOWEL DISEASE (IBD)
- NON-GUT GUT DISORDERS: PARKINSON'S DISEASE, MULTIPLE SCLEROSIS, SCHIZOPHRENIA, AND AUTISM
- FOOD IS THE PROBLEM, AND FOOD IS THE SOLUTION
- EXCLUSION DIETS
- KEY POINTS

Chances are that most readers of this book have either suffered from gut-related symptoms or know someone else who has. The prevalence of GI disorders, such as irritable bowel syndrome (IBS), gastro-esophageal reflux disease (GERD), food allergies and sensitivities, and inflammatory bowel disease (IBD) are collectively high, and seem to be increasing, especially in "Westernized" countries (Ng 2016).

GI disorders are probably the most difficult disorders for which to identify the causes and best management approaches, because they are associated with interrelated psychological, genetic, and physiological factors. Symptoms are often attributed to diet, but the exact role diet plays can vary. One complication is that human experiments are difficult, expensive, and sometimes impossible to do. This ambiguity has led to fad diets and treatments that are not evidence-based and may exacerbate symptoms (Weber 2019).

Although the underlying pathophysiology of the different gut disorders diverges in several ways, and each is considered as a separate diagnostic entity, there are common themes in symptomology that link them. Pathology in the gut seems to involve environmental factors, notably stress and diet-related factors, occurring in the context of genetic and/or epigenetic predisposition. Together these lead to aberrant immune responses and gut barrier permeability. Microbial populations in the gut seem to play a pivotal role, based on their influence on immune homeostasis, gut barrier integrity, and brain-mediated functions, especially mood and cognition (Barber 2021). Symptoms associated with gut disorders are challenging in and of themselves, but perceived or actual stigma, and the general lack of awareness of GI conditions, can increase stress. Even simple things, such as finding and affording food for people with allergies and sensitivities, the need for public restrooms for people with IBD or IBS, and obtaining time off work for people during flare-ups, contribute to the psychological load on people with GI disorders.

Why are gut problems so common? Dysbiosis and the Western Diet

The prevalence of GI disorders has been steadily increasing since the mid-twentieth century (Ng 2017). Although many genetic associations with susceptibility to GI disorders have been identified (e.g., more than 200 gene variants are associated with IBD), rates of gut disorders in the population have increased too rapidly for the increase in prevalence to be solely attributable to genetics (Flynn 2019, Ananthakrishnan 2015). Thus, environmental factors must be principally responsible, and changes in dietary patterns and food production are increasingly implicated as principal culprits in this increased prevalence. Since the 1950's and 1960's food production has been heavily industrialized, with an emphasis in the developed nations of Europe and North America on highly processed, high-energy (fats and refined sugar) food that also tends to be low in fiber as well as in micronutrients (Kopp 2019). At the same time, additives such as preservatives and coloring were introduced to improve the shelf life and appearance of foods. Large-scale agricultural techniques are efficient and economical, but these advantages require the use of herbicides, such as glyphosate, which can remain as residues on grains and other agricultural products. In this way, foods associated with the Western diet can contain ingredients that the gut does necessarily recognize as "foreign" or xenobiotic. These ingredients can induce immune responses and disrupt both gut barrier functions and microbial populations (Barnett 2020). Finally, antibiotic use, more common in Westernized countries, is well-documented to disrupt gut microbial populations, leading to dysbiosis and gut disorders.

How can the Western diet drive GI disorders? The Western diet is based on highly refined carbohydrates, such as wheat flour and sugar, in which many nutrients and non-digestible components or fiber are removed. A serious consequence of such refinement is that these foods do not support the Old Friend microbial populations that provide critical energy sources to the gut epithelial cells, and program the gut immune system to be in a tolerant state (Langgartner 2019, Chen 2018). This can set the stage for inflammation at the gut barrier, reduced microbial diversity, and dysbiosis. Studies have linked the Western diet to all gut disorders, and one of the principal features that gut disorders have in common is microbial dysbiosis (Ananthakrishnan 2015, Singh 2018, Smith 2017, Valitutti 2019). Dysbiosis seems to be a major factor in the onset of IBD, food allergies, and celiac disease (Lewis 2015, Caminero 2019, McKenzie 2017). Similarly, dysbiosis is also a hallmark of IBS, providing one mechanistic explanation for the association of Western diet with gut disorders. Although the link of food additives and pesticides is less well documented, pre-clinical studies have shown that these xenobiotics are capable of causing inflammation and gut barrier dysfunction, which are also mechanistically linked to GI disorders (Di Tommaso, 2021, Ding 2021).

High-fat, high-fructose, processed components of the diet may also contribute to dysbiosis and gut barrier dysfunction. Processed foods contain advanced glycation end-products (AGEs), amino acids that sugars bind to and which form spontaneously, especially at high temperatures such as during manufacturing of processed baked goods or meats (Kellow 2015, Snelson 2019). AGEs can act as DAMPs or alarmins to induce activation of RAGE (receptor of advanced glycation end-products). RAGE is now recognized as a factor in driving inflammatory responses in multiple conditions, including food allergy and neurodegenerative diseases (Jiang 2018, Smith 2017). Pre-clinical studies show that these ingredients can induce inflammation at the gut barrier, as well as change the structure of gut microbial populations. A preliminary study with humans also showed that a diet containing "brown food" was associated with changes in microbes. Brown food refers to food cooked enough that it turns brown and contains glycated amino acids. An earlier study reported that AGEs from the diet can cross into the body and induce biomarkers of inflammation (Uribarri 2015). However, many foods containing glycated proteins, or Maillard reaction products, do not seem to be pro-inflammatory and may in fact be the opposite. Coffee is an example. Much more research needs to be done before specific recommendations can be made, but the findings so far support a mechanistic link between processed foods and inflammation in the gut (Snelson 2019).

Stress, Emotion, and the Gut

Most gut disorders affect more than just the gut (Chapter 15) and are particularly associated with brain-mediated symptoms including fatigue, cognitive "fuzziness," depression, and anxiety that are characteristic of *sickness syndrome.* These symptoms seem to be driven by inflammation and increased gut barrier permeability. At the same time, psychological stress is often expressed in the gut as a consequence of the close bidirectional communication pathways between the gut and brain. It doesn't help that many of the kinds of comfort foods that that are preferred or even craved when people are stressed are sugary, high-fat staples of the Western diet. But the close relationship between stress, diet, and gut problems underlines the importance of managing challenges and increasing our awareness of diet choices.

A hallmark feature of the epigenetic changes following adverse childhood experiences (ACE) is increased inflammation and pain in the gut in adulthood (Liu 2017). Indeed, studies have linked gut disorders with childhood stress, and not only trauma. The most common identified stress was loss of a parent or other close family member. Trauma in adulthood, including rape and war trauma, is associated with gut disorders as well, and the severity of symptoms correlates with severity of trauma (Kolacz 2019). Unfortunately, many traumatic experiences, especially those of a sexual nature, are under-reported. Thus, contributions of trauma to GI symptoms are underappreciated among practitioners.

Although the link between stress and the gut is well-documented, it may not be intuitively obvious why they are linked. It may help to appreciate that the principal roles of the gut, which are to absorb adequate nutrition and alert the body to possible infections, require close communication with the brain. Obtaining food requires behaviors, including seeking food, eating it, and stopping eating, all of which are controlled by the brain. This behavioral control process involves regulation of motivation and reward systems, which are informed by nutritional status and presence of food in the gut. To sustain life, there must be a strong internal motivation to seek food, and the food must be in turn sufficiently rewarding to enable humans to continue to seek adequate nutrition. Similarly, motivation and reward systems need to be informed when the need for food has been met, so that satiety can occur. Close gut-brain connections are critical for life and health, and the link between gut symptoms and mood symptoms is thus unsurprising.

On the other hand, why should stress cause GI disorders? The answer to this seems to lie in the fact that challenge responses are adaptive in the short term; that is, while the challenge is being addressed. Problems occur when the challenge is not met and the responses become chronic. In the case of the gut, challenge responses tip autonomic balance towards sympathetic activity, which leads to reduced blood flow to the gut, changes in gut motility, and increased intestinal permeability (Chapter 15). This is believed to be adaptive in the short term as it redirects resources away from digestion to other organs (e.g., brain or muscle) that are necessary to manage the challenge. But the longer-term effects of unmet challenges on the gut involve inflammation, dysbiosis, motility problems such as constipation or diarrhea, and chronic gut barrier disruption (Konturek 2011). These are the hallmarks of GI disorders. Thus, stress is an extremely important pathophysiological factor in the etiology and course of these disorders.

Gut disorders are particularly challenging, in that they are uniquely disturbing both for people who have these disorders and for others with whom they interact. This may be particularly true for people who have disorders of the colon, or disorders that involve issues with defecation or flatulence. The emotion of disgust is linked to feces and vomit, and their smells (Oaten 2018, van der Geest 2020). Indeed, these odors, as well as blood, are described as "core disgust elicitors." Interestingly, the neural correlates of this emotion overlap with brain networks that process interoceptive information, including the medial prefrontal cortex and anterior insula (Oaten 2018). This suggests that the connection of these gut-related substances and the emotion of disgust may be hard-wired. The link of these body-related stimuli with the emotion of disgust is thought to provide motivation to avoid potential pathogens (Oaten 2011). But this link also leads to avoidance and rejection of the person who is the source of them. For example, feces are considered "unclean" and a likely source of illness. Any person who has an illness that involves defecation problems or vomiting may be rejected, or fear being rejected or avoided, as a result of the disgust that these body products induce. Indeed, people with GI disorders report that lack of awareness and social support contribute to the stress of having these disorders (Bray 2016). It is easy to see how these experiences can drive chronic stress effects on the gut, complicate resolution of the pathology and symptoms, and lead to a vicious cycle, whereby the stress of having a GI disorder exacerbates symptoms, resulting in more stress, and on and on.

In addition to inducing negative emotions, such as the embarrassment, shame, or disgust that originate from the experience of the disorder, GI symptoms can also result in enhanced "gut-brain connections" (i.e., interoception) that can non-specifically drive mood symptoms and fatigue and increase GI symptoms, including pain. Signals from the gut, including inflammation or dysbiosis, can activate sickness syndrome. Interoceptive networks within the brain modulate the activity of vagus and splanchnic nerves that innervate the gut and in turn modulate gut functions and gut barrier integrity (previously discussed in Chapters 15 and 16). In this way gut inflammation and psychological stress interact in a bi-directional way, which has complicated the experiences of people with gut disorders. A lack of understanding of the gut-brain connection tends to lead practitioners and patients to miss the relationship between the gut and mood/ cognitive problems. Historically, the co-occurrence of mood symptoms and gut disorders has led to patients being labeled "psychosomatic," the assumption being that gut pain or other symptoms are "all in the head," or that a patient's "neurotic" personality is causing his or her disorder.

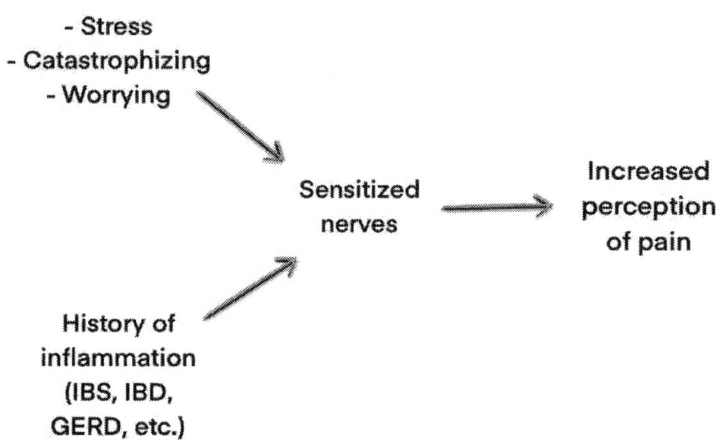

One of the most challenging features of gut disorders is *visceral hyperalgesia*. This involves increased experience of pain, even in response to stimuli that do not normally cause pain (Vermeulen 2014, Woolf 2011). For example, if you have visceral hyperalgesia, the amount of distension within the gut lumen (e.g., bloating) that is painful for you is much less than someone who does not have visceral hypersensitivity. This results from sensitization of nerves in the gut and in brain pathways that normally signal pain in internal tissues (Zhou 2011). Visceral hyperalgesia is a hallmark feature of irritable bowel syndrome (IBS) and heartburn (Barbara 2011, Zhou 2011, Ford 2020). It is also very common in the other bowel disorders including inflammatory bowel disease (IBD) and food allergies and sensitivities (Vermuelen 2014, Tuck 2019). Neuroimaging studies have shown that visceral hyperalgesia involves a potentiation of pain transmission at every level of the nervous system, from spinal cord to cortex (Vermeulen 2014). Pain is part of interoception, and visceral hypersensitivity is associated with mood symptoms and the perception of stress (Enck 2016). Because visceral hyperalgesia involves potentiation of neurological signals, it is highly sensitive to top-down influence, e.g., in the context of stress. This symptom has been linked to both stress and gut barrier dysfunction, specifically paracellular permeability, in pre-clinical models (Greenwood-Van Meerveld 2018). Because the perception of visceral hypersensitivity exaggerates the adverse conditions in the gut, it can provide inaccurate information about potential seriousness of symptoms, making the actual pathology seem worse than it is. This can lead to *catastrophizing*, which in turn increases perception of pain (Enck 2016, Hubbard 2015).

Food Allergies

Although food allergy is the best understood and straightforward of the GI disorders, it has several things in common with other gut conditions. For instance, food allergies, as well as other allergies and asthma, are more common in people who experienced dysbiosis in childhood (e.g., due to antibiotic use or diet). Food allergies are also more common in people who did not grow up with pets or go to daycare (Bunyavanich 2019). These observations have led to the "hygiene hypothesis," which suggests that many allergic or Type 2 immune response conditions follow from insufficient interaction with microbes when we are young (Shu 2019). This idea is reinforced by the fact that food allergies seem to be more common in Westernized countries and urban areas (Loh 2018).

Food allergies involve a process whereby food constituents, such as milk proteins, become perceived as dangerous by the immune system (De Martinis 2020, Valenta 2015). The effects are initially mediated by an immune globulin, IgE, that is responsible for allergies in general, as well as the biogenic amine *histamine*, which is a mediator in both the nervous and immune systems. Activation of IgE and histamine induces inflammation and increased gut barrier permeability. These can lead to nutritional problems due to the inflammation hindering the absorption of food, and to low-grade systemic inflammation, possibly due to the translocation of bacteria from the gut into the body because of the leakiness of the barrier. This leads to mood and cognitive problems, fatigue, and increased inflammation in other parts of the body, including the respiratory system or skin, where it may produce itchiness or hives. Severe reactions can induce a systemic immune response called anaphylaxis, which is life-threatening (Lin 2018).

Non IgE-mediated Allergies and Sensitivities

Non-IgE mediated allergies or sensitivities are conditions in which specific foods induce symptoms including pain, cramping, and bloating or gas, in the absence of immunoglobulin (Ig) responses. Diagnosis can be difficult, as there is no accepted biomarker, and symptoms overlap considerably with irritable bowel syndrome (see below). Indeed, it has been suggested that specific food sensitivities may constitute a sub-type of IBS (Catassi 2017, Soares 2018). The pathophysiology is not well understood clinically, partly due to problems with patient recruitment. People with suspected allergies or sensitivities generally do not want to be exposed to the suspect food, even in an experiment. In addition, while IgE-related conditions can be studied through simple blood sampling, studies of non-immunoglobin sensitivities may require gut tissue biopsies, and few participants are willing to undergo such invasive procedures. Nonetheless, some studies have revealed evidence of rapid inflammatory immune response after exposure to wheat proteins, for instance.

Celiac disease: Although celiac disease is often thought of as a food allergy, it is actually an autoimmune condition in which the immune system attacks a gut barrier protein, called gliadin, in response to the presence of gluten (Elli 2015). Gluten is a protein component of some grains, including wheat, barley, and rye. The classic IgE-mediated allergic pathway is not activated in celiac disease; the response to gluten is a T-cell-mediated inflammatory attack on the gut barrier cells that express gliadin (Caminero 2019). The result is damage to the gut barrier, leading to malabsorption, pain, and brain-mediated symptoms. Celiac disease can also cause inflammation elsewhere in the body, such as in skin (Elli 2015).

Celiac disease is strongly genetic. Nearly all people who develop celiac disease have one of the risk alleles, *HLA-DQ2 or HLA-DQ8,* or a couple of others. However, not everyone with these genes develops celiac disease, indicating environmental factors determine whether the condition occurs. Risks associated with the development of celiac disease include early childhood infections, antibiotic use, and dysbiosis (Caminero 2019, Valititti 2019). Gut barrier function is disturbed in celiac disease and is probably a key part of the pathophysiology (Caminero 2019, Kinashi 2021). Damage to the gut barrier can lead to malnutrition due to malabsorption of food across the barrier. Whereas celiac disease has historically been diagnosed mostly in children, the rates of celiac diagnoses in adults is rising, suggesting that the conditions necessary for gluten to become immunogenic can develop in adulthood (Elli 2015). A mechanistic role for intestinal dysbiosis is suggested by the fact that some microbes can digest gluten, making it less likely to provoke immune responses (Caminero 2019, Valitutti 2019). In the context of low microbial diversity and dysbiosis, gluten-digesting microbes may not be present in sufficient numbers to minimize immune responses in those genetically predisposed to celiac disease.

Non-celiac gluten sensitivity (NCGS): Non-celiac gluten sensitivity is a condition whereby people experience GI symptoms such as pain, bloating, and diarrhea, as well as non-gut symptoms such as fatigue or headaches, after eating wheat products. However, in this condition, people do not have evidence of celiac disease or wheat allergy (Elli 2015). Adhering to a gluten-free diet seems to ameliorate the symptoms, reinforcing the idea that wheat is the source of the problem. This diagnosis has been controversial, however, in part because of the lack of a reliable test that differentiates NCGS from similar disorders, such as IBS.

What is it about wheat? The prevalence of allergies and sensitivities to wheat is rather high, especially when accounting for people who self-diagnose. Estimates are between 5 to 0% of Western populations. The answer to this question is not clear for several reasons. Wheat varieties, and the products made from them, can vary considerably in the possible immunogenic capabilities of different wheat proteins (Elli 2015). In addition, much commercial wheat is sprayed with herbicides, including glyphosate (Round-up®), which has been clearly documented to disrupt the gut barrier and induce inflammation (Ding 2021, Qui 2020). Glyphosate exposure by itself could be responsible for the symptoms, or it could set up the conditions in the gut that lead to a specific inflammatory response to wheat and possibly other foods. Finally, there are individual differences in many of the factors that predispose to allergies and sensitivities (Genius 2010). These include genetics, antibiotic use, diets that influence immune status in the gut and the condition of microbial populations, and the effect of psychological stress on gut function.

Disorders of Brain Gut Interaction

Disorders of Brain Gut Interaction are the most common gut disorders. They constitute a cluster of more than thirty gut-related disorders. In these, the gut is not working properly, but there is no physical obstruction or other obvious organic cause (Rome Foundation 2021, Stanghellini 2017). These disorders share common features, including pain, psychiatric co-morbidities including anxiety, depression, and post-traumatic stress disorder, gut barrier disruption, dysbiosis, evidence of low-grade inflammation, and impairments of enteric nervous system function. In addition, increased gut-brain communication involves the interoceptive drive on brain networks that subserve mood symptoms, and conversely mediate the effects of psychosocial stress on bowel symptoms. Thus, disorders of brain gut interaction exemplify a self-sustaining cycle by which stress in the mind can trigger or worsen stress in the gut, which then feeds forward to increase stress in the mind. Because inflammation contributes to stress, and food both influences inflammation and plays a particularly important role in gut health, diet and challenge management are critical considerations when addressing disorders of brain gut interaction.

The most common of the disorders of brain gut interaction are irritable bowel syndrome (IBS) and functional dyspepsia. These two conditions can be difficult to distinguish, as the symptom patterns overlap (Stanghellini 2017). Furthermore, a significant subpopulation of people with IBS also reports specific food sensitivities, which are also associated with the cramping, bloating, and pain characteristic of IBS. Functional symptoms are also companions of other gut disorders, including inflammatory bowel disease (Aziz 2021, Spiller 2016).

IBS: IBS is the most common disorder of brain gut interaction, affecting more than 30 million people in the United States alone (Defrees 2017, Ford 2020). Prevalence worldwide is around 10%. It affects more women than men, and genes seem to play an as yet undetermined role, based on observations that monozygotic or identical twins are more likely to both have the condition than dizygotic or fraternal twins (Ford 2020). Life experiences including trauma, stress, and family disruption (ACE) increase the risk of developing IBS, as well. Other environmental factors include history of antibiotic use, surgery, and infection (Ford 2020).

IBS is associated with low-grade inflammation in the gut barrier, increased gut barrier permeability, visceral hypersensitivity, dysbiosis, and disordered function of gut neurons leading to constipation (IBS-C), diarrhea (IBS-D), or both (Bhatterai 2017, Defrees 2017). All of this is associated with pain and cramping, bloating, mood symptoms, and fatigue. Visceral hypersensitivity is extremely common in IBS.

IBS develops in childhood or during teenage years and young adulthood, and usually not in people over the age of 50 (Singh 2018). Indeed, IBS-like symptoms appearing in older adults can be a sign of a serious condition, such colon cancer, and should not be ignored. In some people, IBS develops following a bout of food poisoning (post-infective IBS). Post-infective IBS symptoms can persist or months to years after the infection.

Diet and IBS: Food is frequently associated with "flare-ups" of symptoms, and food sensitivities are common among people with IBS (Ford 2020). Indeed, careful studies, including double-blind challenge tests, have found that two-thirds of people with IBS have a food sensitivity, and many have sensitivities to multiple foods. Foods that have been linked IBS include fermentable Fructo-Oligo-Di- and Monosaccharides And Polyols (FODMAPs) which are found in many fruits, vegetables, and grains. Foods containing biogenic amine and histamine-releasing foods (e.g., bananas, alcohol), caffeine, and dairy products have also been linked to IBS (Ford 2020). Spicy or "hot" foods have also been reported to worsen symptoms, especially visceral hypersensitivity. In male IBS sufferers, spicy food may increase diarrhea (Singh 2018).

FODMAPs are non-digestible carbohydrates that may act as "prebiotics", feeding growth of microbe populations. In the context of dysbiosis and low microbial diversity, prebiotics may encourage certain microbes to overgrow, leading to bloating, cramps, low-grade inflammation, and motility problems. Reducing FODMAPs in the diet has generally been found to reduce symptoms of pain and cramping associated in many cases of IBS. FODMAP restriction now being considered a first-line intervention for the disorder (Altobelli 2018, Manning 2020). Because the low-FODMAP diet is deficient in fiber, it is not as effective for constipation as it is for gas and bloating symptoms. The low FODMAP diet is usually followed for not more than 4-6 weeks (Defrees 2017, Manning 2020). However, it is the most effective diet intervention studied so far. Gluten-free diets, while popular, either have no effect or worsen symptoms in people with IBS who do not have celiac disease or NCGS (Singh 2018).

One concern about elimination diets is the effects of reducing diversity of foods and the resulting changes in microbial populations that could exacerbate the dysbiosis usually present in IBS (Catassi 2017). For that reason, some versions of the FODMAP diet are less restrictive. It is worth noting that probiotic yogurts are not excluded on the FODMAP diet. Probiotic formulations have been reported to reduce symptoms in IBS, perhaps by ameliorating the effects of dysbiosis (Defrees 2017). Nonetheless, we are still a long way from being able to make specific recommendations regarding probiotics for IBS symptoms.

Addressing top-down factors: Because of the close functional connections of the brain and the gut, psychological stress has profound effects on gut function and can drive many of the symptoms associated with IBS (Halmos 2017, Weaver 2017). For this reason, developing effective coping styles to manage challenges is imperative for anyone with GI disorders, but especially anyone with IBS. To this end, mindfulness-based stress-reduction training and cognitive behavioral therapy, which address developing attitudes and behaviors that can help in managing challenges, have been shown to also alleviate the gut and brain symptoms of IBS (Naliboff 2020). Similarly, a trial of hypnotherapy was found to be as efficacious in reducing IBS symptoms as the low-FODMAP diet (Peters 2016). Finally, yoga and physical activity have been reported to improve both gut and brain-mediated symptoms (Weaver 2017).

Functional dyspepsia: Functional dyspepsia is a group of syndromes that involve pain, bloating, or delayed gastric emptying (Stanghellini 2017). Post-prandial distress syndrome describes pain or bloating after a meal. It is similar to IBS and may follow from motility problems such as the stomach emptying slowly. Epigastric pain syndrome involves pain and burning in the stomach region that may be similar to heartburn or peptic ulcer (Ford 2020). The pain is not necessarily linked to meals, and perhaps paradoxically, can even be lessened by eating.

Gastroparesis is a condition in which the stomach empties very slowly. It is usually accompanied by nausea, and sometimes vomiting, or early satiety. This condition is associated with loss of gut neurons and of non-neuronal cells that mediate motility (Grover 2019). For reasons that are not understood, there is a higher incidence of gastroparesis in women, especially those who are overweight or obese (Grover 2019). Gastroparesis can occur as a consequence of diabetes, due to vagal nerve neuropathy, and possibly due to persistent hyperglycemia. The vagus nerve functions to control gastric emptying in part by opening the pylorus sphincter that separates the stomach from the small intestine. In the normal course of a meal, hyperglycemia signals that food is being absorbed, and slows down gastric emptying, presumably to allow food that is already in the small intestine to be absorbed before more arrives. Diabetes is associated with persistent hyperglycemia, which may contribute to the delays in gastric emptying seen in diabetic patients. Surgical interventions, such as bariatric surgery, can also lead to gastroparesis due to damage to the vagus nerve, which controls stomach emptying (Camilleri 2018). Gastroparesis can be painful, and some patients are prescribed opiates for pain management. However, opiates themselves slow gastric emptying, and studies indicate that people with gastroparesis taking opiates have more complications and worse prognosis that gastroparesis patients who do not take opiates (Caminlleri 2018). Diet is the first-line treatment for gastroparesis (Camilleri 2018. Patients are advised to limit fats in the diet, as they tend to slow stomach emptying, to eat smaller meals more frequently, and to consume liquids, such as soups.

Cyclic vomiting disorder: This disorder involves episodes of severe nausea, vomiting, and pain that can last days to a week, which are separated by periods of normal health. It can affect both children and adults (Kovacic 2018). Although it is less common than other disorders of brain gut interaction, affecting about 2% of the US population, cyclic vomiting disorder is the most dangerous (Kovacic 2018). Patients often require intravenous fluids during episodes and can require hospitalization. Children typically miss weeks of school per year, and some adults cannot keep working.

The causes of cyclic vomiting disorder are still mysterious, but it shares common features with migraine headache (Kovacic 2018). Indeed, many people with cyclic vomiting disorder go on to develop migraines, and migraine medication can be helpful for some patients. There is clearly autonomic dysfunction that may originate in the brain (Kovacic 2018). Interestingly, a recent diagnostic category, cannabis hyperemesis syndrome (CHS), which is seen in chronic cannabis users, shares many features with cyclic vomiting disorder, and may in fact be a subcategory. Less is known yet about CHS, including whether ceasing cannabis use stops the episodes (Kovacic 2018).

Consistent with other disorders of brain gut interaction, people with cyclic vomiting disorder experience sickness syndrome symptoms, especially anxiety, fatigue, and depression. Similarly, psychological stress seems to contribute to onset of episodes (Kovacic 2018).

Functional Heartburn and Reflux Hypersensitivity

Heartburn is a painful sensation in the esophagus that may or may not be associated with gastro-esophageal reflux disease (Kondo 2017). When occurring with reflux disease, acid in the contents refluxed activates pain-sensing nerves in the esophagus. Visceral hyperalgesia is a key feature, involving *allodynia* and *hyperalgesia.* Allodynia is a state where not-painful stimuli, such as food, feel painful. Hyperalgesia is a state where normally painful stimuli, such as hot peppers, feel more painful. In functional heartburn, these symptoms are experienced in the absence of acid in the esophagus or reflux disease. Not all reflux involves acidic contents, but in reflux hypersensitivity the sensations elicited are painful, and characteristic of visceral hypersensitivity. As with IBS, the evidence of pain in the absence of tissue damage has been perplexing. But like IBS, there is evidence of low-grade inflammation, specifically: the immune cells in the esophagus are in a pro-inflammatory state that activates pain-transmitting nerves and modifies their sensitivity (Kondo 2017). As with IBS, "top-down" factors, including insomnia, stress, and anxiety, cause changes in the sensory function of gut tissue, in this case the esophagus (Kondo 2017). Typical of visceral hypersensitivity, brain responses to esophageal stimuli have been shown to be enhanced in heartburn.

Treating functional heartburn and reflux hypersensitivity is a challenge because these pain conditions do not arise from excess acid. Thus, proton-pump inhibitors, commonly prescribed for GERD (see below) do not alleviate the pain. Because top-down factors contribute to symptoms, coping and stress management approaches similar to those helpful for IBS could also be helpful for functional heartburn and reflux hypersensitivity.

Gastro-Esophageal Reflux Disease (GERD)

GERD is collection of disorders that have in common a dysfunction of the little sphincter at the bottom of the esophagus, the lower esophageal sphincter that keeps things in the stomach (Katzka 2020). The result is that partially digested food and stomach acid, instead of proceeding to the stomach as it is supposed to, gets sent up into lower esophagus, where it can be associated with a painful burning sensation, called "heartburn". This happens when there is increased *gastric pressure*. Gastric pressure occurs when the stomach is full of food or gas. This pressure forces contents back up into the esophagus. Sometime hiatal hernia, in which the top of the stomach can protrude through the diaphragm and into the thoracic cavity, causes GERD (Katztka 2020). Most people "burp" or experience reflux from time to time, especially after drinking bubbly beverages. In GERD, reflux becomes chronic, and the acid from the stomach can damage the esophagus (Katzka, 2020). This damage to the esophagus from acid provides the rationale for the proton-pump inhibitors (PPIs) usually prescribed for GERD.

Acid is normally secreted to facilitate digestion during a meal. PPIs work to block the production of acid into the stomach. This can prevent damage to the esophagus if there is reflux of stomach contents. Unfortunately, PPIs do not treat the actual causes of GERD, and can make them worse. Reducing acid in the stomach changes the pH, which in turn changes gut microbe populations not only in the stomach, but in other parts of the gut (Bruno 2019, Imhann 2017). These changes are associated with small intestinal bacterial overgrowth (SIBO), a type of severe dysbiosis (Su 2018). Because PPIs can have serious side effects, including kidney disease, loss of bone density, micronutrient deficiencies, and gastric and esophageal cancer, PPIs are only intended to be taken for 2-4 weeks at a time to allow the esophagus to heal (Fossmark 2019, Jaynes 2019). But many people take them for years or even decades, even though long-term PPI use can increase the risk of esophageal adenocarcinoma or cancer in some people (Brusselaers 2018). Risk for gastric cancer may also be elevated (Fossmark 2019). In addition, PPI use can cause reductions in stomach emptying or gastroparesis, and predispose to IBS, due to effects on microbial populations (Bruno 2019). One of the biggest risks of PPI use is risk of infection, especially enteric infections, but also hepatobiliary, respiratory, and CNS infections (Martinsen 2019). This risk is believed to be due to the role of gastric acid in killing infectious microorganisms. Many pathogenic microbes are killed at a pH of 4 or lower but survive at the higher pHs that result from use of PPIs or other acid-reducing agents, such as histamine blockers (Martinsen 2019).

Fortunately, lifestyle changes can improve symptoms of GERD (Kahrilas 2013, Katzka 2020, Stein 2020). Eating small meals slowly, and chewing food well before swallowing, can reduce gastric pressure. GERD can be a particular problem at night while lying to sleep. Lying flat can make it easier for food to pass into the esophagus, so elevating the head of the bed or sleeping with pillows to elevate the shoulders and upper chest can relieve pressure on the lower esophageal sphincter. It is also important to have an empty stomach by bedtime, to help keep gastric pressure lower. Overweight and obesity increase the risk of GERD and losing weight can improve symptoms (Katzka 2020, Stein 2020). Finally, symptoms of GERD, especially visceral hypersensitivity, are exacerbated by stress, and stress management approaches such as hypnotherapy can be helpful (Kahrilas 2013).

Inflammatory Bowel Disease (IBD)

As the name implies, IBD involves serious inflammation along the gut. IBD can become life-threatening in its most severe presentation. The main classes of IBD are Crohn's disease, which can affect the entire gastrointestinal tract, ulcerative colitis (UC), which involves inflammation of just the colon, and microscopic colitis. IBD is the result of inborn factors, including genes associated with pathogen-sensing and inflammatory responses, which interact with environmental factors, such as stress and diet, that impact gut barrier function and microbial populations (Ananthakrishnan 2015, Lee 2021, Miehlke 2019, Spiller 2016).

Notably, diet is increasingly recognized as one of the most important environmental factors in the onset of IBD (Rizzello 2019). Diets high in processed meat and low in fiber are associated with increased risk for IBD, and the prevalence of IBD is highest in countries in Europe and North America, both areas where populations tend to consume the Western diet (Rizzello 2019). This diet predisposes to dysbiosis, and to an imbalance that disfavors the microbes that provide butyrate. Therefore, people who are genetically susceptible to gut barrier disfunction and/or poorly regulated inflammation are at greater risk from poor diets.

Although the pathophysiology and genetics of Crohn's and UC are similar, they are now considered different disorders based on slightly differing presenting symptoms, location of inflammation, and response to treatments. An imbalance in microbial populations is characteristic of IBD, but there seem to be subtle differences between Crohn's disease and UC in this regard. For instance, high-fiber diets have been shown to be helpful for people with Crohn's, but not those with UC (Brotherton 2016). In contrast, fecal transplant is more helpful for people with UC than with Crohn's (Lee 2021). Microbes clearly contribute to IBD symptoms, but there is still more to learn about their contributions to develop reliably effective treatments.

When symptoms of IBD emerge under six years of age, it is diagnosed as *Very early onset IBD*. This type of IBD can be associated with immune deficiency syndromes and is often quite severe (Moran 2017). Diagnosis can be delayed because it is frequently attributed to food allergies (Moran 2017).

Crohn's disease: Inflammation in Crohn's disease can affect the entire gastrointestinal tract. It typically presents as abdominal pain, watery and sometimes bloody diarrhea, fatigue, and weight loss (Veauthier 2018). Weight loss occurs due to malabsorption of food due to gut barrier dysfunction, chronic diarrhea, and/or anorexia due to fear of eating. Severe inflammation can cause the formation of fibrous strictures that block the movement of food down the gut. Fistulas, which are little tunnels between organs, such as between the gut and vagina or skin, can also develop as a result of inflammation. The development of strictures and fistulas may require surgery. Because "what happens in the gut does not stay in the gut," Crohn's disease often involves tissues outside the gut, including the heart, kidney, eyes, skin, and joints, where it may cause arthritis or spondylitis (Ott 2013). Inflammation in the gut can also drive symptoms of the brain-mediated sickness syndrome.

Ulcerative colitis: As the name implies, inflammation in ulcerative colitis is restricted to the colon. Like Crohn's, diarrhea is a hallmark of the disease, especially bloody diarrhea. It can develop at any age, but older age of onset is typically associated with less severe disease. The pathophysiology of ulcerative colitis involves dysbiosis, gut barrier dysfunction, and loss of protective mucus (Ungaro 2017), all of which drive inflammation. Ulcerative colitis is most common in Westernized countries, and the link with disordered microbes suggests that the Western diet and an urbanized, overly hygienic lifestyle contribute to the etiology of the disease.

Microscopic or lymphocytic colitis: Inflammation in microscopic colitis is, as the name suggests, only visible in biopsy samples. Because of this, it is often mistaken for IBS (Spiller 2016). Microscopic colitis causes frequent, watery diarrhea and weight loss (Miehlke 2019). Like other IBDs, genetic predisposition contributes to the pathophysiology in concert with gut barrier dysfunction. In addition, the use of certain drugs, including serotonin reuptake inhibitors (SSRIs), NSAIDs, and especially PPIs are linked to microscopic colitis (Miehlke 2019). It is often co-morbid with autoimmune diseases, and like other autoimmune diseases, it disproportionally affects women. Although microscopic colitis is not as severe in terms of threat to life as Crohn's disease and ulcerative colitis, it severely affects quality of life. In addition, damage to gut barrier function and loss of weight indicate a risk for nutritional deficiencies.

Treatment for IBD involves anti-inflammatory medications, including aminosalicylates and sulphasalazine as the first line treatment for UC. These drugs are not as effective for Crohn's disease (Ungaro 2017). More severe cases are treated with steroids or "biological" anti-inflammatory drugs. These work to inhibit pro-inflammatory mediators such as cytokines that are induced as part of the disease process (Moran 2017). Biological drugs have been a breakthrough for the treatment of IBD, but they are not effective for everyone, and they carry serious long-term consequences. The major concern is that because these drugs reduce inflammation, even necessary inflammation, there is a dramatic increase in susceptibility to infections, including fatal infections. Because of these risks, it is important to characterize dietary interventions that can help people with IBD to stay in remission, and thus reduce exposure to the drugs (Day 2012). One diet-based approach for achieving remission in Crohn's disease is called exclusive enteral nutrition (EEN) (Day 2015). This is a liquid diet that is nutritionally complete and seems to help the gut heal (Day 2015, Logan 2020). EEN involves consuming only the diet for a period of 6-12 weeks, and then gradually reintroducing solid foods (Day 2015). In addition, stress management, techniques for learning resilience, and diet approaches are important components of IBD management (Brotherton 2016, Konterek 2011, Oligschlaeger 2019).

Non-gut Gut Disorders: Parkinson's Disease, Schizophrenia and Autism

What happens in the gut does not stay in the gut, and pathology in the gut can affect every other tissue of the body. Interoceptive nerves and gut hormones keep the gut and brain closely linked. The gut influences behavior, especially ingestive behavior, and adverse conditions in the gut drive sickness syndrome symptoms such as fatigue, anxiety, and depression. A possible further link between gut disorders and brain pathology has been suspected for many decades (Brudek 2019). Recent advances in understanding the pathophysiology of neurodegenerative, autoimmune, and neurodevelopmental conditions have spurred increasing recognition that gut problems may contribute either to the etiology of these disorders or to symptomatology, or both (Brudek 2019, Santos 2019).

Parkinson's disease (PD): PD is characterized by accumulation of a protein normally found in neurons, including gut neurons, called alpha synuclein (α-syn). Alpha synuclein becomes misfolded and coalesces into insoluble structures called Lewy bodies. The misfolded protein seems to trigger neuroinflammation that results in the loss of dopaminergic neurons in the brainstem. These neurons are involved in activating movements, thus people with PD have symptoms of muscle rigidity, fatigue, and difficulty initiating movement. Unfortunately, the damage to the neurons does not produce observable impairments until most of the neurons are destroyed, and there is no cure.

Although Parkinson's disease is usually thought of as a brain disorder, gut symptoms are a hallmark of PD (Pfeiffer 2011). Indeed, gut-related symptoms were part of the initial report of the disease by James Parkinson in 1817 (Pfeiffer 2011). Such symptoms affect at least 80% of PD patients and exert marked deleterious effects on quality of life (Caputi 2018). Gut symptoms associated with PD include nausea, slow gastric emptying, and especially constipation. These symptoms are consequences of disordered gut neuron function, possibly due to the Lewy bodies that accumulate in the enteric nervous system (Brudek 2019). The other hallmarks of PD in the gut are gut barrier dysfunction and dysbiosis (Santos 2019).

Clues that gut inflammation may play a role in the pathophysiology of Parkinson's disease derive from observations that gut symptoms appear up to 20 years before motor symptoms. α-syn is expressed in neurons of the enteric nervous system (ENS) and in immune cells, mostly "innate" macrophages and dendritic cells that control inflammation. α-syn seems to accumulate during gut inflammation. Autopsy material from people at different stages of PD reveal that α-syn in the gut appears very early on in the disease. Specifically, α-syn can be found in the gut of people who had not yet reported motor symptoms but showed mild brainstem pathology consistent with PD (Braak 2006).

A key finding from these studies is that the characteristic accumulation of Lewy bodies with neuroinflammation occurs first in the caudal brainstem dorsal motor nucleus of the vagus, where the cell bodies of vagal motor neurons that connect the brain to the gut live. This observation suggests that the misfolded proteins may originate initially in the gut neurons (ENS) (Braak 2006, Brudek 2019, Santos 2019). Some of the misfolded proteins may be taken up by vagal motor neurons and transported into the brain. Misfolding of the protein may occur as a consequence of inflammation, as this induces upregulation of synuclein, or it may occur secondary to gut barrier disruption (Brudek 2019). Dysbiosis is associated with both gut barrier disruption and alpha synuclein in the gut early on in PD. Gut microbes can be a source of misfolded proteins. Thus, one hypothesis regarding the early pathophysiology of PD is that alpha synuclein gets into the body via increased paracellular permeability, is taken up by cells of the enteric nervous system and vagus nerve, which transports it to the brain, and induces inflammation and propagation further into the brain (Brudek 2019).

A key issue for neurodegenerative diseases is early detection, as by the time that movement symptoms are evident the damage is irreversible. Because GI issues precede the motor impairments, these symptoms could be a prodromal biomarker for PD risk. Early detection might allow interventions to prevent neurodegeneration, and instituting measures that support gut health might also be preventive for PD (Santos 2019). These misfolded proteins also occur in IBD (Brudek 2019). Whereas most people with IBD do not go on to develop PD, IBD is a risk factor, and it is suggested that people with IBD be monitored for the development of PD symptoms.

Schizophrenia: Schizophrenia is a brain disorder that is characterized by disorganized thoughts and behaviors, and experiences that seem out of touch with reality, including hallucinations and delusions (Severance 2016). The causes of schizophrenia are not known, but there seems to be an interaction of genetic susceptibility with environmental factors (Nemai 2015). Gene-linkage studies implicate immune system gene alleles with schizophrenia, including those that also contribute to brain development and plasticity. As in PD, gut disorders have long been recognized to be commonly associated with schizophrenia, including a high rate of gut inflammation found at autopsy (Severance 2016).

One typical finding in people with schizophrenia is abnormal or enhanced immune responses to food antigens (Severance 2016). Celiac disease and NGCS are more common among people with schizophrenia compared to the general population. People with schizophrenia also have high rates of immune responses to wheat and other food-related antigens (Severance 2016). Such food intolerances may drive systemic inflammation, and via gut-brain connections influence brain function, including cognition. Although antipsychotic medications can influence gut function, gut pathology, especially increased gut barrier permeability, is seen early in the course of the disease, and in medication-naïve patients (Dickerson 2017). Although it is not clear what accounts for gut barrier disruption, DAMPs, notably those associated with *Toxoplasma gondii*, correlate with symptoms and may drive inflammation (Dickerson 2017).

Although the gut-brain link to schizophrenia is still not well understood, the recent link to gut microbes and brain development, specifically their still mysterious role in programming neural populations involved in cognition, raises hope for better understanding and possibly new treatment for this challenging and devastating condition (Bastiannssen 2018, Langgartner 2019).

Autism: Autism is a neurodevelopmental disorder characterized by deficits in social behavior and cognition, with a wide spectrum of severity. The causes of autism are not known, but like schizophrenia, the condition likely emerges as an interaction between genetic and environmental factors. Autism is associated with high rates of comorbid gut symptoms (e.g., 40%) including chronic gut pain and dysmotility. The severity of these symptoms correlates with the severity of cognitive and behavioral symptoms (Fattorusso 2019). As in other gut disorders, dysbiosis and increased gut barrier permeability are typical features (Fattoruusso 2019). The possible mechanistic contributions of dysbiosis and gut permeability to the symptoms of autism are not established. But, as in schizophrenia, gut-brain communication may be contributing to brain dysfunction, perhaps via inflammation. Another common feature observed in autism is *hyperserotonemia,* or elevated serotonin in blood. More than 90 percent of circulating serotonin originates in the gut, suggesting this system is dysregulated. The meaning of this is not clear and may well be related to the gut-related symptoms experienced in autism. But because the vagus nerve contains serotonin receptors, elevated gut serotonin may also influence interoceptive networks in the brain, thereby influencing behavior and cognition.

Although dysbiosis is common among people with autism, and dysbiosis has been linked to a wide variety of brain disorders, the relationship of altered microbes to the pathophysiology is not clear. Microbial populations are strongly influenced by diet, and many people with autism are "weird" about food, for example, eating only a limited variety of foods, rejecting fruits and vegetables, or having strong emotional reactions to food they do not like. Such eating behaviors may well contribute to dysbiosis. Nonetheless, there are several possible ways that dysbiosis could influence the expression of autistic symptoms. Certain microbes produce substances such as butyrate and other short-chain fatty acids that keep the gut barrier healthy, as well as program immune cells, supporting anti-inflammatory activity. Missing these microbes could lead to increased inflammation and gut barrier dysfunction. Further, neurotransmitters produced by gut microbes can interact with gut immune cells and neurons, as well as with the extrinsic nerves (e.g., vagus) that connect the gut and brain. This could provide a connection between gut function and symptoms associated with autism. The link of autism with dysbiosis suggests that probiotics might be helpful, but findings in that regard have been mixed. However, a recent small study of children with autism found that fecal transplant led to about a 50 percent improvement in both social behavior and cognitive function, reinforcing the idea that whatever the actual cause of autism, gut dysbiosis may contribute to symptom severity (Kang 2019).

Multiple sclerosis (MS): MS is an autoimmune disease in which the immune system attacks the myelin sheaths that insulate neuronal axons, inducing neuroinflammation. Neuronal damage leads to motor deficiencies and can also lead to cognitive impairment. Although the precise causes of multiple sclerosis are not clearly established, recent observations from clinical and pre-clinical studies implicate gut-related factors in driving the nervous system inflammation that is the hallmark of the disease (Buscainu 2019, Ochoa-Reparaz 2018, Parodi 2021).

Like the other non-gut gut disorders, MS is associated with dysbiosis, gut barrier disruption, and increased intestinal permeability (Buscarinu 2019). There is evidence that this permeability may drive the neuroinflammation by several possible mechanisms (Buscarinu 2019). A key feature of multiple sclerosis is that, as in other autoimmune diseases, immune system homeostasis is disrupted, leading to uncontrolled inflammation and destruction of brain tissue (Ochoa-Reparaz 2018). At the same time, pro-inflammatory antigens from gut bacteria (microbe-associated molecular patterns; MAMPs), presumably consequent to translocation across a leaky gut, can been found in the blood of MS patients. MAMP level correlate with levels of pro-inflammatory cytokines and disability status (Buscarinu 2019).

One key feature of multiple sclerosis is Treg dysfunction, in that Treg fails to suppress inflammation. Because immune homeostasis is regulated by gut microbes, in part via programming of T cells and regulatory cells, disruption of the immune balance in the gut could lead to inflammatory phenotypes of T cells associated with multiple sclerosis. Pre-clinical models of multiple sclerosis implicate gut microbes in aberrant programming of these cells (Ochao-Raparaz 2018).

A potentially important consequence of dysbiosis for multiple sclerosis is reduction in butyrate production. In addition to serving as a key fuel source for gut barrier cells, the short-chain fatty acid butyrate also functions to regulate inflammation, both in the gut and in the brain. Neuroinflammation is a key feature of the pathophysiology of multiple sclerosis. In addition, microbe-derived short-chain fatty acids (SCFAs) act to protect the blood-brain barrier. There is evidence that people with multiple sclerosis have fewer gut microbes that produce these SCFAs (Ochoa-Reparaz 2018). These findings emphasize the importance of gut barrier function in regulating the neurological symptoms associated with MS and suggest that dietary approaches could be beneficial in helping regulate neuroinflammation.

Food is the Problem, and Food is the Solution

Of all the tissues of the body, the gut is uniquely sensitive to diet. It is the first place food arrives, thus it has a high potential exposure to toxins in food or water, was well as to pro-inflammatory oxidized lipids and advanced glycation end-products (Urribari 2005). Gut health relies on certain microbial populations that provide butyrate, which serves as the major energy source for gut barrier cells, and other short-chain fatty acids that modulate immune functions (Vital 2015). Microbes also provide other nutrients, including vitamin K. Diets deficient in the kinds of foods that nourish these microbes lead to dysbiosis, low-grade inflammation, and gut barrier dysfunction, including malabsorption of food and increased gut permeability. The challenge then is: How to ameliorate an unhealthy gut?

The jury is still out. Practices that keep the gut healthy are better understood than those that can support a gut in distress. The weight of the epidemiological, observational, and clinical evidence points to a Mediterranean-style diet based heavily on vegetables, fruit, grains, olive oil, beans/legumes, nuts, and good-quality dairy and meat, as important for gut health (Antoniussen 2921, Mentella 2020, Paduano 2019, Sugihara 2021). Good-quality dairy and meat largely means probiotic fermented dairy products, and poultry and fish, rather than red/mammal meat. However, there are potential issues with this diet when it comes to certain gut disorders.

For example, both whole wheat and dairy are "prebiotic" for many commensal microbes known to be beneficial to the gut. However, many people are intolerant to wheat products and sometimes other grains, such as barley and rye, that contain gluten. Fortunately, there are many gluten-free or low-gluten grains such as oats, whole rice, and grain-like plants like quinoa, that can be part of a healthy diet for wheat/gluten-sensitive people. As yet, the complete picture of wheat intolerance is not yet understood. It may be the case that some kinds of wheat, notably "ancient wheat," can be tolerated by people who can't manage the modern varieties (Rizzello 2019).

Although dairy products are also a staple of the Mediterranean diet, many people are intolerant or allergic to the sugars or proteins in milk. One of the sugars in milk, lactose, needs to be enzymatically broken down in order be absorbed into the body, but many people lose activity of the enzyme by the time they reach adulthood. Lactose that is not absorbed into the body is then fermented by microbes, leading to gas and bloating. However, the microbes in fermented dairy product such as yogurt and kefir break down the lactose, thus allowing some lactose-intolerant people to tolerate fermented dairy products. People with demonstrated milk allergies do need to avoid dairy, and because dairy is an important source of bioavailable calcium, people with these allergies or intolerance need to be mindful to include other sources of calcium in their diets.

For people with IBD, dietary factors that support gut health are less clear. IBD is closely associated with microbial dysbiosis, and it would seem that dietary fiber would be important, especially, to heal the gut barrier, and keep it healthy. Paradoxically, however, during flare-ups when the gut is overtly inflamed, low-fiber diets are most beneficial. For instance, essential enteral nutrition (EEN, e.g., products like

Ensure®), which involves a low-fiber, nutritionally complete liquid meal, used exclusively for 6-8 weeks, has been shown in several studies of children with IBD to result in remission in 80% of cases (Day 2015). This rate is comparable to that obtained by treatment with steroids, the usual care for pediatric IBD. Whether or not EEN is efficacious in adults has not been addressed. Although high fiber in the diet during frank inflammation is problematic, many practitioners recommend adopting a plant-based or Mediterranean diet when remission is obtained (Saez-Gonzalez 2019). In particular, and contrary to previous recommendations, including fiber in the diet when in remission is associated with fewer flare-ups (Brotherton 2016).

A number of diets are popular among IBD patients for addressing the reduction of inflammation during a flare-up, including the *specific carbohydrate diet* (SCD) and the low-FODMAP diet (see above), which are similar, as well as the "anti-inflammatory diet" gluten-free diets, and other elimination diets. The SCD and low-FODMAP diets to seem to improve symptoms, but one concern is that these elimination diets can lead to micronutrient deficiencies, including calcium, zinc, vitamin D, the B vitamin group, and protein (Mentella 2020). Lack of protein is of particular concern because sufficient protein intake is necessary for healing the gut during periods of inflammation (Antoniussen 2021). Thus, these diets should only be followed for defined time periods, e.g., 6-8 weeks, with gradual reintroduction of specific foods after that. In general, although there is very good reason to believe diet is important for achieving a healthy gut in IBD, there are few well-designed studies that support the efficacy of these diets.

Exclusion Diets

The emerging recognition of the link between diet, the gut, and inflammation has encouraged some practitioners to blame specific types of foods, usually wheat and grain, dairy, nightshade vegetables (e.g., tomatoes, peppers, eggplants, potatoes) and lectins (found in beans). Exclusion diets have become increasing popular as a way to address sickness syndrome symptoms (fatigue, depression, anxiety) and gastro-intestinal problems (IBS, reflux), based on claims that the excluded foods are naturally inflammatory. However, this approach is NOT evidence-based, and from what we know about triggers of inflammation, and the role of a diverse microbial population, these diets may worsen rather than ameliorate problems.

As noted previously, microbial dysbiosis has been linked to a wide variety of disorders, including mood disorders, autism, and neurodegenerative diseases. Dysbiosis is usually a consequence of reduced diversity, often linked to antibiotic use. However, it has become clear now that diet is the single most important influence on the health and diversity of gut microbial populations (Garcia-Mantrana 2018, Vital 2015). A diverse diet containing many different foods is necessary for maintaining a diverse microbial population, and thus a dramatic exclusion diet, for instance such as one that is restricted to lettuce and meat while excluding dairy, grains, beans, and nightshade vegetables, and sometimes many fruits, can result in dysbiosis and increased inflammation.

In addition to what exclusion diets imply for overall microbial diversity, the types of foods typically excluded, especially red-pigmented, polyphenol-rich members of the nightshade family, beans (lectins) and whole grains (gluten) may be particularly important for the microbes that produce butyrate (Fan 2019,

Rodriguez-Daza 2021). Because butyrate provides the principal source of energy for gut barrier cells, gut barrier cells that are already struggling with the effects of chronic inflammation will find it difficult to heal without butyrate.

Another risk involves changes in gut immune responses to foods that have been excluded. There is some evidence that people who eliminate foods they are not actually allergic to, can lose tolerance to the eliminated or restricted foods over time. Symptoms can develop after periods of exclusion, making it very difficult to reintroduce foods. Currently, it is not clear how to reinstate food tolerances in adults, meaning that people who go on exclusion diets may find it very difficult to resume eating the excluded foods, setting the stage for long-term risk of dysbiosis and gut barrier inflammation.

Finally, it can be difficult to ascertain the connection between specific foods and symptoms, when there is not an evident pathophysiological consequence, such as an observable antibody response in the case of food allergy. Humans and other animals are hard-wired to associate symptoms of illness, such as gastrointestinal distress, with the last thing they ate (Garcia 1974). This has an obvious survival advantage, in that a major way for poisons, toxins, or pathogenic microbes to enter our bodies is through food. Learning to associate feelings of sickness with food helps us avoid possible poisoning, but it is unfortunately non-specific. The food does not have to actually cause illness for this "conditioned taste aversion" learning to induce us to link the food to the symptoms. In fact, many of us have had the experience of developing a "stomach flu" and associating it with the last thing we ate before becoming ill, even though we know consciously that the food did not cause the illness. This is extremely powerful learning. For instance, it has been shown in animals that they do not even have to be conscious when made ill to develop a food aversion (Garcia 1974). Because there are several factors, including dysbiosis, stress, "gut brain," and gut barrier dysfunctions that can cause symptoms, it is difficult to know whether a specific food is interacting with these factors, or if it just happened to be the last thing we ate. Given the risks of exclusion diets, it is important to consider that the symptoms might be more effectively addressed in view of the other objectively observed factors that can drive gastrointestinal disturbances.

Key Points

- The Western diet, consisting of high-energy, low-nutrient processed foods, is associated with all gut disorders, emphasizing the important role of diet for gut health.
- Another key feature common to gut disorders is dysbiosis. This is an imbalance in microbes caused by antibiotics and/or a diet poor in "prebiotic" foods, such as fiber, fresh fruit, and vegetables.
- New findings now indicate that brain disorders, including Parkinson's disease, autism, schizophrenia, and multiple sclerosis, seem to be either initiated by conditions in the gut or are worsened by pro-inflammatory immune cell programming of gut immune cells.
- "Top-down" influences on the gut, for instance stress, can act to enhance visceral hyperalgesia, which is a chronic pain condition of the gut.
- The intimate and bidirectional character of gut and brain interactions can complicate accurate association of specific foods with gut-related symptoms. For instance, we naturally associate symptoms with the last thing we ate, and the symptoms can be re-experienced via classical conditioning as a "conditioned food aversion."

References

Altobelli E, Del Negro V, Angeletti PM, Latella G. Low-FODMAP Diet Improves Irritable Bowel Syndrome Symptoms: A Meta-Analysis. Nutrients, 9:940, 2017.

Ananthakrishnan AN. Epidemiology and risk factors for IBD. Nature Reviews Gastroenterology and Hepatology,12:205-217, 2015.

Antoniussen CS, Rasmussen HH, Holst M, Lauridsen. Reducing disease activity of inflammatory bowel disease by consumption of plant-based foods and nutrients. Frontiers in Nutrition, 8:733433, 2021.

Aziz I, Simren M. The overlap between irritable bowel syndrome and organic gastrointestinal diseases. Lancet Gastroenterology and Hepatology, 6:139-148, 2021.

Barbara G, Cremon C, De Giorgio R, Dothel G, Zecchi L, Bellacosa L, et al. Mechanisms underlying visceral hypersensitivity in irritable bowel syndrome. Current Gastroenterology Reports, 13L:308-315, 2011.

Barber TM, Valsamakios G, Mastorakos G, Hanson P, Kyrou I, Randeva HS, Weickert MO. Dietary influences on the microbiota-gut-brain axis. International Journal of Molecular Sciences, 22:3502, 2021.

Barnett JA, Gibson DL. Separating the empirical wheat from the pseudoscientific chaff: A critical review of the literature surrounding glyphosate, dysbiosis and wheat-sensitivity. Frontiers in Microbiology, 11:556729, 2020.

Bastiaanssen TFS, Cowan CSM, Claesson MJ, Dinan TG, Cryan JF. Making sense of ... the microbiome in psychiatry. International Journal of Neuropsychopharmacology, 22:37-52, 2019.

Bhatterai Y, Muniz Pedrogo DA, Pashnat PC. Irritable bowel syndrome: a gut microbiota-related disorder? American Journal of Physiology Gastrointestinal and Liver Physiology, 312:G52-G62, 2017.

Braak H, de Vos RAI, Bohl J, Del Tredici K. Gastric a-synuclein inclusions in Meissner's and Aurbach's plexuses in cases staged for Parkinson's disease-related brain pathology. Neuroscience Letters, 396:67-72, 2006.

Bray J, Fernandes A, Nguyen GC, Otley AR, Heatherington J, Stretton J, et al. The Challenges of Living with Inflammatory Bowel Disease: Summary of a Summit on Patient and Healthcare Provider Perspectives. Canadian Journal of Gastroenterology and Hepatology, 2016:9430942, 2016.

Brotherton CS, Marin CA, Long MD, Kappelman MD, Sandler RS. Avoidance of fiber is associated with greater risk of Crohn's Disease flare in a 6-month period. Clinical Gastroenterology and Hepatology, 14:1130-1136, 2016.

Brudek T. Inflammatory Bowel Diseases and Parkinson's Disease. Journal of Parkinson's Disease 9:S331-S344, 2019.

Bruno G, Zaccari P, Rocco G, Scalese G, Panetta C, Porowska B, Pontone S, Severi C. Proton pump inhibitors and dysbiosis: Current knowledge and aspects to be clarified. World Journal of Gastroenterology, 25:2706-271, 2019.

Brusselaers N, Engstrand L, Lagergren J. Maintenance proton pump inhibition and the risk of oesophageal cancer. Cancer Epidemiology, 53:172-177, 2018.

Bunyavanich S, Berin MC. Food allergy and the microbiome: Current understandings and future directions. Journal of Allergy and Clinical Immunology, 144:1468-1477, 2019.

Buscarinu MC, Fornasiero A, Romano S, Ferraldeschi M, Mechelli R, Renie R, et al. The contribution of gut barrier changes to multiple sclerosis pathology. Frontiers in Immunology,10:1916, 2019.

Camilleri M, Chedid V, Ford AC, Haruma K, Horowitz M, Jones KL, Low PA, Park SY, Parkman HP, Stanghellini V. Gastroparesis. Nature Review Disease Primers. 4(1):41, 2018.

Caminero A, Verdu EF. Celiac disease: should we care about microbes? American Journal of Physiology Liver and Gastrointestinal Physiology, 317:G161-G170, 2019.

Caputi V, Giron MC. Microbiome-Gut-Brain Axis and Toll-Like Receptors in Parkinson's Disease. International Journal of Molecular Sciences, 19:1689, 2018.

Catassi G, Elena Lionetti E, Gatti S, Catassi C. The Low FODMAP Diet: Many Question Marks for a Catchy Acronym. Nutrients, 9:292, 2017.

Catassi C, Alaedini A, Bojarski C, Bonaz B, Bouma G, Carroccio A, et al. The Overlapping Area of Non-Celiac Gluten Sensitivity (NCGS) and Wheat-Sensitive Irritable Bowel Syndrome (IBS): An Update. Nutrients, 9:1268, 2017.

Chen J, Vitetta L, Inflammation-modulating effect of butyrate in the prevention of colon cancer by dietary fiber. Clinical Colorectal Cancer, 17: e541-4, 2018.

Creekmore AL, Hong S, Zhu S, Xue J, Wiley JW. Chronic stress-associated visceral hyperalgesia correlates with severity of intestinal barrier dysfunction. Pain, 159:1777-1789, 2018.

Day AS, Ledder O, Leach ST, Lemberg DA. Crohn's and colitis in children and adults. World Journal of Gastroenterology, 18:5862-5869, 2012.

Day AS, Lopez RN. Exclusive enteral nutrition in children with Crohn's disease. World Journal of Gastroenterology, 21:6809-6816, 2015.

Defrees DN, Bailey J. Irritable Bowel Syndrome: Epidemiology, Pathophysiology, Diagnosis, and Treatment. Primary Care Clinic and Office Practice, 44:655-671, 2017.

Di Martinis M, Sirufo MM, Suppa M, Ginaldi L. New perspectives in food allergy. International Journal of Molecular Sciences, 21:1474, 2020.

Di Tommaso N, Gasbarrini A, Ponziani FR. Intestinal barrier in health and disease, International Journal of Environmental Research and Public Health, 18:12836, 2021.

Ding W, Shangguan Y, Zhu Y, Sultan Y, Feng Y, Zhang B et al. Negative impacts of microcystin-LR and glyphosate on zebrafish intestine: Linked with gut microbiota and microRNAs? Environmental Pollution, 286:117685, 2021.

Elli L, Branchi F, Tomba C, Villalta D, Norsa L, Ferretti F, et al. Diagnosis of gluten related disorders: Celiac disease, wheat allergy and non-celiac gluten sensitivity. World Journal of Gastroenterology, 21:7110-7119, 2015.

Enck P, Aziz Q, Barbara G, Farmer AD, Fukudo S, Mayer E, et al. Irritable bowel syndrome. Nature Review Disease Primers, 2:16014, 2016.

Fan Y, Zhang J. Dietary modulation of intestinal microbiota: Future opportunities in experimental autoimmune encephalomyelitis and multiple sclerosis. Frontiers in Microbiology, 10:740, 2019.

Fattorusso A, Di Genova L, Battista Dell'Isola G, Mencaroni E, Esposito S. Autism Spectrum Disorders and the Gut Microbiota. Nutrients, 11:521, 2019.

Flynn S, Eisenstein S. Inflammatory Bowel Disease Presentation and Diagnosis. Surgery Clinics of North America, 99:1051-1062, 2019.

Ford AC, Mahadeva S, Carbone MF, Lacy BE, Talley NJ. Functional dyspepsia. Lancet, 396:1689-1702, 2020.

Ford AC. Sperber AD, Corsetti M, Camilleri M. Irritable bowel syndrome. Lancet, 396:1675-1688, 2020.

Fossmark R, Martinsen TC, Waldum HL. Adverse effects of proton pump inhibitors- evidence and plausibility. International Journal of Molecular Sciences, 20:5203, 2019.

Freedman SN, Shahi SK, Mangalam AK. The "Gut Feeling": Breaking Down the Role of Gut Microbiome in Multiple Sclerosis. Neurotherapeutics, 15:109-125, 2018.

Fumery M, Singh S, Dulai PS, Gower-Rousseau C, Peyrin-Biroulet L, Sandborn WJ. Natural History of Adult Ulcerative Colitis in Population-based Cohorts: A Systematic Review. Clinical Gastroenterology and Hepatology, 16:343, 2018.

Garcia J, Hankins WG, Rusiniak KW. Behavioral regulation of the milieu interne in man and rat. Science, 185:824-831, 1974.

Garcia-Mantrana I, Selma-Royo M, Alcantara C, Collado MC. Shifts on gut microbiota associated to Mediterranean diet adherence and specific dietary intakes on general adult population. Frontiers in Microbiology, 9:980, 2018.

Genius SJ. Sensitivity-related illness: The escalating pandemic of allergy, food intolerance and chemical sensitivity. Science of the Total Environment, 408:6047-6061, 2010.

Gracie DJ, Hamlin PJ, Ford AC. The influence of the brain-gut axis in inflammatory bowel disease and possible implications for treatment. Lancet Gastroenterology and Hepatology, 4:632-642, 2019.

Greenwood-Van Meerveld B, Johnson AC. Mechanisms of stress-induced viscerla pain. Journal of Neurogastroenterology and Motility, 24:7-18, 2018.

Grover M, Farrugia G, Stanghellini V. Gastroparesis: A turning point in understanding and treatment. Gut, 68:2238-2250, 2019.

Halmos EP. When the low FODMAP diet does not work. Journal of Gastroenterology and Hepatology, 32:69-72, 2017.

Hubbard CS, Hong J-Y, Jiang A, Ebrat B, Suyenobu B, Smith et al. Increased attentional network functioning related to symptom severity measures in females with irritable bowel syndrome. Neurogastroenterology and Motility, 27:1282-1294, 2015.

Imhann F, Vich Vila A, Jan Boder M, Lopez Manosalva AG, Koonen DPY, Fu Y, et al. The influence of proton pump inhibitors and other commonly used medication on the gut microbiota. Gut Microbes, 8:351-358, 2017.

Jaynes M, Kumar AB. The risks of long-term use of proton pump inhibitors: a critical review. Therapeutic Advances in Drug Safety, 10:1-13, 2019.

Jiang X, Wang X, Tui M, Ma J, Xie A. RAGE and its emerging role in the pathogenesis of Parkinson's disease. Neuroscience Letters, 672:65-69, 2018.

Kahrilas PJ, Boeckxstaens G, Smout AJPM. Management of the patient with incomplete response to PPI therapy. Best Practices Research in Clinical Gastroenterology, 27:401-414, 2013.

Katzka DA, Pandolfino JE, Kahrilas, PJ. Phenotypes of gastroesophageal reflux disease: When Rome, Lyon, and Montreal meet. Clinical Gastroenterology and Hepatology, 18:767-776, 2020.

Kondo T, Miwa H. The Role of Esophageal Hypersensitivity in Functional Heartburn. Journal of Clinical Gastroenterology, 51:571-578, 2017.

Kano M, Dupont P, Aziz Q, Fukudo S. Understanding Neurogastroenterology From Neuroimaging Perspective: A Comprehensive Review of Functional and Structural Brain Imaging in Functional Gastrointestinal Disorders. Journal of Neurogastroenterology and Motility, 24:512-527, 2018.

Kellow NJ, Coughlin MT. Effect of diet derived advanced glycation end products on inflammation. Nutrition Reviews, 73:737-759, 2015.

Kinashi Y, Hase K. Partners in leaky gut syndrome: intestinal dysbiosis and autoimmunity. Frontiers in Immunology, 12:673708, 2021.

Konturek PC, Brzozowski T, Konturek SJ. Stress and the gut: pathophysiology, clinical consequences, diagnostic approach and treatment options. Journal of Physiology and Pharmacology, 20:591-599, 2011.

Kolacz J. Kovacic KK, Porges SM. Traumatic stress and the autonomic brain-gut connection in development: Polyvagal Theory as an integrative framework for psychosocial and gastrointestinal pathology. Developmental Psychobiology, 61:796–8 2019.

Kopp W. How Western diet and lifestyle drive the pandemic of obesity and civilization diseases. Diabetes, Metabolic Syndrome and Obesity: Targets and Therapy, 12:2221-2236, 2019.

Kovacic K, Manu Sood M, Venkatesan T. Cyclic Vomiting Syndrome in Children and Adults: What Is New in 2018? Current Gastroenterology Reports, 20:46, 2018.

Langgartner D, Lowry CA, Reber SO. Old Friends, immunoregulation, and stress resilience. Pflügers Archive - European Journal of Physiology, 471:237-269, 2019.

Lee M, Chang EB. Inflammatory bowel diseases and the microbiome: Searching the crime scene for clues. Gastroenterology, 160:524-537, 2021.

Lewis JD, Chen EZ, Baldassano RN, Otley AR, Griffiths AM, Dale Lee D, et al. Inflammation, Antibiotics, and Diet as Environmental Stressors of the Gut Microbiome in Pediatric Crohn's Disease. Cell Host Microbe, 18: 489-500, 2015.

Lin CH. Food allergy: What it is, and what it is not. Current Opinion in Gastroenterology, 35:144-188, 2019.

Loh W, Tang MLK. The epidemiology of food allergy in the global context. International Journal of Environmental Research and Public Health, 15:2043, 2018.

Liu S, Hagiwara, SI Hagiwara, Bhargava A. Early-life adversity, epigenetics, and visceral hypersensitivity. Neurogastroenterology and Motility, 29:10.1111/nmo.13170, 2017.

Manning LP, Yao CK, Biesiekierski JR. Therapy of IBS: Is a low FODMAP diet the answer? Frontiers in Psychiatry,11:865, 2020.

Martinsen TC, Fossmark R, Waldum HL. The Phylogeny and Biological Function of Gastric Juice—Microbiological Consequences of Removing Gastric Acid. International Journal of Molecular Sciences, 20:6031, 2019.

McCoy KD, Ignacio A, Geuking MB. Microbiota and Type 2 immune responses. Current Opinion in Immunology, 54:20-27, 2018.

McKenzie C, Tan J, Macia L, Mackay CR. The nutrition-gut microbiome-physiology axis and allergic diseases. Immunological Reviews, 278:277-295, 2017.

Mentella MC, Scaldaferri F, Pizzoferrato M, Gasbarrini A, Miggiano GAD. Nutrition, IBD and the gut microbiota: A review. Nutrients, 12:944, 2020.

Miehlke S, Verhaigh B, Tontini GE, Madisch A, Langner C, Munch A. Microscopic colitis: pathophysiology and clinical management. Lancet Gastroenterology and Hepatology, 4:305-314, 2019.

Moran CJ. Very early onset inflammatory bowel disease. Seminars in Pediatric Surgery, 26:356-359, 2017.

Naliboff BD, Smith SR, Serpa JG, Laird KT, Stain J, Connolly LS, Labus JS, Tillisch K. Mindfulness-based stress reduction improves irritable bowel syndrome (IBS) symptoms via specific aspects of mindfulness. Neurogastroenterology & Motility, 32: e13828, 2020.

Namani K, Ghomi RH, McCormick B, Fan X. Schizophrenia and the gut-brain axis. Progress in Neuro-Psychopharmacology and Biological Psychiatry, 56:155-160, 2015.

Nazarenkov N, Seeger K, Beeken L, Ananthakrishnan AN, Khalili H, Lewis JD, Gupta Konijet G. Implementing Dietary Modifications and Assessing Nutritional Adequacy of Diets for Inflammatory Bowel Disease. Gastroenterology & Hepatology, 15:133-144, 2019.

Ng SC, Shi HY, Hamidi N, Underwood FE, Tang W, Benchimol EI, et al. Worldwide incidence and prevalence of inflammatory bowel disease in the 21st century: a systematic review of population-based studies. Lancet, 390:2769-2778, 2017.

Oaten M, Stevenson RJ, Case TI. Disease avoidance as a functional basis for stigmatization. Philosophical Transactions of the Royal Society B, 366:3433-3452, 2011.

Oaten M, Stevenson RJ, Williams MA, Rich AN, Butko M, Case T. Moral violations and the experience of disgust or anger. Frontiers in Behavioral Neuroscience, 12:179, 2018.

Ochoa-Reparaz J, Kirby TO, Kasper LH. The gut microbiome and multiple sclerosis. Cold Spring Harbor Perspectives in Medicine, 8:a029017, 2018.

Oligschlaeger Y, Yadati T, Houben T, Condello Olivan CM, Shiri-Sverdlov R. Inflammatory bowel disease: A stressed "gut/feeling." Cells, 8:659, 2019.

Ott C, Scholmerich J. Extraintestinal manifestations and complications in IBD. Nature Reviews Gastroenterology and Hepatology, 10:585-595, 2013.

Parodi B, Kerlero de Rosbo N. The gut-brain axis in multiple sclerosis. Is its dysfunction a pathological trigger or a consequence of the disease? Frontiers in Immunology, 12:718220, 2021.

Peters SL, Yao CK, Philpott H, Yelland GW, Muir JG, Gibson PR. Randomised clinical trial: The efficacy of gut-directed hypnotherapy is similar to that of the low FODMAP diet for the treatment of irritable bowel syndrome. Alimentary Pharmacotherapy and Therapeutics, 44:447-459, 2016.

Pfeiffer RF. Gastrointestinal dysfunction in Parkinson's disease. Parkinsonism and Related Disorders, 17:10-15, 2011.

Qiu S, Fu H, Zhou R, Yang Z, Bai G, Shi B. Toxic effects of glyphosate on intestinal morphology, antioxidant capacity and barrier function in weaned piglets. Ecology and Environmental Safety, 187:109846, 2020.

Rizzello F, Spisni E, Giovanardi E, Imbesi V, Salice M, Alvisi P, et al. Implications of the Westernized diet in the onset and progression of IBD. Nutrients, 11:1033, 2019.

Rome Foundation, Rome IV Criteria, theromefoundation.org/rome-iv/rome-iv-criteria/, 2021.

Santos SF, de Oliveira HL, Yamada ES, Neves BC, Pereira A Jr. The Gut and Parkinson's Disease—A Bidirectional Pathway, Frontiers in Neurology, 10:574, 2019.

Soares RLS. Irritable bowel syndrome, food intolerance and non-celiac gluten sensitivity. A new clinical challenge. Arquivo Gastroenterology, 55:417-422, 2018.

Severancea EG, Yolkena RH, Eaton WW. Autoimmune diseases, gastrointestinal disorders and the microbiome in schizophrenia: More than a gut feeling. Schizophrenia Research,176(1):23-35, 2016.

Shu S-A, Yuen AWT, Woo E, Chu K-H, Kwan H-S, Yang G-X, Yang Y, Leung PSC. Microbiota and Food Allergy. Clinical Reviews in Allergy and Immunology, 57:83-97, 2019.

Singh R, Salem A, Nanavati J, Mullin GE. The Role of Diet in the Treatment of Irritable Bowel Syndrome: A Systematic Review. Gastroenterology Clinics of North America, 47:107-137, 2018.

Smith PK, Masilamamani M, Li X-M, Sampson HA. The false alarm hypothesis: Food allergy is associated with high dietary advanced glycation end-products and glycating dietary sugars that mimic alarmins. Journal of Allergy and Clinical Immunology, 139:429-437, 2017.

Snelson M, Coughlin MT. Dietary advanced glycation end products: Digestion, metabolisms and modulation of gut microbial ecology. Nutrients, 11:215, 2019.

Spiller R, Major G. IBS and IBD- separate entities or on a spectrum? Nature Reviews: Gastroenterology and Hepatology, 13:613-621, 2016.

Stein E, Sloan J, Sonu I, Kathpalia P, Jodorkovsky D. GERD for the nongastroenterologist: successful evaluation, management, and lifestyle-based symptom control. Annals of the New York Academy of Sciences, 1482:106-112, 2020.

Su T, Lai S, Le, A, He X, Chen S. Meta-analysis: proton pump inhibitors moderately increase the risk of small intestinal bacterial overgrowth. Journal of Gastroenterology, 53:27-36, 2018.

Sugihara K, Kamada N. Diet-microbiota interactions in inflammatory bowel disease. Nutrients, 13:1533, 2021.

Sundin J, Öhman L, Simrén M. Understanding the Gut Microbiota in Inflammatory and Functional Gastrointestinal Diseases. Psychosomatic Medicine, 79:857-867, 2017.

Tuck CJ, Biesiekierski JR, Schmid-Grendelmeier P, Pohl D. Food intolerances. Nutrients, 11:1684, 2019.

Ungaro R, Mehandru S, Allen PB, Peyrin-Biroulet L, Colobel F. Ulcerative colitis. Lancet, 389:1756-1770, 2017.

Uribarri J, Cai Q, Sandu O, Peppa M, Goldberg T, Vlassara H. Diet-Derived Advanced Glycation End Products Are Major Contributors to the Body's AGE Pool and Induce Inflammation in Healthy Subjects. Proceedings of the National Academy of Sciences, 1043:461-466, 2005.

Valenta R, Hochwallner H, Linhard B, Pahr S. Food allergies: the basics. Gastroenterology, 148:1120-1131.e4. 2015.

Valitutti F, Cucchiara S, Fasano A. Celiac Disease and the microbiome. Nutrients, 11:2403, 2019.

van der Geest S, Zaman S. 'Look under the sheets!' Fighting with the senses in relation to defecation and bodily care in hospitals and care institutions. Medical Humanities, 0:1-9, 2020.

Veauthier B, Hornecker JR. Crohn's Disease: Diagnosis and management. American Family Physician, 11:662-669, 2018.

Vermeulen W, De Man JG, Pelckmans PA, De Winter BY. Neuroanatomy of lower gastrointestinal pain disorders. World Journal of Gastroenterology, 20:1005-1020, 2014.

Vital M, Gao J, Rizzo M, Harrison T, Tiedje JM. Diet is a major factor governng the fecal butyrate-producing community structure across *Mammalia*, *Aves*, and *Reptilia*. The ISME Journal, 9:832-843, 2015.

Weaver KR, Melkus GD, Henderson WA. Irritable Bowel Syndrome: A review. American Journal of Nursing, 117:48-55, 2017.

Weber AT, Shah ND, Sauk J, Limketkai BN. Popular Diet Trends for Inflammatory Bowel Diseases: Claims and Evidence. Current Treatment Options Gastroenterology 17:564-576, 2019.

Witges KM, Bernstein CN, Sexton KA, Afifi T, Walker JR, Nugent Z, Lix LM. The Relationship Between Adverse Childhood Experiences and Health Care Use in the Manitoba IBD Cohort Study. Inflammatory Bowel Disease, 25:700-710, 2019.

Woolf CJ. Central sensitization: Implications for the diagnosis and treatment of pain. Pain, 152:S2-15, 2011.

Zhou QQ, Vern GN. New insights into visceral hypersensitivity—clinical implications in IBS. Nature Reviews Gastroenterology and Hepatology, 8:349-355, 2011.

- FEATURES OF DEPRESSION CAN BE ADAPTIVE

- DEPRESSION, INFLAMMATION, AND NEUROPLASTICITY

- FOOD AND MOOD

- DIET, INFLAMMATION, AND ANXIETY

- MECHANISMS OF PAIN

- CHRONIC PAIN IS CHALLENGING TO TREAT

- MOOD, PAIN, AND THE GUT

- PSYCHOBIOTICS

- KEY POINTS

Along with obesity, mood symptoms and pain occupy central positions in the self-sustaining cycle by which stress and poor diet choices perpetuate feelings of being unwell. These symptoms are highly co-morbid, so much so that historically they have been considered part of the same disorder (Croqc 2019). Between 60 to 80 percent of people with depression report physical pain symptoms (Jaracz 2016). Moreover, co-morbid pain and depression are associated with more severe depression, worse physical condition, and higher body-mass index (BMI). Together these symptoms form the core of a syndrome of inflammation, psychological, and physiological distress. As we will see, a poor diet is a key feature of this syndrome.

Mood and pain disorders exact a high toll on individuals and society. Mood and pain disorders worsen personal well-being, cause lost productivity, and increased health care expenses. Compounding these negative outcomes, mood and pain disorders can confer increased risk of other conditions such as dementia. But despite considerable research and development effort, pharmacological treatments for mood and pain disorders are only partially effective (Miller 2013). Many people do not respond to antidepressant drugs (Miller 2013). Even among responders, relapse rates are high. Similarly, pharmaceutical approaches for chronic pain may confer initial relief, but can cause serious long-term negative effects including toxicity, addiction, and increased pain (Tick 2018).

This is worrisome because anxiety and depression are the top two most common psychiatric diagnoses, and along with "unspecified" pain conditions, anxiety and depression are among the top five causes of disability in the world (Global Health Collaborators, 2017). Unspecified pain conditions include non-cancer chronic painful conditions such as migraine and fibromyalgia. Mood symptoms commonly accompany medical conditions including cardiometabolic disorders, autoimmune disorders, gastrointestinal disorders, and eating-related disorders. Why are these disorders so common?

The most fundamental function of the brain is to respond appropriately to conditions in the internal and external world. The brain must coordinate physiological adjustments with psychological and behavioral states to meet challenges. In the context of a challenge, signals from the body and the external world converge on overlapping brain networks that integrate this information with memories, emotions, and cognitions to generate appropriate physiological, behavioral, and emotional responses. Successful behavioral or cognitive responses to challenges require flexibility. This means that the brain must be capable of *neuroplasticity*. Neuroplasticity is the ability of the brain to change its functions, and even structure, to adapt to changes in the environment and other challenges. Neuroplasticity is the basis of learning, and thus of cognitive and behavioral flexibility. As we will see, mood and pain disorders are strongly associated with deficits in neuroplasticity.

Emotions are a normal part of our psychological experience of perceiving challenges, especially threats (McEwen 2020). Emotions can be considered adaptive in that they signal that something is wrong. Emotions motivate us to address the challenge. However, if a challenging situation is not successfully addressed, negative emotions can persist and become an integral part of the experience of stress. This is particularly common when the threat or stressor is uncontrollable due to the situation or to the lack of skills necessary to control the threat. Thus, mood and pain disorders are common because many individuals are faced with challenges, such as those associated with interpersonal problems or socio-economic conditions, they are unable to directly control. Uncontrollable challenges become stress, leading to persistence of the otherwise integral and adaptive emotional responses to challenge. Repeated exposure to uncontrollable challenges leads to chronic stress responses.

Emotional responses are intertwined with metabolic and immune responses that are also part of the comprehensive reaction to challenges. These functional interrelationships are reflected in the neural substrates that receive shared feedback about physiological conditions, emotion, and pain. For example, interoceptive pathways in the brain bring information about blood pressure, metabolic status, and inflammation to limbic brain regions that process information about emotion, threat, and pain. Behavioral responses to threats can induce the fight-or-flight" response, which signals brain and muscle cells to increase energy to carry out these behaviors. Fighting and fleeing both involve risk of tissue damage. Thus, metabolic regulation, and by association, eating behaviors, are a key component of the integrated response to challenges. In the context of stress, dysregulation of emotions can result in dysregulation of eating behavior, including over-eating, anorexia, and stress/emotional eating (Konttinen 2010). These behaviors may provide short-term relief, but due to longer-term effects, such as obesity, they ultimately serve to prolong the dysfunctional mood and pain experiences.

Features of depression can be adaptive

The core features of *major depressive disorder* are depressed mood and anhedonia, an inability to experience pleasure (Truschel 2020). Increases or decreases in appetite can also occur, along with other "vegetative" symptoms such changes in sleep and energy levels. Major depression may also cause cognitive impairment. At first glance it may be hard to imagine how these symptoms could be adaptive when attempting to meet a challenge. Certainly, they are not helpful for fighting or fleeing. However, the aftermath of surviving a challenge may involve *recuperation*. After a fight or flight, one may need to take time to replenish metabolic fuels and heal any injuries sustained. This recuperation involves an inward focus and avoidance of external stimulation.

The classic example of recuperative behavior is the sickness syndrome experienced during illness. During sickness it is common to experience fatigue, low mood, social withdrawal, anhedonia, and cognitive "fuzziness." These symptoms encourage rest to conserve metabolic resources and potentially reduce contagion. In this way, recuperation is either key to recovering from a challenge or an integral part of meeting it. In the face of uncontrollable challenges that can provoke chronic stress, these symptoms may emerge or persist as the brain's attempt to prevent further injury, and may ultimately prevent successful coping with the challenge.

Changes in neural network activity in depressed brains illustrate key features of depression (Price 2020). Neuroimaging studies comparing connectivity of brain networks of depressed with non-depressed individuals show a consistent pattern associated with depression. In depressed individuals, prefrontal cortex regions are less connected to other brain networks, including the mesolimbic motivation/reward components of the Salience Network. Within the prefrontal cortex, medial and lateral regions are also less connected. At the same time, there is increased connectivity with the Default Mode Network. This pattern indicates less executive control on mood, emotions, and motivation (Price 2020, Drevets 2008, Cosgrove 2020, Felger 2016). In "neurosymphonic" terms, depression is associated with a weak Conductor (prefrontal cortex) that allows or enables preoccupation with negative emotions and cognitions, and an inability to disconnect from them, leading to "rumination." The increased connectivity within the Default Mode Network is consistent with an inward, self-focused activity pattern characteristic of "recuperation."

The disconnection of the motivation/reward network from the prefrontal executive function, combined with impairments in the arousal system, inhibits attempts to engage in behaviors that could improve mood (Felger 2016). This facilitates the development of self-sustaining preoccupation with negative thoughts and anhedonia. In this way, depression becomes a cognitive/emotional "loop." What factors sustain this loop?

Depression, inflammation, and neuroplasticity

The marked similarities between recuperative/sickness behavior and pathological depression (e.g., Major Depressive Disorder) raises the question of whether inflammation may contribute to the pathophysiology of depressive disorders (Maes 1995, Dantzer 2008, Miller 2009, Pariente 2017, Keicolt-Glaser 2015). To review, sickness behavior is induced by pro-inflammatory cytokines released in the context of injury or illness. These cytokines activate interoceptive pathways leading to mood symptoms, fatigue, and cognitive impairment. Human experimental studies consistently show that inducing peripheral inflammation by administering PAMPs, such as bacterial lipopolysaccharide or cytokines, induces depressive symptoms in healthy people (Miller 2009), demonstrating that cytokines or inflammation can cause symptoms of depression. Subsequent studies have demonstrated links of inflammation with depression, most closely with treatment-resistant and more severe depression (Savitz 2020, Miller 2013). A substantial proportion of people with major depressive disorder (MDD) have elevated levels of pro-inflammatory cytokines and other inflammatory mediators in their blood (Maes 2012, Bauer 2019, Miller

2009). Inflammation has been specifically linked to anhedonia in people with MDD, along with suppression of dopaminergic arousal/reward pathways (Felger 2017). Notably, social stress, which seems to be the most pro-inflammatory type of stress, is linked to depression, especially in women (Slavich 2019). Inflammation is also associated with key pathophysiological features of depression: hippocampal dysfunction and deficits in neuroplasticity (McEwen 2020, Miller 2013).

The hippocampus regulates emotional and neuroendocrine responses to challenges. Impairment of its functions under conditions of stress leads to a cascade of consequences that can serve to perpetuate the "depressive loop" (McEwen 2020). The hippocampus expresses cortisol receptors, and the binding of cortisol to these receptors leads to the inhibition of HPA axis activity in a classic "negative feedback" loop. Dysfunction of the hippocampus can lead to persistently elevated levels of cortisol, which causes cells to become resistant to its effects, a state called *glucocorticoid resistance*. Cortisol normally acts as a brake on inflammation by reducing the expression of pro-inflammatory mediators, including cytokines, in immune cells. When these cells become resistant to cortisol, they release pro-inflammatory cytokines, inducing chronic low-grade inflammation in the body and in the brain. Dysfunction of the hippocampus and the HPA axis, along with the resulting increase in inflammation, provides one avenue of association with depression. Impairments of hippocampal function are also associated with more severe and recurrent depression (McEwen 2020). Because the hippocampal complex is part of the Default Mode Network, which regulates emotions, sense of self, and autonomic functions, dysfunction of the hippocampus can lead to mood and coping deficits.

Evidence of neuroinflammation has been found in people with depression. Neuroinflammation can induce oxidative stress and impair the cellular mechanisms that mediate neuroplasticity. Oxidative stress can damage neurons and other cells in the brain (Black 2015). The brain is the most metabolically active organ in the body and is therefore already at risk for oxidative stress. High rates of metabolism can lead to excessive production of reactive oxygen and nitrogen species that cause damage. Further, the brain is enriched in polyunsaturated fatty acids (PUFAs) that are easy targets for oxidation. PUFAs reside in cell membranes and in the myelin sheaths that insulate neuronal axons. Damaged or altered PUFAs can lead to impairment of neuronal function. The link between inflammation and oxidative stress is also supported by findings of lipid peroxidation and DNA damage in patients with anxiety and depressive disorders (Black 2015, das Gracas Fedoce 2018). Oxidative stress can also lead to mitochondrial dysfunction, further impairing the ability of neurons to generate energy to perform their functions, and further driving neuroinflammation.

Neuroinflammation inhibits neuroplasticity, which is associated with the cognitive impairment and mental inflexibility that are key features of depression (Donofrey 2016, Price 2020, Miller 2013). For instance, deficits in neuroplasticity prevent the brain from disconnecting from negative thought processes and rumination. This cognitive and behavioral rigidity can also prevent depressed people from engaging in behaviors such as exercise and improved diet that can help alleviate symptoms (Donofrey 2016), thus further impeding the ability to escape the "depressive loop."

Inflammation is directly linked to impairments in neuroplasticity via dysregulation of the brain's glutamate system. Dysfunction in glutamate systems in the brain are linked to depression (Miller 2013, Haroon

2020). The anesthetic drug ketamine acts on this system and has recently emerged as an effective treatment for depression. Glutamate is a neurotransmitter that has long been linked to memory and neuroplasticity via two receptors (Gerhard 2016): NMDA and AMPA. NMDA receptors are linked to long-term memory formation, while AMPA receptors activate cellular mechanisms that enable changes in synapses. Binding of glutamate to AMPA receptors triggers the release of brain-derived neurotrophic factor (BDNF) and activates a protein, called mTOR, that signals production of proteins needed for this growth. Thus, AMPA receptor function is critical to neuroplasticity. At the same time, excessive activation of NMDA receptors seems to inhibit AMPA's ability to activate BDNP and mTOR, impairing neuroplasticity. Ketamine, however, is an NMDA receptor antagonist. Ketamine's ability to block NMDA receptor activation is believed to contribute to its antidepressant actions. In short, ketamine takes the brake off neuroplasticity, a key to relieving depression.

How does inflammation impair glutamate receptor function? During inflammation, immune cells need energy. One energy source is a derivative of the amino acid tryptophan called quinolinic acid (Miller 2013, Savitz 2019, Haroon 2020). Quinolinic acid can be broken down into NAD, an energy substrate, but it can also induce oxidative stress and activate NMDA receptors. Elevated quinolinic acid levels in cerebrospinal fluid have been linked to suicide. Evidence of high quinolinic acid levels in key brain regions (e.g., medial PFC) have been reported for depressed patients (Miller 2013, Savitz 2019). The idea that quinolinic acid is a key link between inflammation, neuroplasticity, and depression has also been supported by pre-clinical studies showing that ketamine can prevent depressive behaviors normally induced by inflammation (Miller 2013, Savitz 2019). Ketamine does not influence the level of inflammation (e.g., cytokines). Instead, ketamine's ability to prevent depression symptoms in response to inflammation was shown to be dependent on glutamate receptors. Taken together, these findings link these two pathophysiological factors to the development of depression.

A causative relationship between inflammation and depression is further illustrated by recent clinical trials with anti-inflammatory drugs. Drugs including NSAIDs, steroids, and anti-cytokine "biological drugs" have been reported to reduce depressive symptoms (Kohler 2019). The antidepressant effects of NSAIDS are similar in size to standard antidepressant drugs, and when an NSAID and an antidepressant were administered together, the effects were additive. This connection between inflammation, oxidative stress, and depression is the major link between food and mood.

Food and Mood

When we think about mood and food, stress and emotional eating come to mind (Marx 2021). But do these types of eating behaviors actually influence the course of depression? That is, why is "stress eating" bad? The reason is that stress eating typically involves pro-inflammatory, high-energy, sugary, processed foods that can exacerbate oxidative stress and impair brain functioning (Marx 2021, Attuquayefio 2017). These foods can also contribute to the development of overweight or obesity, and the attendant risks for inflammation and metabolic diseases. Thus, the inflammatory consequences of eating these foods can exacerbate depressive symptoms.

Indeed, it has been well-documented that poor diets and malnutrition are linked with mood disorders (Firth 2020, Huang 2019, Li 2017, Marx 2021, Wang 2018). Many studies from all over the world have found correlations of diet with both anxiety and depression (Knuppel 2017, Li 2017, Nakamura 2019). People who eat diets rich in fresh fruits and vegetables, whole grains including wheat, probiotic foods, olive oil, not too much meat, and moderate amounts of red wine report low levels of depression, particularly compared to people who eat diets low in vegetables and mostly based on refined carbohydrates and processed foods that are low in vitamins and minerals (Marx 2021).

The idea that nutrition contributes to mood is supported by clinical trials of Mediterranean diet-type interventions. These studies have shown benefits on several measures, including both inflammation and mood (Oliviero 2015, Parletta 2019). Indeed, many participants in the SMILES trial found that when they replaced high-energy Western diet foods with whole/intact grains, fruits, vegetables, and fiber for twelve weeks, they no longer met diagnostic criteria for major depressive disorder (Chatterton 2018, Jacka 2017). Similar findings were reported in another clinical trial (Parletta 2019). These dramatic findings support the idea that diet affects mood, rather than a poor diet being simply the consequences of depression or anxiety on food choices. Anecdotally, several people have related to me how they suffered for years with depression, taking anti-depressant medications but not really feeling better. Finally, they decided to seriously address their diets, mostly by getting the sugar, soda, and processed "junk food" out of their diets. They began eating whole grains and vegetables, mostly cooking at home. Each person told me that after about two weeks their moods lifted and they felt better than they had in years.

Diet as "global support" for neuroplasticity

The cognitive and behavioral flexibility required for meeting challenges requires chemical building blocks such as amino acids to make the proteins that are necessary for building and maintaining new synapses that support neuroplasticity. The brain is a highly metabolically active organ and requires sufficient protein and vitamins to support this activity. Poor nutrition is linked to oxidative stress, possibly because many vitamins, including B vitamins, are antioxidants. Oxidative stress can lead to damage of brain cells, driving loss of function, inflammation, and thus depression. Chronic severe mood disorders are associated with evidence of brain impairment and neuroinflammation (Haroon 2020, Maes 2012, Miller 2013, McEwen 2020). Thus, a diet that is deficient in nutrients fails to provide the necessary building blocks and metabolic fuels for proper brain function and neuroplasticity, while also inducing inflammation. In this way, a poor diet acts to further impair the ability to break out of a "depressive loop."

Malnutrition is commonly associated with mood symptoms, particularly depression. One possible reason involves the link of B vitamins to monoamine synthesis (Kennedy 2016). Folate and B12, which are often lacking in malnutrition, are key. Monoamines, including dopamine, serotonin, and norepinephrine, are neurotransmitters associated with the brain's arousal systems. They mediate activity in reward pathways that support coping behaviors. Dysfunction of monoamine neurotransmitters is associated with depression and these neurotransmitter systems are targets of several antidepressant drugs.

B vitamin deficiencies are less common than in the past, partly due to supplementation in flour and other processed food products. However, recent changes in dietary habits, and certain interventions for weight loss, have been found to lead to B vitamin deficiency (Tsao 2017). Because meat is a good source of B vitamins, vegetarians and vegans must be particularly conscientious about food choices to ensure sufficient intake of B complex vitamins, or possibly consider supplementation. Interventions that affect gut function, including bariatric surgery for weight loss, have led to a form of Wernicke's encephalitis due to lack of thiamine (Kennedy 2016). The surgical reduction in the absorptive surface of the gut leads to thiamine uptake. This condition involves mood, cognitive, and motor impairments that can be permanent. The use of proton-pump inhibitors (PPIs), which reduce the acidity of the stomach, can also be associated with B vitamin deficiencies (Kennedy 2016). Finally, the drug metformin, which is used to treat type 2 diabetes, can reduce the absorption of vitamin B12, which has been linked to mood symptoms, cognitive impairment, and peripheral nerve damage (Bieman 2015).

Other consequences of malnutrition can potentially contribute to mood symptoms as well. Low-protein diets can fail to provide the amino acids that are precursors for the monoamines. Vitamin D deficiency has also been linked to depression, as well. Taken together, findings of protein and micronutrient deficiencies associated with depression underline the importance of consuming a nutrient-rich diet, especially for anyone struggling with mood symptoms.

Diet, Inflammation, and Anxiety

Like depression, anxiety symptoms are linked by many lines of evidence to a poor diet (Kris-Etherton 2021, Li 2017, Masana 2019). This may simply follow from the high rates of co-morbidity of the two syndromes. Yet, there are reasons to suppose that the neurobiological underpinnings of anxiety may uniquely contribute to inflammation and diet choices that can sustain cognitive and behavior loops associated with the symptoms of anxiety.

Anxiety is characterized as the response to a real or imagined threat (Crocq 2019). Such threats can involve physical or psychological danger ("top-down") or they can involve internal threats, such as inflammation or difficulty breathing ("bottom-up"). The responses to these threats range from psychological discomfort or dread to acute activation of autonomic and neuroendocrine stress/challenges, such as in panic disorder and post-traumatic stress disorder (PTSD). Anxiety is considered fundamentally adaptive in the face of threat, because it drives motivation to either address the threat or to avoid it (Crocq 2019). Thus, anxiety is a normal, necessary emotion that can become pathological when it persists.

The brain neurocircuitry that supports challenge responses engages both behavioral activation networks and hedonic/reward networks (Berridge 2018, Porrecca 2017). In a normal psychological challenge situation, the Salience Network (SN, including the amygdala, insula, and dorsal anterior cingulate cortex) determines the importance of the key components of the situation and interacts with the Executive Control Network to determine the responses to it. These responses will involve the Central Autonomic Network to coordinate physiological adjustments that may be necessary. The SN also induces neurological arousal and motivation via dopaminergic mesolimbic pathways, supporting behaviors necessary to cope with challenge/threat. Hedonics, or pleasure and pain effects, play key roles in the motivation to manage challenges. Anxiety is an uncomfortable experience, and relief from it can serve as a major reward for managing a challenge (Berridge 2018). The link between anxiety and reward may well be important in the context of stress eating. When a challenge is not met and becomes bona fide stress, the lack of reward may drive appetite for high-energy, sugary foods that, while providing a short-term feeling of pleasure, in fact can drive inflammation to further exacerbate negative mood.

Inflammation is an important type of bottom-up/physiological stress, and neuroimaging studies demonstrate that inflammation activates the same neural networks as acute stress and anxiety (Felger 2018). Marked overlap in activation patterns between acute stress and anxiety, and inflammation, is seen particularly in the amygdala, insula, and dorsal anterior cingulate cortex. These are key components of the SN. These findings suggest that inflammation may "prime" the neurocircuitry that subserves the experience of anxiety, making anxiety more likely or more intense. An example of the inflammation-anxiety link is the finding that one of the first conscious experiences during experimental immune challenge is anxiety (Reichenberg 2001). Many pre-clinical studies have linked inflammation, measured as elevated levels of circulating cytokines, to anxiety (Mehta 2018). Inflammation also seems to play a role in PTSD, where inflammation seems to be associated with more severe symptoms (Michopoulos 2017). Thus, like depression, anxiety is closely tied to inflammation.

This link between anxiety and depression implies that even in the absence of an experience of top-down psychological stress, a habit of consuming pro-inflammatory high energy sweets, and fried and processed foods, could predispose individuals to the development of anxiety. In this way, diet could be an environmental stressor (Felger 2018). Inflammation-related drive on interoceptive pathways can activate neural processes that are experienced as anxiety (Felger 2018). This may contribute to the higher incidence of anxiety disorders among those consuming the Western diet.

Mechanisms of Pain

Pain is a noxious psychological experience that is generated in the context of damage or dysfunction in bodily tissues, or infection. The purpose of pain is to activate avoidance responses to limit damage and to encourage recuperative behavior that will allow the body to heal. Examples of these protective pain-induced behavior include pulling a hand away from a hot stove burner or not walking on a sprained ankle. In this way, like depression and anxiety, pain is both adaptive and necessary for survival, but it can become pathological when it becomes chronic (Ji 2016).

Inflammation is the trigger for pain: When damage to tissue occurs, immune and other cells in the vicinity of the damage release damage-associated molecular patterns (DAMPs) and pro-inflammatory hormones, including prostaglandins and cytokines (Matsuda 2019). These mediators activate local inflammatory cells, induce NFkB activity and inflammasomes, and recruit immune cells to the area, to both fight a potential infection, and to direct the process of healing. The initial response involves acute inflammation, with swelling and the experience of tenderness or pain. These responses serve to immobilize tissues to protect them and to localize potential infection and fight potential pathogens. For example, the swelling around a sprain prevents movement and isolates potential pathogens from the rest of the body.

The neural pathway that gives rise to our perception of pain begins with the peripheral sensory neurons, called _nociceptors_, that innervate bodily tissues. There are two types of nociceptors. The _Ad_ nociceptors respond to conditions such as heat or pressure that could cause tissue damage. They are responsible for initiating protective reflexes, such as withdrawing a hand from a hot stove. The *c-fiber* nociceptors respond to actual tissue damage or inflammation, as signaled by prostaglandins and cytokines. C-fibers also contain and release the pro-inflammatory neuropeptides Substance P and CGRP. These neuropeptides contribute to the local inflammatory response, increasing pain and causing vasodilation. Vasodilation is why injuries often look red. The inflammation caused by activation of c-fibers and release of neuropeptides is called *neurogenic inflammation* (Matsuda 2019). Nociceptor neurons live in collections of other neurons, glia, and immune cells, called dorsal root ganglia. The dorsal root ganglia are located just outside of the spinal cord. Nociceptors have two axons. One axon extends into bodily tissues and monitors local conditions, and the other extends into the *dorsal horn* region of the spinal cord.

In the spinal cord dorsal horn, local neurons and glia modulate the pain signals, either enhancing them or inhibiting them. This modulation enables our perceptions of pain to be responsive to environmental situations such as threats, where being less sensitive to pain may enable fighting or fleeing. On the other hand, being more sensitive to pain can enable protective reflexes and encourage recuperative behavior. Thus, early processing of pain signals allows for flexibility in responses to pain.

From the spinal cord, *projection neurons* convey the information to the brainstem, where they can influence autonomic function and arousal systems. Information from the spinal cord is also sent to the thalamus, which "sorts" the different aspects of the pain, and then to brain regions including somatosensory cortex, insula, and other areas that process the different features of pain (Khera 2021, Porreca 2017, Wang 2021). Activation of this pathway gives rise to our perception of pain, and our physiological and emotional responses to it. Because pain can signal potentially life-threatening situations, it exerts a strong influence on the Salience Network. SN activation of especially the insula, anterior cingulate cortex, and amygdala ensure that we pay attention to the pain. Pain is a multidimensional experience, involving mood and cognitive features, such as suffering and worry. Thus, pain also recruits components of the Default Mode Network and Executive Control Network. These networks integrate the sensory signals related to pain with the demands of ongoing behavior, mood states, previous experience, and expectations. Considering these all together, these networks organize behavioral responses.

The outcomes of brain processing of pain signals can also include regulation of the sensory experience of pain. The brain can turn the volume of pain up or down via signals in the descending neural pathways, targeting the early, spinal transmission of the signals. For instance, pathways producing analgesia or a reduction in pain are associated with endogenous opiates and endocannabinoids. Drugs that interact with these systems are used to treat pain. Modulation of these pathways can also lead to increased intensity of pain, known as hyperalgesia. Via this top-down regulation, mood, stress, cognition, and attitudes can influence our perception of pain.

Chronic pain: After the initial phase of response to injury or infection, the healing phase begins. Rather like a switch being flipped, immune cells transition from releasing pro-inflammatory mediators to releasing anti-inflammatory mediators, such as interleukin-10, and growth factors. These anti-inflammatory mediators recruit cells capable of re-building damaged tissues to the area (Goehler 2019). Pain diminishes as healing occurs.

What happens when the switch does not get flipped? In many cases the injury appears to heal, but inflammation continues (Matsuda 2019, Ji 2016). For example, 20% of post-surgical patients show signs of ongoing inflammation and pain (Glare 2019). In this case, immune cells in the nociceptor axons and the dorsal root ganglia up-regulate inflammatory mediators, resulting in hyperalgesia, and often, a phenomenon called allodynia (Ji 2016). Allodynia describes the condition whereby stimuli that are not usually painful, such as movement or light touch, become painful. This occurs because other sensory neurons now drive the activity of pain-conducting neurons in the spinal cord (Ji 2016). Activity in Ad neurons, which respond to temperature and touch, may now be interpreted as painful. Through this mechanism, persistent inflammation in peripheral nerves can produce an experience of chronic pain (Pinho-Ribeiro 2017).

This persistent activation of pain signals also leads to neuroplastic changes in pain-responsive neurons. That is, the increase in activity in pain pathways leads to changes in synaptic function, such that neurons that process pain information are more easily and more strongly activated (Ji 2016, Woolf 2011). This central sensitizaicn, also known as *wind-up*, occurs throughout the pain pathway, from the spinal cord up to cortex (Khera 2021, Woolf 2011, Matsuda 2019, Boadas-Vaello 2016). Central sensitization may occur especially in the Salience Network components: insula, amygdala and anterior cingulate cortex. Central sensitization is a learning-like phenomenon. It is activity-dependent and involves changes in receptors for the neurotransmitter glutamate (Glare 2019). Glutamate is used by nociceptors and modulates activity in many brain networks. Essentially, the nervous system "learns" to more efficiently transmit pain signals. It is important to note that persistent neuroinflammation and central sensitization can occur even after an injury seems to have healed. Similarly, neuroinflammation and central sensitization may be the basis of *unexplained pain*, a diagnostic category for conditions including fibromyalgia, visceral hypersensitivity (e.g., heartburn, irritable bowel syndrome, pelvic pain, etc.) and migraine headache (Matsuda 2019).

Chronic Pain is Challenging to Treat

Chronic pain is defined as pain that persists for three months or more. By this time, neuroplastic changes have occurred that enhance pain transmission, compromising the effects of analgesic drugs. Chronic pain conditions have been classified separately as "neuropathic," "inflammatory," or "unexplained pain." Neuropathic pain describes conditions in which there is evidence of damage to or dysfunction of nerves. Diabetic neuropathy, post-herpetic neuralgia or shingles, and chemotherapy-induced pain are examples of conditions categorized as neuropathic. Despite separate categorization, it is becoming clear that all chronic pain conditions involve both neural and inflammatory features (Ji 2016). For instance, in many cases of fibromyalgia, an "unexplained" class of pain, there is evidence of Ad and c-fiber sensory neuron neuropathy and low levels of systemic inflammation (Martinez-Lavin 2021).

Pharmacological treatments target either peripheral mechanisms, such as inflammation, or they target the central nervous system pathways that convey or modulate pain perception. Drugs targeting peripheral nervous system mechanisms and inflammation include steroids, NSAIDs, and local anesthetics such as lidocaine, capsaicin, or botulinum toxin. Opiates, cannabinoids, serotonin-norepinephrine re-uptake inhibitor (SNRI) antidepressants, NMDA receptor antagonists (e.g., ketamine), and anti-seizure drugs that target glutamatergic systems (e.g., pregabalin and gabapentin) influence central nervous system pain pathways. All of these drugs can provide relief from pain, but the effect sizes are small, and side effects are of concern. In particular, opiates are well-recognized for their risks of tolerance and addiction. Prolonged use of opiates can lead to a condition called *opiate-induced hyperalgesia*, in which prolonged use of opiates actually enhances pain. Thus, by both training in unhelpful pain responses and behaviors, and worsening pain experience, chronic use of opiates can render management of pain even more difficult (Glare 2019, Salduker 2019, Tick 2018).

Whereas the interactions of stress and pain have long been recognized, recent studies elucidate some of the more perplexing aspects of the chronic pain experience. Top-down influences, notably negative emotions associated with stress, and attitudinal habits such as catastrophizing, enhance the experience of pain and are associated with worse outcomes (Crettaz 2013). Unfortunately, this has often led to practitioners and others to blame people for their pain. Blaming responses do nothing to address the pathophysiological underpinnings that mediate stress effects on pain. This has been especially true for cases of unexplained pain, such as fibromyalgia or visceral hypersensitivity associated with IBS. However, the recent recognition of the relationships between stress and inflammation, and of the pivotal role of cortisol dysregulation and inflammation in chronic pain, strengthens the case for multimodal treatment approaches for chronic pain (Hannibal 2014, Tick 2018). Further, neuroimaging studies now consistently demonstrate long-term changes in brain networks, particularly the Salience and Default Mode networks, in the context of chronic pain (Wang 2021). These changes are consistent with enhanced experience of pain, as well as increased sensitivity to stress.

Because stress is associated with increased inflammation, it can also contribute to bottom-up drive on pain experiences. This enhanced inflammation may explain, at least in part, the marked gender difference in the epidemiology of chronic pain. Women are much more likely to suffer chronic pain than men, and female sex hormones, especially estrogen, have been linked to greater inflammation (Martinez-Lavin 2021). Hormonal effects on immune function are highly complex, but gender differences in regulation of inflammation and endocrine responses to stress seem to play role in the sensitivity of women to developing chronic pain.

Other bottom-up, interoceptive signals can enhance pain as well. For instance, dehydration is associated with increased pain and may be especially associated with headache (Tan 2020). Hypoglycemia induces acute pain, at least in part by causing oxidative stress (Zhang 2016). Like inflammation, other interoceptive signals can drive the activity of brain networks responsive to pain, as well as trigger the mood symptoms that are commonly comorbid with pain (Zick 2020). Thus, treatment approaches for chronic pain need to address both top-down (e.g., mood and coping) and bottom-up (e.g., inflammation) contributors to this highly complex array of conditions (Tick 2018). Cognitive behavior therapy can address both attitudes and habits in efforts to improve coping and stress. More recently, mindfulness-based therapies have shown benefits for chronic pain (Tick 2018). Such programs have the advantage of addressing both top-down (emotion-regulation) and bottom-up (vagal influence on interoceptive pathways and inflammation) contributions to pain.

The association of pain with inflammation means that weight and diet need to be addressed. Overweight and obesity are common among people with chronic pain. Key reasons for this relationship include that fact that pain can impair the ability and motivation for exercise, and that the elevated inflammation associated with obesity can enhance pain, as well as comorbid mood symptoms and fatigue (Zick 2020). Thus, pain and obesity reinforce each other.

Pain and food: Pain is an exceptionally stressful experience, and one way that many people cope with it is by "comfort eating." Indeed, three-fifths of a sample of people with chronic pain reported consuming high-energy sweets and fats specifically because of pain (O'Laughlin 2019). Pain-induced comfort eating seems to be more associated with stress than exacerbation of pain or experiencing a pain episode. This emphasizes the important link between stress and eating behaviors. In the short term, sweets and fats do seem to relieve stress, based on self-report and cortisol levels. Sweets have analgesic properties as well, likely because they activate endogenous opiate systems in the brain. The pain-relieving effect of sugar is robust enough that sucrose is given to infants in neonatal intensive care units to alleviate procedural pain (Janke 2016).

Whereas occasional bouts of comfort eating may not impact inflammation enough to exacerbate pain, poor-quality diets were shown in a study of chronic spinal pain to be strongly associated with more pain (Zick 2020). "Poor quality" was defined as low in fresh fruits, vegetables, whole grains, and protein, but high in sweets, fats, and refined carbohydrates.

In contrast, foods containing antioxidants, like colorful fruits and vegetables, are recommended to address pain conditions. These antioxidants may reduce pain by preventing oxidative stress and mitochondrial damage (Tick 2018, Philpot 2019). Similarly, NSAID-like anti-inflammatory components of foods and spices, especially curcumin, but also ginger, resveratrol, and quercetin, are used as analgesics, and are common in fresh fruit and vegetables (Tick 2018). Foods rich in minerals and vitamins reduce the levels of inflammatory mediators in the blood and are associated with reports of less pain (Rodrigues Mendonca 2020). Magnesium regulates NMDA receptors and may be particularly helpful for reducing pain. Vitamins D and E, and B complex vitamins, may be particularly helpful for inflammation. Notably, the diet strategy recommended for pain overlaps with the Mediterranean diet. In several small trials of people with rheumatoid arthritis, patients following a Mediterranean diet experienced reductions in both pain and inflammation biomarkers compared to those on a control diet (Oliviero 2015).

Mood, Pain, and the Gut

Moods and emotions are fundamentally psychological experiences, and we tend to attribute them to things that are going on in our psychological world. But if something is not right in the body, we can experience a general feeling of uneasiness that is hard to attribute to an understandable cause. We usually try to attribute it to something in the mind, even if we cannot determine what it is. One of the most common places in the body where things can be felt as "not right" is the gut. Whereas neuroinflammation in brain and/or sensory neurons contributes to chronic pain, severe depression, and PTSD, recent findings highlight contributions from disturbances of microbes and barrier functions of the gut in driving or modulating both pain and mood symptoms (Guo 2019, Marx 2021). Thus, whereas our conscious experiences of depression, anxiety, and pain are produced by specific activity patterns in the brain, these patterns are strongly influenced by interoceptive, bottom-up inputs, notably related to inflammation. These conditions are very much mind-body disorders.

Gut hormones activate interoceptive pathways: Hormones released in the gut are nutrient-related signals, but they are also able to influence stress and mood-related pathways in the brain. To review, endocrine cells in the gut respond to nutrient-related signals by releasing peptide hormones, including ghrelin, neuropeptide Y (NPY) family members, glucagon-like peptide (GLP), and other hormones and neurotransmitters, such as serotonin. These local signals interact with enteric neurons in the gut to control gut motility and secretion of digesting enzymes. They also signal gut immune cells, modifying inflammation. In addition, many endocrine cells line the epithelium and can interact directly with microbes or microbial products, such as butyrate or neurotransmitters such as GABA (reviewed in Lach 2018). Gut-derived peptides and neurotransmitters also interact with interoceptive nerves, particularly the vagus nerve, to transmit information about conditions in the gut to the brain. Many of these signals concern food and serve to modulate appetite. Several of these, however, including the NPY family, GLP, and ghrelin, have been shown in pre-clinical work to also enter the circulation and act in the brain directly, where they can influence mood, motivation, and stress-related behaviors. Thus, the activity of gut endocrine cells can directly link diet to mood and behavior.

Gut barrier contributions to mood and pain: The term "gut barrier" refers to the complex collaboration of the several types of cells residing in the gut. The epithelial cells that line the lumen of the gut produce pathogen-fighting molecules and protective mucus. Commensal gut microbes provide energy for the epithelial cells that absorb nutrients and help control the growth of potentially pathogenic other microbes. Immune cells and neurons in the gut also contribute by releasing molecules that influence tightness of the barrier as well as other protective functions. The critical function of the barrier is to control gut permeability. That is, the barrier must absorb nutrients but keep out toxins, such as food additives or agricultural chemicals such as glyphosate, and microbes or microbe products, such as the PAMP lipopolysaccharide (LPS). Dysfunction of this barrier leads to local inflammation, with ramifications for the other tissues of the body, and especially the brain. For instance, translocation of LPS from the gut lumen through the gut barrier has been linked to both chronic pain and major depressive disorder (Lagomarsino 2021, Maes 2012, Berk 2013). Inflammation of the gut barrier is associated with malabsorption of nutrients, compromising brain function, including coping and neuroplasticity.

The fact that top-down neuroendocrine factors also exert influence on gut barrier function is particularly relevant for pain and disorders. For instance, the hormone cortisol, which is typically dysregulated in depression, down-regulates adhesion proteins that help maintain the integrity of the gut barrier (Wiley 2016). In this way, stress and depression lead to gut barrier dysfunction.

Dysbiosis contributes to pain and mood disorders: Since the early reports by my team and others, it has become increasingly evident that the populations of microbes in our gut play remarkable roles in brain function and mental health (Goehler 2007, Dinan 2013). Because inflammation plays a central role in the pathophysiology of both mood disorders and chronic pain, much subsequent work has focused on microbe-immune system interactions. However, in the context of dysbiosis, microbial products can directly influence the function of brain, spinal cord, and dorsal root ganglion cells (Lagomarsino 2021, Chiu 2013). Thus, dysbiosis can play a pivotal role in the development of mood and pain-related disorders (Koopman 2017).

Inflammation: absence of protective factors: As noted in Chapters 17 and 18, many of the Old Friends microbes are gram-positive bacteria that ferment foods containing fiber to produce short-chain fatty acids (SCFA) such as butyrate. These SCFAs can travel via the blood to enter the brain, where they act to down-regulate inflammation by binding to aryl hydrocarbon receptors on glia (Lagomarsino 2021). In this way, SCFAs act as a "brake" on neuroinflammation. Thus, one way the Western diet, which tends to be low in the kinds of foods that support SCFA-producing microbes, can facilitate or enable inflammation is to not provide this "brake" on neuroinflammation, In a study of people with anorexia nervosa, the idea that low levels of SCFAs can influence mood is supported by reports that levels of butyrate are inversely correlated with symptom severity of depression and anxiety (Borgo 2017).

Gut-derived PAMPs such as LPS contribute to inflammation: One common feature of dysbiosis is that it tends to involve overgrowth of gram-negative bacteria, which produce the PAMP, lipopolysaccharide (LPS). LPS interacts with pattern recognition receptors to directly induce inflammation. Because dysbiosis is usually accompanied by gut barrier dysfunction or "leakiness," LPS can enter the circulation and directly interact with peripheral nerves, driving pain by sensitizing dorsal root ganglion neurons (Chiu 2013, Guo 2019, Lagomarsino 2021). LPS-induced inflammation can impair permeability of the blood-brain barrier, contributing to neuroinflammation. Notably, circulating LPS been reported in both depressed and chronic pain patients, supporting this mechanism of gut dysbiosis as contributing to mood and pain (Lagomarsino 2021, Maes 2012).

Microbial metabolites can induce oxidative stress and inflammation: Another consequence of dysbiosis and impaired gut barrier integrity is the overgrowth of bacteria that produce potentially toxic metabolites. For example, trimethylamide-N-oxide (TMAO) is a microbial product derived from nutrients (e.g., carnitine, lysine, and choline) in red meat, eggs, fish, and dairy. Higher levels of TMAO are linked to heart disease and neurodegeneration based on its ability to induce oxidative stress and impair neuroplasticity (Zhang 2020, Govidarajaluji 2020). It has also been linked to the development of PTSD in the aftermath of heart attack (Baranji 2021). Thus, TMAO may provide another mechanism by which diet contributes to the pathophysiology of mood disorders and chronic pain. Interestingly, a study assessing the effects of the Mediterranean diet on microbial products found that TMAO levels were inversely correlated with adherence to the diet (De Filipas 2016). This finding suggests that one way the Western diet conveys risks for health in general, and for mood and pain symptoms, may be through elevated production of TMAO.

Psychobiotics

Microbe-based therapeutic approaches for mood and pain disorders: This consistent association of microbial dysbiosis and gut barrier inflammation or leaky gut with brain-related disorders has given rise to the proposal of a new field of "psychobiotics" (Fond 2015, Bastiaansson 2018). The idea that manipulating gut microbes might improve mood and brain function is not actually new. In 1910, Dr. George Porter Philips reported that live lactobacillus in whey improved melancholic depression (Philips

1910). Since then, many studies in non-humans show probiotic bacteria improve depressive and anxiety-like behavior. A few studies have addressed their potential effects in depressed or anxious humans (Huang 2016, Liu 2018). So far, the effects seem to be most helpful for mild symptoms (Yang 2019).

One reason that probiotics may only exert mild effects on mood symptoms is that they may not have a large enough influence on the composition of microbial populations. They may even induce dysbiosis by enriching the population with a high number of only one or a few species. A more dramatic approach involves replacing the microbial population with one from a healthy person, via a *fecal transplant*. Fecal transplants do seem to improve symptoms of both depression and anxiety, however the improvements do not last more than a few months (Meyyappan 2020). It was not reported whether the post-transplant diet was monitored or whether it would support the new population of microbes. One possible reason for the lack of persistence of benefits could be that the participants continued with their previous Western diet type, which would not support the healthy new gut microbes. Given that the single most important determinant of gut microbe population is diet, any long-term efficacy of a treatment would be dependent on post-treatment diet. Disturbances in gut microbes are also associated with chronic pain (Guo 2019, Lagomarsino 2021). The PAMP LPS can sensitize nociceptors, and several other mechanisms have been identified for microbe effects on pain (Lagomarsino 2021). Currently, most of the mechanistic studies have been performed in animals. Understanding the microbe influences in human pain conditions is limited largely to visceral pain. Similarly, studies of microbe-manipulating therapies are still scarce and targeted towards visceral pain. An exception is migraine headache, which is highly comorbid with gastrointestinal conditions (Guo 2019). Probiotics do seem to improve pain symptoms for both visceral pain and migraine (Guo 2019). Such findings support optimism for other such microbe-targeted approaches and underline the importance of diet for pain as well as mood.

Depression, anxiety, and pain are highly comorbid conditions that emerge from overlapping physiological, inflammatory, and neurological mechanisms. Key features are oxidative stress and dysregulated neuroplasticity that drive neuroinflammation and cognitive/emotional "loops" in brain network activity, reinforcing symptoms and impairing recovery. Diet can exacerbate these mechanisms by inducing or enhancing inflammation and oxidative stress. Likewise, diet can help healing and recovery by providing necessary vitamins, minerals, and macronutrients for proper brain function, as well as antioxidant or anti-inflammatory food constituents that ameliorate oxidative stress and inflammation. Further, diet can induce dysbiosis and its deleterious effects, or support health through maintaining diverse microbial populations that regulate immune function and neuroplasticity. Thus, diet is a critical factor that must be addressed if lasting relief from mood and pain conditions is to be attained.

<table>
<tr><td>

Key Points

- In the short term, depression, anxiety, and pain are adaptive in that they serve to either motivate us to address challenges, or to recuperate from physical or emotional damage due to threats or challenges.

</td></tr>
</table>

- If challenges go unmet, however, anxiety or depressive symptoms can persist. Persistence of symptoms can, in severe cases, be associated with lasting changes in brain function, neuroinflammation, and cognitive impairment.
- Dysfunction of the hippocampus and the HPA axis results in increases in inflammation. This stress-induced inflammation links stress to depression.
- Inflammation is consistently associated with depression, both in the brain, called neuroinflammation, and in the body. Inflammation by itself is capable of inducing symptoms of depression.
- Both the Salience Network, with key nodes in the insula, striatum, and amygdala, and the Default Mode Network, especially medial prefrontal cortical areas that process emotions and sense of self, are key targets of interoceptive signals and are dysfunctional in mood disorders and chronic pain syndromes.
- A poor diet contributes to mood disorders in several ways, such as failing to provide adequate nutritional support for the brain, and by increasing inflammation that can drive mood symptoms.
- Gut barrier dysfunction is commonly associated with mood disorders. A "leaky gut" may drive inflammation via programming of the immune system, or by allowing microbes to cross the barrier and induce inflammation via their release of PAMPs.
- The field of psychobiotics is inspired by the association of dysbiosis and gut barrier inflammation with psychiatric disorders. Its goal is to develop treatment approaches to psychiatric disorders using diet, probiotics, or other ways to work with our gut microbes to improve brain function.
- Mediterranean type diets are associated with lower incidence of depressive, anxiety, and pain symptoms compared to Western diets, and adopting a Mediterranean type diet improves symptoms, linking food to mood.

References

Attuquayefio T, Stevenson RJ, Oaten MJ, Francis HM. A four-day Western-style dietary intervention causes reductions in hippocampal-dependent learning and memory and interoceptive sensitivity. PLoS ONE 12(2):0172645, 2017.

Baranyi A, Enko D, von Lewinski D, Rothenhausler H-B, Amouzadeh-Ghadikolai O, Harpt H, Harpf L, Traninger, H et al. Assessment of trimethylamine N-oxide (TMAO) as a potential biomarker of severe stress in patients vulnerable to posttraumatic stress disorder (PTSD) after acute myocardial infarction. Journal of Psychotraumatology, 12:1920201, 2021.

Bastiaanssen TFS, Cowan CSM, Claesson MJ, Dina TG, Cryan JF. Making sense of … the microbiome in psychiatry. International Journal of Neuropsychopharmacology, 22(1):37-52, 2019.

Bauer ME, Teixeira AL. Inflammation in psychiatric disorders: what comes first? Annals of the New York Academy of Sciences, 1437:57-67, 2019.

Berk M, Williams LJ, Jacka FN, O'Neil A, Pasco JA, Moylan S, Allen NB, Stuart AL, Hayley AC, Byrne ML, Maes M. So depression is an inflammatory disease, but where does the inflammation come from? BMC Medicine, 11:200, 2013.

Berridge KC. Evolving concepts of emotion and motivation. Frontiers in Psychology, 9:1647, 2018.

Bieman, E, Hart HE, Rutten GEHM, Cuellar Renteria VG, Kooijman-Buiting AMJ, Beulens JWJ. Cobalamin status and its relation with depression, cognition and neuropathy in patients with type 2 diabetes mellitus using metformin. Acta Diabetologia 52:383-393, 2015.

Black CN, Bota M, Scheffer PG, Cuijpers P, Penninx BWJH. Is depression associated with increased oxidative stress? A systematic review and meta-analysis. Psychoneuroendocrinology, 51:164-175, 2015.

Boadas-Vaello P, Castany S, Homs J, Alvarez-Perez B, Deulofeu M, Verdu E. Neuroplasticity of ascending and descending pathways after somatosensory system injury: reviewing knowledge to identify neuropathic pain therapeutic targets. Spinal Cord, 54:330-340, 2016.

Borgo F, Riva A, Benetti A, Casiraghi MC, Bertelli S, GarbossaS, et al. Microbiota in anorexia nervosa: The triangle between bacterial species, metabolites and psychological tests. PLOS ONE, 12(6):e0179739, 2017.

Chatterton ML, Mihalopoulos C, O'Neil A, Itsiopoulos C, Opie R, Castle D, Dash S, Brazionis L, Berk M, Jacka F. Economic evaluation of a dietary intervention for adults with major depression (the "SMILES" trial). BMC Public Health, 18:599, 2018.

Chiu IM, Heesters BA, Ghasembou N, Von Hehm CA, Zhao Z, Tran J, et al. Bacteria activate sensory neurons that modulate pain and inflammation. Nature, 501:52057, 2013.

Cosgrove KT, Burrows K, Avery JA, Deville DC, Aupperle RL, Teague TK, Drevets WC, Simmons WK. Appetite change profiles in depression exhibit differential relationships between systemic inflammation and activity in reward and interoceptive neurocircuitry. Brain, Behavior, and Immunity, 83:163-171, 2020.

Crettaz B, Marziniak M, Willeke P, Young P, Hellhammer D, Stumpf A, Burgmer M. Stress-induced allodynia — evidence of increased pain sensitivity in healthy humans and patients with chronic pain after experimentally induced psychosocial stress. PLOS ONE, 8:e69460, 2013.

Crocq M-A. A history of anxiety: from Hippocrates to DSM. Dialogues in Clinical Neuroscience, 17:310-325, 2019.

das Graças Fedoce A, Ferreira F, Bota RG, Bonet-Costa V, Sun PY, Davies KJA. The role of oxidative stress in anxiety disorder: cause or consequence? Free Radical Research, 52: 737-750, 2018.

Dantzer R, O'Connor JC, Freund GG, Johnson RW, Kelley KW. From inflammation to sickness and depression: when the immune system subjugates the brain. Nature Reviews Neuroscience, 9:46-56, 2008.

De Filippis F, Pellegrini N, Vannini L, Jeffery IB, La Storia, Laghi C, et al. High-level adherence to a Mediterranean diet beneficially impacts the gut microbiota and associated metabolome. Gut, 65:1812-1821, 2016.

Dinan TG, Cryan JF. Melancholy microbes: A link between gut microbiota and depression? Neurogastroenterology and Motility, 25:713-719, 2013.

Donofry SD, Roecklein KA, Wildes JE, Miller MA, Erickson KI. Alterations in emotion generation and regulation neurocircuitry in depression and eating disorders: A comparative review of structural and functional neuroimaging studies. Neuroscience and Biobehavioral Reviews, 68:911-927, 2016.

Drevets WC, Price JL, Furey ML. Brain structural and functional abnormalities in mood disorders: implications for neurocircuitry models of depression. Brain Structure and Function, 213:93-118, 2008.

Felger JC, Li Z, Haroon E, Woolwine BJ, Jung MY, Hu X, Miller AH. Inflammation is associated with decreased functional connectivity within corticostriatal reward circuitry in depression. Molecular Psychiatry, 21:1358-1365, 2016.

Felger JC, Treadway MT. Inflammation effects on motivation and motor activity: role of dopamine. Neuropsychopharmacology Reviews, 42:216-241, 2017.

Felger JC. Imaging the Role of Inflammation in Mood and Anxiety-related Disorders. Current Neuropharmacology,16:533-558. 2018.

Firth J, Gangwisch JE, Borsini B, Wootton RE, Mayer EA. Food and mood: how do diet and nutrition affect mental wellbeing? BMJ, 360:m2382, 2020.

Fond G, Boukouaci W, Chebavier G, Regnault A, Erberl G, Hamdani N, et al. The "psychomicrobiotic": Targeting microbiota in major psychiatric disorders: A systematic review. Pathologie Biologie 63:35-42, 2015.

Gerhard DM, Wohleb ES, Duman RS. Emerging treatment mechanisms for depression: focus on glutamate and synaptic plasticity. Drug Discovery Today, 21:454-464, 2016.

Glare P, Aubrey KR, Myles PS. Postoperative pain management and opioids 1. Transition from acute to chronic pain after surgery. Lancet, 393:1537-1546, 2019.

Global Health Collaborators. Global, regional, and national incidence, prevalence, and years lived with disability for 328 diseases and injuries for 195 countries, 1990–2016: a systematic analysis for the Global Burden of Disease Study 2016. Lancet, 390:1211-1259, 2017.

Goehler LE. Flipping the switch on chronic pain. Brain Behavior and Immunity, 79:6-7, 2019.

Goehler LE, Lyte M, Gaykema RPA. Infection-induced viscerosensory signals from the gut enhance anxiety: implications for psychoneuroimmunology. Brain, Behavior and Immunity, 21:721-726, 2007.

Govindarajulu M, Pinky PD, Steinke I, Bloemer J, Ramesh S, Kariharan T, et al. Gut metabolite TMAO induces synaptic plasticity deficits by promoting endoplasmic reticulum stress. Frontiers in Molecular Neuroscience, 13:138, 2020.

Guo R, Chen L-H, Xing C, Liu T. Pain regulation by gut microbiota: molecular mechanisms and therapeutic potential. British Journal of Anaesthesia, 123:637-654, 2019.

Hannibal KE, Bishop MD. Chronic Stress, Cortisol Dysfunction, and Pain: A psychoneuroendocrine rationale for stress management in pain rehabilitation. Physical Therapy, 94, 1816-1825, 2014.

Haroon E, Raison CL, Miller AH. Psychoneuroimmunology meets neuropsychopharmacology: translational implications of the impact of inflammation on behavior. Neuropsychopharmacology Reviews, 37,137-162, 2012.

Haroon E, Wele JR, Woolwine BJ, Goldsmith DR, Baer W, Patel T, Felger JC, Miller AH. Associations among peripheral and central kynurenine pathway metabolites and inflammation in depression. Neuropsychopharmacology, 45:998-1007, 2020.

Huang R, Wang K, Hu J. Effect of probiotics on depression: a systematic review and meta-analysis of randomized controlled trials. Nutrients, 8:2016.

Huang Q, Huan Liu H, Suzuki K, Ma S, Liu C. Linking What We Eat to Our Mood: A Review of Diet, Dietary Antioxidants, and Depression. Antioxidants, 8:376, 2019.

Jacka FN, O'Neil A, Opie R, Itsiopoulos C, Cotton S, Mohebbi M, et al. A randomised controlled trial of dietary improvement for adults with major depression (the 'SMILES' trial). BMC Medicine, 15:23, 2017.

Janke EA, Jones E, Hopkins CM, Ruggieri M, Hruska A. Catastrophizing and anxiety sensitivity mediate the relationship between persistent pain and emotional eating. Appetite, 103:64-71, 2016.

Jaracz J, Gattner K, Jaracz K, Gorna K. Unexplained painful physical symptoms in patients with Major Depressive Disorder: Prevalence, pathophysiology and management. CNS Drugs, 293-304, 2016.

Ji R-R, Chamessian A, Zhang Y-Q. Pain regulation by non-neuronal cells and inflammation. Science, 354:572-577, 2016.

Kennedy DO. B Vitamins and the Brain: Mechanisms, Dose and Efficacy-A Review. Nutrients, 8:68, 2016.

Kiecolt-Glaser JK, Derry HM, Fagundas CP. Inflammation: Depression fans the flames and feasts on the heat. American Journal of Psychiatry, 172:1075-1091, 2015.

Khera T, Rangasamy V. Cognition and pain: a review. Frontiers in Psychology, 12:673962, 2021.

Knüppel A, Shipley MJ, Llewellyn CH, Brunner EJ. Sugar intake from sweet food and beverages, common mental disorder and depression: prospective findings from the Whitehall II study. Scientific Reports, 7:6287, 2017.

Kohler-Forsberg O, Lydholm CN, Hjorthoj C, Nordentoft M, Mors O, Benros ME. Efficacy of anti-inflammatory treatment on major depressive disorder or depressive symptoms: meta-analysis of clinical trials. Acta Psychiatrica Scandinavica, 139:404-419, 2019.

Konttinen H, Silventoinenen K, Sario-Lahteenkorva S, Mannisto S, Haukkala A. Emotional eating and physical activity self-efficacy as pathways in the association between depressive symptoms and adiposity indicators. American Journal of Clinical Nutrition, 92:1031-1039, 2010.

Koopman M, , El Aidya S, MIDtrauma consortium. Depressed gut? The microbiota-diet-inflammation trialogue in depression. Current Opinion in Psychiatry, 30:369-377, 2017.

Kris-Etherton PM, Petersen KS, Hibbeln JR, Hurley D, Kolick V, Peoples S, et al. Nutrition and behavioral health disorders: depression and anxiety. Nutrition Reviews, 79:247-260, 2021.

Lach G, Schellekens H, Dinan T, Cryan J. Anxiety, depression, and the microbiome: A role for gut peptides. Neurotherapeutics, 15:36-59, 2018.

Lagomarsino VN, Kostic AD, Cjiu IM. Mechanisms of microbial-neuronal interactions in pain and nociception. Neurobiology of Pain, 9:100056, 2021.

Li Y, Lv M-R, Wei Y-J, Sun L, Zhang J-X, Zhang H-G, Li B. Dietary patterns and depression risk: A meta-analysis. Psychiatry Research, 253:373-382, 2017.

Liu B, Yunan He Y, Wang M, Liu J, Ju Y, Zhang Y, Liu T, Li L, Li, Q. Efficacy of probiotics on anxiety—A meta-analysis of randomized controlled trials. Depression and Anxiety, 35(10):935-945, 2018.

Maes M. Evidence for an immune response in Major Depression: A review and hypothesis. Progress in Neuro-psychopharmacology and Biological Psychiatry, 19:11-38, 1995.

Maes M, Berk M, Goehler L, Song C, Anderson G, Gałecki P, Leonard B. Depression and sickness behavior are Janus-faced responses to shared inflammatory pathways. BMC Medicine, 10:66, 2012.

Martinez-Lavin M. Fibromyalgia in women: somatisation or stress-evoked, sex-dimorphic neuropathic pain? Clinical and Experimental Rheumatology, 39:422-425, 2021.

Marx W, Lane M, Hockey M, Aslam H, Berk M, Walder K et al. Diet and depression: exploring the biological mechanisms of action. Molecular Psychiatry, 26:134-150, 2021.

Masana MF, Tyrovolas S, Kollia N, Chrysohoou C, Skoumas J, Haro JM, et al. Dietary Patterns and Their Association with Anxiety Symptoms among Older Adults: The ATTICA Study. Nutrients, 11:1250, 2019.

Matsuda M, Huh Y, Ji RR. Roles of inflammation, neurogenic inflammation, and neuroinflammation in pain. Journal of Anesthesiology, 33:131-139, 2019.

Mayyappan AC, Forth E, Wallace CJK, Miley R. Effect of fecal microbiota transplant on symptoms of psychiatric disorders: a systematic review. BMC Psychiatry, 20:299, 2020

McEwen BS, Akil H. Revisiting the stress concept: Implications for affective disorders. Journal of Neuroscience, 40:12-21, 2020.

Mehta ND, Haroon E, Xu X, Bobbi J. Woolwine BJ, Li Z, Felger JC. Inflammation negatively correlates with amygdala-ventromedial prefrontal functional connectivity in association with anxiety in patients with depression: preliminary results. Brain Behavior and Immunity, 73:725-730, 2018.

Mendonca CR, Noll M, Rezende Castro MC, Silveira EA. Effects of nutritional interventions in the control of musculoskeletal pain: An integrative review. Nutrients, 17, 3075, 2020.

Micholoulos V, Powers A, Gillespie CF, Ressler KJ, Jovanovic T. Inflammation in fear- and anxiety-based disorders: PTSD, GAD, and beyond. Neuropsychopharmacology Reviews, 42:254-270, 2017.

Miller AH. Conceptual Confluence: The Kynurenine Pathway as a Common Target for Ketamine and the Convergence of the Inflammation and Glutamate Hypotheses of Depression. Neuropsychopharmacology, 38:1607-1608, 2013.

Miller AH, Maletic V, Raison CL. Inflammation and Its Discontents: The Role of Cytokines in the Pathophysiology of Major Depression. Biological Psychiatry, 65:732-741, 2009.

Nakamura M, Miura A, Nagahata T, Shibata Y, Okada E, Ojima T. Low zinc, copper, and manganese intake is associated with depression and anxiety symptoms in the Japanese working population: Findings from the eating habit and well-being study. Nutrients, 11, 847, 2019.

Oliviero F, Spinella P, Fiocco U, Ramonda R, Sfriso P, Punnzi L. How the Mediterranean diet and some of its components modulate inflammatory pathways in arthritis. Swiss Medical Weekly, 145: w14190, 2015.

O'Loughlin I, Newton-John TRO. 'Dis-comfort eating': An investigation into the use of food as a coping strategy for the management of chronic pain. Appetite, 140:288-297, 2019.

Pariante CM. Why are depressed patients inflamed? A reflection on 20 years of research on depression, glucocorticoid resistance and inflammation. European Neuropsychopharmacology, 27:554-559, 2017.

Parletta N, Zarnowiecki D, Cho J, Wilson A, Bogomolova S, Villani A et al. A Mediterranean-style dietary intervention supplemented with fish oil improves diet quality and mental health in people with depression: A randomized controlled trial (HELFIMED). Nutritional Neuroscience, 22:474-487, 2019.

Philips J. The treatment of melancholia by the lactic acid bacillus. Journal of Mental Sciences 56:422-31, 1910.

Philpot U, Johnson MI. Diet therapy in the management of chronic pain: better diet less pain? Pain Management, 9:335-338, 2019.

Pinho-Ribeiro FA, Verri WA Jr, Chiu IM. Nociceptor sensory neuron-immune interactions in pain and inflammation. Trends in Immunology, 38:5-19, 2017.

Porreca F, Navratilova E. Reward, motivation and emotion of pain and its relief. Pain, 158:S43-S49, 2017.

Price RB, Duman R. Neuroplasticity in cognitive and psychological mechanisms of depression: An integrative model. Molecular Psychiatry, 25:530-543, 2020.

Reichenberg A, Yirmiya R, Schuld A, Kraus T, Haack M, Morag A, et al. Cytokine-associated emotional and cognitive disturbances in humans. Archives of General Psychiatry, 58:44, 2001.

Salduker S, Allers E, Bechan S, Hodgson RE, Meyer F, Meyer H, et al. Practical approach to a patient with chronic pain of uncertain etiology in primary care. Journal of Pain Research, 12:2651-2662, 2019.

Savitz J. The kynurenine pathway: a finger in every pie. Molecular Psychiatry, 25:131–147, 2020.

Simmons WK, Burrows K, Avery JA, Kerr KL, Bodurka J, Savage CR, Drevets WC. Depression-related increases and decreases in appetite reveal dissociable patterns of aberrant activity in reward and interoceptive neurocircuitry. American Journal of Psychiatry, 173:418-428, 2016.

Slavich GM, Sacher J. Stress, sex hormones, inflammation, and major depressive disorder: Extending Social Signal Transduction Theory of Depression to account for sex differences in mood disorders. Psychopharmacology, 236:3063-3079, 2019.

Tan B, Philipp M, Hill S, Che Muhamed AM, Mundel T. Pain across the menstrual cycle: considerations of hydration. Frontiers in Physiology, 11:585667, 2020.

Tick H, Nielsen A, Pelletier KR, Bonakdar R, Simmons S, Glick R, Ratner E, Lemmon RL, Wayne P, Zador V. Evidence-based nonpharmacologic strategies for comprehensive pain care: the consortium pain task force white paper. Explore, 14:177-211, 2018.

Truschel J. Depression definition and DSM-5 diagnostic criteria. Psycom, https://www.psycom.net/depression-definition-dsm-5-diagnostic-criteria/ , 2020

Tsao W-C, Ro2 L-S, Chen C-M, Chang H-C, Kou H-C. Non-alcoholic Wernicke's encephalopathy with cortical involvement and polyneuropathy following gastrectomy. Metabolic Brain Disease, 32:1649-1657, 2017.

Wang J, Zhou Y, Chen K, Jing Y, He J, Sun H, Hu X. Dietary inflammatory index and depression: a meta-analysis. Public Health Nutrition, 22(4):654-660, 2018.

Wang N, Zhang Y-H, Wang J-Y, Luo F. Current understanding of the involvement of the insular cortex in neuropathic pain: a narrative review. International Journal of Molecular Science, 22:2648, 2021.

Wiley JW, Higgins GA, Athey BD. Stress and glucocorticoid receptor transcriptional programming in time and space: Implications for the brain–gut axis. Neurogastroenterology and Motility, 28:12-25, 2016.

Woolf CJ. Central sensitization: Implications for the diagnosis and treatment of pain. Pain, 152: S2-15, 2011.

Yang B, Wei J, Ju P, et al. Effects of regulating intestinal microbiota on anxiety symptoms: A systematic review. General Psychiatry, 32:e100056, 2019.

Zhang YP, Mei S, Yan J, Rodriguez Y, Candiotti KA. Acute Hypoglycemia Induces Painful Neuropathy and the Treatment of Coenzyme Q10. Journal of Diabetes Research, 2016:4593052, 2016.

Zhang Y, Wang Y, Ke B, Du J. TMAO: how gut microbiota contribute to heart failure. Translational Research, 228:109-125, 2020.

Zick SM, Murphy SL, Colacino J. Association of chronic spinal pain with diet quality. Association of chronic spinal pain with diet quality. Pain Reports, 5:e837, 2020.

- WHAT IS SLEEP?

- WHY WE NEED TO SLEEP

- SLEEP, RHYTHMICITY, AND METABOLISM

- WHY ARE METABOLIC FUNCTIONS RHYTHMIC?

- "SLEEP HYGIENE" IS MORE THAN CRUMBS IN BED: LIFESTYLE HABITS AND ACTIVITY AFFECT SLEEP

- SLEEP AND THE IMMUNE SYSTEM: PARTNERS IN HOMEOSTASIS

- BIDIRECTIONAL INTERACTIONS OF STRESS AND SLEEP

- THE INSOMNIA TRAP: "HURRY UP AND GO TO SLEEP"

- SLEEP CHANGES AS WE AGE

- DIET EFFECTS ON SLEEP

- KEY POINTS

We spend about a third of our lives asleep, or at least we should. How much we sleep and how well we sleep are closely linked to how we feel during the day. Sleep is generally measured as sleep duration and sleep quality. Sleep quality assesses how long it takes to go to sleep and whether there are episodes of awaking. Both sleep duration and sleep quality have been found to be associated with health and wellness. Further, lack of sleep is associated with increased risks of disease and even mortality (Opp 2015). Low sleep duration has been particularly associated with increased risk of metabolic disease, and poor sleep quality has been linked to mood symptoms (Irwin 2019). Indeed, how we feel relies on a complex interplay between biological rhythms, metabolic and immune function, and sleep. What and when we eat strongly influence these rhythms. Understanding what sleep is can provide a basis for explaining how sleep exerts widespread influences on the mind and body. Sleep is a central component of daily, circadian rhythms that coordinate brain and body functions. Learning how our lifestyle habits influence these circadian rhythms is crucial if we are to effectively address problems with sleep.

What is Sleep?

The phenomenon of sleep involves a prolonged period of unconsciousness occurring at a similar time each 24-hour period. Although we are unconscious while sleeping, the brain is quite active. Brain activity is divided into "sleep cycles" and characterized by different brain wave patterns. These different brain wave patterns can be measured by electroencephalography (EEG) and EEG patterns serve as biomarkers for different states of sleep.

When we first fall asleep, we are in "non-rapid eye movement," or NREM, sleep. NREM consists of three stages of successively "deeper" sleep. These stages are followed by a bout of rapid eye movement (REM) sleep. During REM sleep, the EEG pattern looks like brain wave patterns that occur when we are awake. Because of this similarity, REM sleep was called "paradoxical sleep" in early studies. REM sleep is now so named because during this phase of sleep the eyes move rapidly, which can be seen through closed eyelids. In contrast to this rapid eye movement, during REM, movement of the rest of the body is suppressed. Dreams can occur in both REM and NREM sleep. REM sleep is associated with dreams with a clear, if sometimes bizarre, narrative. NREM dreams are more amorphous and may consist of purely emotions. For instance, the "night terrors" that can affect toddlers are associated with NREM sleep. Although they can be challenging for parents, night terrors are common and normal. They usually peak around age three, and then go away. A full sleep cycle takes about 90 minutes, but over the course of a full night's sleep, the time spent in REM sleep is increased. This why we often "wake out of a dream" in the morning.

Why We Need to Sleep

Disturbances of sleep are associated with both subjective feelings of distress or impairment (e.g., fatigue, cognitive "fuzziness"), and performance deficits in memory, motor, or other tasks. As such, sleep plays a critical role in maintaining physical and mental health. How exactly sleep affects health is still debated, but recent research is illuminating some of the mechanisms by which sleep supports so many bodily functions.

Early hypotheses about the function and benefits of sleep centered on the "restorative" aspects of sleep. Sleep could relieve the feeling of fatigue, and regular rest-activity cycles could help conserve energy (Krueger 2016). If occurring in a protected location at the same time that predators are active, sleep could help avoid predation (Krueger 2016).

The most obvious effects of sleep, and sleep disturbances, are seen in brain function. Poor sleep is associated with cognitive impairment and memory problems as well as deficits in motor function (Krueger 2016). These deficits are associated with the subjective feeling of fatigue and "sleepiness." The brain is a very metabolically active place, and sleep is associated with replenishment of brain energy stores (Krueger 2016). The link of brain activity to sleep is also supported by the fact that adenosine, which is a product of energy generation in cells, is a potent inducer of sleep. Because it is made from metabolic activity in the brain, adenosine is a reliable marker of brain activity. This positions adenosine to act as a helpful signal of brain activity levels.

More recently, research has uncovered specific mechanisms that underlie the effects of sleep loss. During sleep, glial cells in the brain interact with neurons to support "neuroplastic" rewiring of brain connections due to activity or experiences (Krueger 2016). Without this glia-supported brain restructuring, learning would be impaired. Sleep has also been linked to function of the brain's "glymphatic system," a portmanteau of "glia" and "lymphatic." The glymphatic system consists of glia and lymphatic cells that function to remove potentially toxic metabolites and other molecules, such as beta-amyloid, from the brain's circulatory system (Krueger 2016). This function is rather like "taking out the garbage." The glymphatic system is active during sleep. Restriction of this glymphatic function is hypothesized to link sleep problems with the risk of neurological disorders, including Alzheimer's disease (Krueger 2016). By supporting required brain restructuring for learning, and cleaning up the messes left by brain activity during waking periods, sleep serves as a homeostatic process that supports the overall health and function of the brain.

Sleep, Rhythmicity, and Metabolism

Sleep cycles are part of a larger, highly integrated system of circadian rhythms that coordinate physiological functions according to the time of day. These sleep cycles are sometimes called "homeostatic sleep." Hormone levels, for example, fluctuate in a regular way according to the time of day (Skene 2018). The principal signals that entrain these rhythms are light, behavior, and activity. For example, nutrient intake entrains rhythmicity of some endocrine and physiological functions (Bae 2019, Gopalakrishnan 2021). Cortisol is a prime example of a hormone whose levels are entrained by daily patterns of light and behavior. Light-entrained rhythms are referred to as *photic rhythms*. Activity-related patterns are called *non-photic behavioral rhythms*. To stay healthy, the "clocks" in individual organs and tissues must be synchronized. When body clocks become misaligned, risk increases for metabolic disorders such as diabetes, cardiovascular disease, and other diseases associated with dysregulated inflammation (Bae 2019, Morris 2017, Skene 2018). This desynchronization of body clocks may occur with poor "sleep hygiene" or shift work.

Circadian rhythms dependent upon ambient light are governed by a brain region in the hypothalamus called the suprachiasmatic nucleus (SCN). This "master clock" coordinates the expression of *clock genes* in peripheral tissues, such as the liver, that serve as tissue-specific clocks in the body (Skene 2018). One of the ways the SCN synchronizes clock genes all over the body is by influencing cortisol rhythms and the autonomic nervous system (Flanagan 2021, Skene 2018). These cortisol and autonomic nervous system signals coordinate metabolism and immune function in turn.

Behavioral rhythms include light/dark exposure, sleep/wakefulness, rest/activity, and eating/fasting. These rhythms influence the activity of brain arousal systems. Here, brain networks activate and coordinate other brain regions to enable behavior and cognition (Bai 2019, Saper 2006). Eating behaviors also influence insulin and metabolic rhythms. Thus, biological rhythms are closely intertwined with daily activities, and help control metabolism.

Why are Metabolic Functions Rhythmic?

The control of metabolism usually means that the "fuel" that provides for the energy needs for the cells of the body is made available to cells in a coordinated and efficient way (Gopalakrishan 2021, Johnston 2014). The more active cells are, the more energy they need. Thus, metabolic fuels should be available when cells are active, usually in the daytime. Likewise, fuel should not be present when not needed, for example when cells are less active and not absorbing nutrients. If cells are not absorbing nutrients, fuels such as glucose or lipids continue to circulate in the blood, leading to hyperglycemia or hyperlipidemia. This extra circulating fuel increases risk for conditions such as diabetes.

Because cortisol is closely involved in metabolic control, metabolic rhythms track closely with cortisol rhythms (Bai 2019, Bhat 2018). Thus, levels of cortisol are normally higher during the day. Metabolic efficiency is higher, too. Metabolic efficiency includes, for example, how well cells take up glucose from the blood (Pogiogalle 2018). In the evening, glucose tolerance, even in non-diabetic people, is similar to pre-diabetes (Pogiogalle 2018). Here, cells are reducing metabolic efficiency in preparation for sleep. This diurnal variation in glucose tolerance is related to clock-gene function within cells, as well as to the diurnal rhythms of the hormone insulin. Like cortisol, insulin peaks during the day and is low at night.

Biological rhythms associated with activity, including sleep and waking, are linked to meals (Saper 2006). Overlapping mechanisms in the hypothalamus control both feeding and arousal/wakefulness. These shared mechanisms intrinsically tie together feeding and sleep rhythms. This makes sense because we need to be awake to eat, and behavior and arousal require metabolic fuels. Thus, periods of the circadian cycle that are associated with activity co-occur with increased food-related motivation and more efficient metabolism. The hypothalamus coordinates these rhythmic behavioral functions with the metabolic endocrine systems (e.g., cortisol, insulin). In this way, the hypothalamus plays a key role in the regulation of behavioral rhythms.

The pineal hormone melatonin is also released in a rhythmic way (Zisapel 2018), in a pattern opposite to cortisol and insulin. Levels are low during the daytime but start to rise about 2 hours before normal bedtime. Melatonin levels stay up until the middle of the night, and then decline to daytime levels. Thus, melatonin seems to play a role in preparing the brain and body for sleep, and for maintaining sleep (Zisapel 2018). Melatonin levels are sensitive to light. Light inhibits melatonin release. Working at night, such as during shift work, can lead to lower levels of melatonin. Melatonin is a potent antioxidant as well as a signaling hormone. Melatonin is implicated in the regulation of many physiological functions, ranging from modulation of lipid metabolism, gut microbe populations, and neuroplasticity.

"Sleep Hygiene" is More than Crumbs in Bed: Lifestyle Habits and Activity Affect Sleep

In addition to our daily circadian rhythms, when we sleep depends on the level of brain activity we have engaged in. During our usual awake time, we may engage in activity that requires more than the usual metabolic activity in the brain. Some products of that increased metabolism, such as adenosine, are potent sleep inducers. The greater the brain activity, the more adenosine and other factors are produced. These metabolic products increase the drive for sleep (Krueger 2019). This is why, after studying or working hard on a problem, we may have a strong urge for a nap.

In addition to coordinating functions and organ systems of the body, circadian rhythms also influence a network of brain regions that govern the activity or arousal levels of the brain. This network regulates the onset and maintenance of sleep, as well the distinctive stages of sleep. The neurons in this network use a variety of neurotransmitter systems, including norepinephrine, serotonin, acetylcholine, histamine, and orexin (Scamell 2017, Saper 2006). In addition to controlling sleep, this network helps coordinate our ability to engage in thoughts and cognitions and behavior. In general, engaging in activities that induce arousal, such as eating or exercise, tend to keep us awake. It is largely through this network that our lifestyle habits affect our sleep.

The term *sleep hygiene* refers to lifestyle habits associated with bedtime and other activities that influence sleep. These habits include activities carried out shortly before bedtime, level of daily exercise, and the regularity of meals and bedtime. Poor sleep hygiene is linked to mood symptoms (Bhat 2018, Van Dyk 2019). Sleep hygiene seems to be especially important for children and adolescents (Jodi 2018).

The brain needs to wind down before falling asleep. Thus, engaging in arousing activities such as exercise or computer use is associated with poor sleep. Sleep specialists also counsel against engaging in activities other than sleep, or sex, in bed (Jansson-Frojmark 2019). In this way the brain will be trained to associate bed with sleep specifically, rather than more arousing activities, such as eating meals or working on a computer. Nicotine use before bedtime is associated with persistent insomnia, as is ambient light and noise (Jansson-Frojmark 2019, Yazdi 2016). Similarly, exercise should not be undertaken right before bedtime. However, regular daily exercise is associated with better sleep (Yazdi 2016).

Given the close links between circadian rhythmicity, metabolism and sleep, meal timing plays an important role in good sleep hygiene and the synchronicity of rhythms necessarily for good sleep and good health. Recently, the 24/7 availability of food and the habit of many people to eat "around the clock" has been linked to cardiovascular disease and obesity (Flanagan 2021). *Night eating syndrome* describes a pattern of eating whereby people routinely consume many calories at night, often waking up to eat (Berketvedt 1999). This is a sleep disorder, but it is also associated with mood disorders and metabolic disease (Lee 2019, Goel 2009, Lee 2019).

One possible mechanism linking disease to eating at night involves disruption of cortisol rhythms. Cortisol levels are highest in the morning and decline throughout the day to a low level at night. Cortisol levels are especially low during sleep (Liiyanarachchi 2017). They rise again in the morning, and this is thought to contribute to awaking. One problem with eating late at night is that eating induces cortisol release, leading to higher-than-normal cortisol levels during the night (Berketvedt 1999). Night-time eating also lowers levels of melatonin. Low cortisol levels at night seem to be important to facilitate immune functions that occur during that time, such as healing and clearing toxins (Krueger 2016). Higher levels of cortisol may also influence arousal systems in a way that does not support good sleep.

Consuming calories at night dramatically raises the risk of obesity, compared with consuming calories in the morning (Zarrinpar 2016). One reason may be that foods eaten at night tend to be high-energy, low-fiber, low-nutrition foods. Skipping breakfast, and thus taking a greater percentage of calories later in the day, also raises risk of type 2 diabetes (Flanagan 2021). This effect of skipping breakfast may result from misalignment of the circadian rhythms of metabolic hormones.

Because of the evident importance of consistent mealtimes and risks of late-night eating, a protocol called "time-restricted eating" is becoming popular (Longo 2016). Time-restricted eating is just that: eating is limited to specific time periods during the day, allowing a long period of fasting time during the evening and night. Time-restricted eating is a variation on intermittent *fasting*, where a daily 8-to-10 hour period of eating is alternated with a 14-to-16 hour period of fasting. People who practice restricted eating report that it is easier to control their eating behavior. In a controlled study with overweight adults, participants consumed fewer calories, lost weight, and reported better sleep after restricting their nutrient intake to

10 hours per day (Melkani 2017). The beneficial effects of time-restricted eating likely follow at least in part from preventing night-time eating and thereby realigning circadian rhythms of light, activity, and food with endocrine rhythms (e.g., cortisol, insulin, melatonin). Overall, these findings underline the importance of maintaining good sleep hygiene that can support well-synchronized behavioral rhythms for sleep and metabolism.

Sleep and the Immune System: Partners in Homeostasis

Both sleep and the immune system play pivotal roles in maintaining homeostasis by regulating physiological function. Sleep and immune system function are closely linked (Irwin 2019). Normal daily immune functions follow circadian rhythms that are regulated by cortisol (Shimba 2020). One way that cortisol regulates rhythmicity of immune function is by influencing clock gene expression in immune cells (Shimba 2020). In general, immune rhythms are the opposite of cortisol rhythms. For instance, based on pre-clinical models, microglia in the brain seem more active during sleep (Choudury 2020). Levels of circulating cytokines in humans peak in the middle of the night and early hours of the morning when cortisol levels are normally low. Whereas the significance of this is not fully established, animal studies have implicated pro-inflammatory cytokines, released as part of homeostasis (i.e., not in response to infection), in triggering growth and re-modeling of neuronal networks in the brain (Krueger 2019). During sleep, numbers of circulating immune cells decrease. This implies that during sleep the immune cells move from blood into tissue (Besedovsky 2019). What they are doing there is unknown, but based on evidence that immune cells seem to have restorative effects and housekeeping roles in the brain, it may be that during sleep, immune cells are also cleaning up tissues or healing any damage in the rest of the body. Pro-inflammatory cytokines may also contribute to regulation of normal sleep, along with other immune-derived substances such as prostaglandins, specifically PGD_2 (Besedovsky 2019). Conversely, metabolism-related molecules such as adenosine also signal immune cells suggesting common regulation of both sleep and immune function in the brain (Krueger 2019). Thus, sleep seems necessary for normal immune function, and normal immune function contributes to the regulation of sleep.

Sleep also seems to be a prominent part of the body's response to infection. Inflammation, the body's first response to infection, contributes to *interoception*. This immune-to-brain communication induces the sickness response, which includes changes in sleep. This can involve increases in sleep, as well as changes in the relative amount of REM and NREM sleep. The exact role of sleep for the immune response is not well-established, but sleep loss is associated with impaired immune function and increased risk of infection (Besedovsky 2019, Irwin 2019). Indeed, studies of people after vaccination show that sleep seems necessary for an optimal generation of antibodies. In fact, in one study, sleep-deprived people had to receive an extra inoculation because the titers of antibody they produced were too low to provide protection (Besdovsky 2019). Normal sleep duration was found to double the response to vaccination compared to sleep restriction (Besdovsky 2019). Conversely, chronic infections such as AIDS, hepatitis C, Epstein-Barr virus mononucleosis, and chronic fatigue syndrome, are associated with sleep disturbances, as are chronic inflammatory diseases, including autoimmune diseases such as inflammatory bowel disease, Sjogren's syndrome, rheumatoid arthritis, and multiple sclerosis. Further, sleep disturbance is linked to Alzheimer's disease, which is increasingly being recognized as an inflammatory condition (Irwin 2019).

Laboratory studies report that sleep deprivation is associated with elevated levels of cytokines and NFkB upregulation (Besedovsky 2019). This sleep deprivation effect is more pronounced in women than in men (Dolson). This may at least partly explain why insomnia or chronic short sleep duration raises the risk for mood disorders, type 2 diabetes, chronic pain, and cardiovascular disease. All these conditions are associated with elevated inflammation. Immune disturbances likely interact with lifestyle factors that influence inflammation and immune function. This, again, underlines the importance of good sleep hygiene.

Bidirectional Interactions of Stress and Sleep

Psychological stress is recognized to be one of major contributors to poor sleep (McEwen 2015). Sleep loss/deprivation or "misalignment" due to shift work or air travel can also act as stressors (McEwen 2015). Sleep disruption causes neuroendocrine, metabolic, and immune disruption in both animal models and epidemiological studies of humans, who experience routine misalignment of circadian signals, such as that experienced with "jet lag." These can result in increased weight, pre-diabetes, and elevated inflammation. Sleep loss encourages poor food choices (Greer 2013, St. Onge 2019). Even people who normally prefer healthy food will choose and tend to overconsume sugary and fatty foods when sleep-deprived. This also likely contributes to the relationship between sleep problems and metabolic disorders, such as diabetes. Further, stress increases inflammatory mediators and could disrupt sleep by dysregulating cytokine roles in homeostatic sleep. Thus, stress has a bidirectional relationship with sleep that has serious implications for health.

Stress dysregulates the hypothalamic-pituitary-adrenal axis, and therefore impacts circadian rhythms. The clock genes that coordinate function of the autonomic nervous system, and the brain regions that mediate responses to challenges, such as the hypothalamus and amygdala, are under control of cortisol and depend on normal cortisol rhythms. Disruption of these rhythms contributes to allostatic load (i.e., the price paid for not managing challenges). Allostatic load contributes to the cognitive and mood symptoms that can accompany disrupted sleep or misalignment of circadian signals (McEwen 2015). This close relationship between stress and sleep problems means that people suffering from sleep problems need to address stress. Fortunately, there are several mind-body modalities, including mindfulness meditation and restorative yoga, that have been found to help people suffering from sleep problems (Black 2016). These modalities can facilitate relaxation and reduce the brain arousal that can impair sleep. They may also teach skills to help learn to "address the challenge" and banish stress.

The Insomnia Trap: "Hurry Up and Go to Sleep"

Many of us attempt to go to bed and find ourselves unable to turn off our brains. We lie there, wide awake, thinking about things that have happened during the day, and things we are afraid may happen tomorrow. No matter how we try, we cannot stop thinking. Meanwhile, the minutes and hours tick away. Hurry up and go to sleep! Soon it will be morning, and we will have to get up and face another day. We know the dangers of not getting enough sleep. We will be tired all day, and at more risk for Alzheimer's disease. Hurry up and go to sleep!

Anxiety is associated with sleep problems (Gould 2018, Rice 2019). Worries can contribute to arousal that inhibits falling asleep. Awareness of the risks of sleep loss can exacerbate anxiety, ironically making it harder to go to sleep.

But do we really "not sleep a wink all night"? This issue has been addressed by sleep studies. Here, people who feel they haven't slept in days spend the night in a sleep lab trying to sleep, while their brain EEG activity is recorded. Although people typically report that they did not sleep at all, their EEG over the night actually reflects normal sleep. The interpretation of this phenomenon is that people were dreaming they were awake when they were not.

I experienced this phenomenon a few years ago when my husband was out of town. For the first time in many years, I was alone in the house at night. I was not worried about that, but I was not able to fall asleep. I just kept thinking and thinking, until I heard my husband breathing. But it couldn't be him. He's in Holland. Who's breathing?! I tried to sit up but realized I couldn't. I had the feeling of trying to surface from the deep end of a swimming pool. Clearly, I had been asleep. Or, at least, a large part of my brain was asleep.

Recent sleep research has cast doubt on the idea that sleep necessarily involves the whole brain (Krueger 2019, Vantomme 2019). Local brain regions may sleep after intense activity, independently from other regions or from systemic circadian or arousal regulation (Kruger 2019, Vantomme 2019). Thus, it is possible for part of our brain, the "conscious" part, to be awake and thinking while much of the rest of our brain is asleep. That is, we may not be losing as much sleep as we think. Knowing this has helped me to let go of my anxiety about needing to hurry up and go to sleep. Consequently, I fall asleep more readily.

Sleep Changes as We Age

How much we sleep changes over the lifespan. How well we sleep can change too, in the context of lifestyle and overall health (Li 2018, Mattis 2016). In general, time spent sleeping decreases as we age, but the biggest difference is between infancy and adulthood. Babies sleep the most, but there is not much difference among healthy adults of all ages in how much we sleep. However, many older adults experience "phase advance" (Li 2018), which means that people tend to feel sleepy and go to bed earlier than when they were younger. I have noticed this effect with pets as well as they get older. Older adults are also reported to nap more than younger people (Mattis 2016. Li 2018), but that may be related to lifestyle factors. For example, older people when retired just may have more opportunity to nap. In addition, older people have more difficulty adjusting to time changes, such as jet lag (Li 2018).

Endocrine function changes over the lifespan in ways that can contribute to sleep problems. For instance, during the night, when we are sleeping, cortisol levels are typically low and rise in the morning immediately prior to awakening. However, in some older people, cortisol levels increase in the middle of the night (Li 2018). This could plausibly explain the phenomenon of waking up at 3 AM, and feeling "wide awake." In addition, changes in gonadal hormones associated with menopause may affect one's ability to fall asleep and stay asleep (Li 2018). In addition, melatonin levels drop with aging and may not become high enough to support a full night of sleep, contributing to sleep problems in older people (Li 2018).

That said, studies show that healthy older adults do not suffer from more sleep disorders than younger people (Li 2018). Rather, sleep problems, including sleep apnea, REM behavior disorder, restless legs syndrome, and other primary sleep disorders that are more common in older people are associated with co-morbid chronic disease (Li 2018, St Louis 2017). Thus, older people are more likely to have chronic illnesses that have bidirectional interactions with sleep. As we age, we normally experience increased inflammation, and lifestyle factors including diet, physical activity, and social interaction can influence inflammation and perhaps effect the quality of sleep (Li 2018).

Sleep problems are particularly common in neurodegenerative diseases, including Alzheimer's disease (AD), Parkinson's disease (PD), Lewy body dementia, and Huntington's disease (Mattis 2016). Circadian rhythms are disrupted in AD, possible due to degeneration of the SCN. One common consequence of this is nighttime awakening where people with AD awaken in the night, become confused, and sometimes wander. Sleep problems affect about two-thirds people with PD (Mattis 2016, St Louis 2017). Sleep disruption in PD is correlated with hallucinations, but not motor symptoms. Interestingly, more than ninety percent of people who have REM behavior disorder, in which people "act out their dreams," go on to develop PD (Mattis 2016). Normally during REM sleep, motor movement is inhibited; this inhibition is impaired in REM behavior disorder. Thus, REM behavior disorder may represent a prodromal impairment in the coordination of arousal and motor systems that characterize PD.

What are the mechanisms that mediate the link between sleep problems and neurodegenerative disease? Neurodegenerative diseases are characterized by neuroinflammation and oxidative stress that lead to the destruction of neurons. What triggers this inflammation is not firmly established, but diets high in sugar and other refined carbohydrates are linked to AD (Pistollato 2018). The accumulation of pro-inflammatory misfolded proteins is found in all type of neurodegenerative disease. Sleep loss can induce preferences for sugary, high-calorie foods, and potentially impair the ability of the glymphatic system to remove pro-inflammatory misfolded proteins (Greer 2013, Mattis 2016). Sleep loss is associated with signs of stress, including oxidative stress, which could further drive inflammation (Mattis 2016, McEwen 2015).

Diet Effects on Sleep

Given the links between circadian rhythms, metabolism, and inflammation, what is the evidence that diet can influence sleep?

Currently, good studies investigating specific foods or diet effects on sleep are still rather rare. The complex interplay of stress, inflammation, and diet can complicate interpretation of studies that manipulate diet or attempt to correlate diet with specific sleep symptoms. Early studies focused on specific macronutrient content (e.g., high-carbohydrate versus low-carbohydrate) but the results were inconsistent and hard to interpret. Recent studies are now addressing overall dietary patterns. Based on current insights into the role of inflammation in symptoms of disease and in regulation of sleep, several studies have addressed possible relationships between intake of anti-inflammatory or antioxidant foods, such as fresh vegetables and whole grains, compared to highly refined carbohydrate and/or processed foods, including processed meats (Muscigiuri 2020). Indeed, cross-sectional and epidemiological studies now support the idea that diets based on mostly plants (e.g., Mediterranean diet) and that limit processed foods and refined carbohydrates are associated with better and longer sleep (St-Onge 2016).

As one might predict, diets that are associated with less inflammation, such as the Mediterranean or keto diet, seem to improve sleep (Castro-Diehl 2018). For instance, diabetes, which is characterized by chronic inflammation and hyperglycemia, is associated with high rates of sleep problems (Siegmann 2019). A low-carbohydrate keto diet improved subjective reports of several sleep parameters in people with type 2 diabetes or pre-diabetes (Siegmann 2019). This supports the idea that high-carbohydrate diets may affect sleep, possibly by effects on inflammation.

What foods have been specifically linked to sleep quality or duration? It seems that some single ingredients (e.g., tart cherries, valerian or chamomile, or malted milk) may help sleep for some people, but the effect sizes are small. Interestingly, high-fiber diets are reported to be associated with better sleep, and it has been proposed that this effect may be mediated at least in part by gut microbes (Krueger 2016, St-Onge 2019). Given the association between oxidative stress, inflammation, and sleep problems, the antioxidant and anti-inflammatory properties of Mediterranean diet foods such as fresh fruits and vegetables should be helpful for sleep problems. Indeed, a recent study in a large sample of adults found that adherence to the Mediterranean diet was strongly associated with better sleep quality (Muscogiuri 2020). The study also found that low adherence to the Mediterranean diet was associated with both obesity and poor sleep. These findings reinforce the relationship between sleep and metabolism and suggest that a key linking factor concerns quality of diet.

Key Points

- Sleep provides time for resting the body, but also for "housekeeping" functions such as removal of cellular debris. This is particularly important for the brain, because much of the physical remodeling of neuronal connections necessary for neuroplasticity is done by immune cells in the brain during sleep.
- Sleep is one of the circadian rhythms, which also govern the endocrine and immune systems and metabolism. Regulating physiological activities within rhythmic cycles enables these activities to be effectively coordinated to maintain optimum physiological functioning (homeostasis).
- The importance of adequate sleep is reflected in the wide-ranging consequences of sleep disorders or disruption, which include metabolic disease (type 2 diabetes), mood disorders, and increased risk for neurodegenerative diseases.
- Sleep has a bi-directional relationship with stress, in that stress disrupts sleep and sleep loss is a potent stressor. Like chronic stress, sleep loss is associated with increased inflammation.
- Sleep patterns are enmeshed with metabolic regulation and eating behavior, such that circadian rhythms of eating behavior help time both metabolism and sleep.
- Night-time eating disrupts metabolic regulation, because metabolic systems are more sensitive and efficient earlier in the day. This may be why people who eat breakfast have lower risks for obesity and diabetes.
- Night-time eating can also disrupt sleep, possibly by disrupting cortisol and melatonin rhythms.

- Diets high in energy but low in nutrients (e.g., Western diet) are associated with poor sleep, whereas diets such as the Mediterranean diet improve sleep. Diets associated with better sleep provide fresh fruit and vegetables, plenty of fiber, and avoid refined carbohydrates.
- "Time-restricted eating," where eating is limited to an 8-to-10-hour period, can also improve sleep. This is particularly true if the period is earlier in the day.

References

Bae S-A, Fang MZ, Rustgi V, Zarbl H, Androulakis IP (2019) At the Interface of Lifestyle, Behavior, and Circadian Rhythms: Metabolic Implications. Frontiers in Nutrition, 6:132, 2019.

Berketvedt GS, Florholmen J, Sundsfjord J, Osterud B, Dinges D, Bilker W, Stunkard A. Behavioral and neuroendocrine characteristics of the night-eating syndrome. JAMA, 282:657-663, 1999.

Besedovsky L, Lange T, Haack M. The sleep-immune crosstalk in health and disease. Physiological Reviews, 99:1325-1380, 2019.

Bhat S, Pinto-Zipp G, Upadhyay H, Polos PG. "To sleep, perchance to tweet": in-bed electronic social media use and its associations with insomnia, daytime sleepiness, mood, and sleep duration in adults. Sleep Health, 4:166-173, 2018.

Black DS, O'Reilly GA, Richard Olmstead R, Breen EC, Irwin MR. Mindfulness Meditation and Improvement in Sleep Quality and Daytime Impairment Among Older Adults with Sleep Disturbances: A Randomized Clinical Trial. JAMA Internal Medicine. 175:94-501, 2016.

Castro-Diehl C, Wood AC, Redline S, Reid M, Johnson DA, Maras JE, Jacobs, DR, Shea S, Crawford A, St-Onge M-P. Mediterranean diet pattern and sleep duration and insomnia symptoms in the Multi-Ethnic Study of Atherosclerosis. Sleep Journal, 4:1-10, 2018.

Choudhury ME, Miyanishi K, Takeda H, Islam A, Matsuika N, Kubo M, et al. Phagocytic eliminations of synapses by microglia during sleep. Glia, 64:44-59, 2020.

Flanagan A, Bechtold DA, Pot GK, Johnstone JD. Chrono-nutrition: From molecular and neuronal mechanisms to human epidemiology and timed feeding patterns. Journal of Neurochemistry, 157:53-72, 2021.

Jansson-Fröjmark M, Evander J, Alfonsson S. Are sleep hygiene practices related to the incidence, persistence and remission of insomnia? Findings from a prospective community study. Journal of Behavior Medicine, 42:128-138, 2019.

Goel N, Stunkard AJ, Rogers NL, Van Dongen HPA, Allison KC, O' Reardon JP, Ahima RS, Cummings DE, Heo M, Dinges DF. Circadian rhythm profiles in women with Night Eating Syndrome. Journal of Biological Rhythms, 24:85-94, 2009.

Gopalakrishnan S, Kanna NN. Only time will tell: The interplay between circadian clock and metabolism. Chronobiology International, 38:149-167, 2021.

Gould CE, Spira AP, Liou-Johnson V, Cassdy-Eagle E, Kawai M, Mashal N, et al. Association of Anxiety Symptom Clusters with Sleep Quality and Daytime Sleepiness. Journal of Gerontology B: Psychological Science and Social Sciences, 73:413-420, 2018.

Greer SM, Goldstein AN, Walker MP. The impact of sleep deprivation on food desire in the human brain. Nature Communications, 4: 2259, 2013.

Irwin MR. Sleep and inflammation: partners in sickness and health. Nature Reviews Immunology, 19:702-715, 2019.

Jodi A, Mindell JA, Williamson AA. Benefits of a bedtime routine in young children: Sleep, development, and beyond. Sleep Medicine Review, 40: 93-108, 2018.

Johnston JD. Physiological links between circadian rhythms, metabolism and nutrition. Experimental Physiology, 99:1133-1137, 2014.

Krueger JM, Frank M, Wisor J, Sandip Roy S. Sleep Function: Toward Elucidating an Enigma. Sleep Medicine Review, 28: 46-54, 2016.

Krueger JM, Opp MR. Sleep and Microbes. International Review of Neurobiology, 131: 207-225, 2016.

Krueger JM, Nguyen JT, Dykstra-Aiello CJ, Taishi P. Local sleep. Sleep Medicine Reviews, 43:14021, 2019.

Lee KW, Shin D. Association of night eating with depression and depressive symptoms in Korean women. International Journal of Environmental Research and Public Health, 16:4831, 2019.

Li J, Vitiello MV, Gooneratne N. Sleep in Normal Aging. Sleep Medicine Clinics, 13:1-11, 2018.

Liyanarachchi K, et al. Human studies on hypothalamo-pituitary-adrenal (HPA) axis. Best Practice & Research Clinical Endocrinology & Metabolism, 31: 459e473, 2017.

Longo VD, Panda S. Fasting, circadian rhythms, and time restricted feeding in healthy lifespan. Cell Metabolism, 23:1048-1059, 2016.

Mattis J, Sehgal A. Circadian Rhythms, Sleep, and Disorders of Aging. Trends in Endocrinology and Metabolism, 7:92-203, 2016.

McEwen BS, Karatsoreos IN, Sleep Deprivation and Circadian Disruption: Stress, Allostasis, and Allostatic Load. Sleep Medicine Clinics, 10:1-10, 2015.

Melkani GC, Panda S. Time-restricted feeding for prevention and treatment of cardiometabolic disorders. Journal of Physiology, 595: 3691-3700, 2017.

Morris CJ, Purvis TE, Mistretta J, Hu K, Scheer FAJL. Circadian misalignment increases C-reactive protein and blood pressure in chronic shift workers. Journal of Biological Rhythms, 32: 154-164, 2017.

Muscogiuri G, Barrea L, Aprano A, Lydia Framondi L, Di Matteo R, Laudisio D, Pugliese G, Savastano S, Colao A, and on behalf of the OPERA PREVENTION Project. Sleep quality in obesity: does adherence to the Mediterranean diet matter? Nutrients, 12: 1364, 2020.

Opp MR, Krueger JM. Sleep and Immunity: A Growing Field with Clinical Impact. Brain, Behavior and Immunity, 47:1-3, 2015.

Postollato F, Calderon Iglesias R, Ruiz R, Aparicio S, Crespo J, Dzul Lopez L, Pia Manna P, Giampieri F, Battino M. Nutritional patterns associated with the maintenance of neurocognitive functions and the risk of dementia and Alzheimer's disease: A focus on human studies. Pharmacology Research, 131:32-43, 2018.

Poggiogalle E, Jamshed H, Peterson CM. Circadian Regulation of Glucose, Lipid, and Energy Metabolism in Humans. Metabolism, 84:11-27, 2018.

Rice VJB, Schroedert PJ. Self-Reported Sleep, Anxiety, and Cognitive Performance in a Sample of U.S. Military Active Duty and Veterans. Military Medicine, 184:488-497, 2019.

Saper CB. Staying awake for dinner: hypothalamic integration of sleep, feeding, and circadian rhythms. Progress in Brain Research, 153:243-252, 2006.

Scammell TE, Arrigoni E, Lipton J. Neural Circuitry of Wakefulness and Sleep. Neuron, 22:747-765, 2017.

Shimba A, Ikuta K. Glucocorticoids regulate circadian rhythm of innate and adaptive immunity. Frontiers in Immunology, 11:2143, 2020.

Siegmann MJ, Athinarayanan SJ, Hallberg SJ, McKenzie AL, Bhanpuri NH, Campbell WW, McCarter JP, Phinney SD, Volek JS, Van Dort CJ. Improvement in patient-reported sleep in type 2 diabetes and prediabetes participants receiving a continuous care intervention with nutritional ketosis. Sleep Medicine, 55:92-99, 2019.

Skene DJ, Skornyakov E, Chowdhurya NR, Gajula RP, Middleton B, Satterfield BC, Porter KI, Dongen HPA, Gaddameedhi S. Separation of circadian- and behavior-driven metabolite rhythms in humans provides a window on peripheral oscillators and metabolism. Proceedings of the National Academy of Sciences, 115:7825-7830, 2018.

St Louis EK, Boeve BF. REM Sleep Behavior Disorder: Diagnosis, Clinical Implications, and Future Directions Mayo Clinic Proceedings. 92:1723-1736, 2017.

St-Onge M-P, Mikic A, Pietrolungo CE. Effects of Diet on Sleep Quality. Advances in Nutrition, 7:938-49, 2016.

St-Onge M-O, Zuraikat FM. Reciprocal roles of sleep and diet in cardiovascular health: a review of recent evidence and a potential mechanism. Current Atherosclerosis Reports, 21:11, 2019.

Van Dyk TR, Becker SP, Byars KC. Rates of Mental Health Symptoms and Associations With Self-Reported Sleep Quality and Sleep Hygiene in Adolescents Presenting for Insomnia Treatment. Journal of Clinical Sleep Medicine, 15:1433-1442, 2019.

Vantomme G, Osorio-Forero A, Lüthi A, Fernandez LMJ. Regulation of Local Sleep by the Thalamic Reticular Nucleus. Frontiers in Neuroscience, 13:576, 2019.

Yazdi Z, Loukzadeh Z, Moghaddam P, Jalilolghadr S. Sleep Hygiene Practices and Their Relation to Sleep Quality in Medical Students of Qazvin University of Medical Sciences. Journal of Caring Sciences, 5:153-160, 2016.

Zarrinpar A, Chaix A, Panda S. Daily Eating Patterns and Their Impact on Health and Disease. Trends in Endocrinology and Metabolism, 27:69-83, 2016.

Zisapel N. New perspectives on the role of melatonin in human sleep, circadian rhythms and their regulation. British Journal of Pharmacology, 175:3190-3199, 2018.

- THE BRAIN IS DIRECTLY VULNERABLE TO INFLAMMATION: NEUROINFLAMMATION

- THE HIGH ACTIVITY LEVEL OF THE BRAIN REQUIRES EXTRA ENERGY AND PUTS IT AT RISK FOR OXIDATIVE STRESS: PROTECTION BY MICRONUTRIENTS

- THE BRAIN NEEDS BUILDING BLOCKS FOR PROTEINS, NEUROTRANSMITTERS/SIGNALING MOLECULES, AND MEMBRANES

- WHICH IS BEST: SINGLE SUPPLEMENT AND "SUPERFOODS" OR DIET PATTERNS?

- DIET PATTERNS DESIGNED FOR BRAIN HEALTH: MIND AND KETOGENIC DIETS

- "HEALTHY GUT, HEALTHY BRAIN"

Because the brain mediates our perceptions of how we feel, it is an obvious target for dietary strategies to improve symptoms such as fatigue, mood disorders, sleep problems, pain, and "cognitive fuzziness." Indeed, the marketplace is filled with products advertised as "brain-boosters" and superfoods. Food constituents that may act as nootropic or cognitive-enhancing, "smart drugs" raise hopes for improving brain function directly (Onaoplalo 2019, Napoletano 2020). These "smart drugs" may exert their effects through boosting of neurotransmitter systems or growth factors such as brain-derived neurotrophic factor (BDNF) that contribute to learning and memory. This idea is attractive because the brain faces particular challenges to its ability to stay healthy. Most neurons are long-lived and can accumulate damage that impairs their functioning and leads to aging-related cognitive impairment.

The idea that brain function is affected by the foods we eat is supported by recent studies linking diet to performance on cognitive tests. One large study, entitled REGARDS, compared five different diet patterns. REGARDS demonstrated the opposing effects of a "Southern" dietary pattern, characterized by processed meats, fried food, and high-energy sugary foods, and two Mediterranean-type diets, referred to as "plant-based" and "alcohol and salads" (Pearson 2018). The more closely people followed the Southern dietary pattern, the worse were their scores on cognitive tests. In contrast, people who strongly adhered to the plant-based or alcohol and salads dietary patterns performed much better. The alcohol and salads diet seemed to protect against cognitive impairment. The reasons for this could not be determined from the study but could well relate to consumption of green leafy vegetables and tomatoes, which contain antioxidant polyphenols and are often found in salads. The role that alcohol may play also seems surprising, but it should be noted that intake was moderate. Any benefits from alcohol could follow from, for instance, antioxidant and anti-inflammatory constituents in wine. It might simply reflect the fact that the participants in this diet group were not drinking soda. The idea that green vegetables may indeed be protective for the brain is supported by another study that followed diet in people 58-99 years of age (Morris 2018). This study found that high consumption of green vegetables, defined as several servings daily, was associated with better cognitive function. Interestingly, people who consumed the most green vegetables also consumed more alcohol, albeit still at moderate levels, similar to those in the REGARDS study. Importantly, differences in cognitive function were correlated with diet, even when other factors, such as socioeconomic status, were accounted for in the analysis (REGARDS, Morris 2018). The findings from these and other studies strongly reinforce the importance of diet in brain health and function (Jennings 2020, Rajaram 2019).

How can dietary constituents or foods, such as green leafy vegetables, protect or improve brain function? To answer this question, we first need to review basic features of the challenges related to brain health and diet.

The Brain is Directly Vulnerable to Inflammation: Neuroinflammation

For many years the brain was considered to be "immune-privileged," because the blood-brain barrier keeps out large proteins such as antibodies. Thus, the brain was thought to be entirely separate from the immune system. In the last few decades, however, it has become clear that not only does the brain have a close functional relationship with the immune system, but it contains its own local network of immune cells including microglia, T cells, and even mast cells. Microglia are similar to monocytes and macrophages. This means that inflammation can be induced within the brain, and in fact this is typical in the context of head injuries, strokes, infections, and neurodegenerative diseases (Bar 2020). This type of inflammation is called *neuroinflammation*.

Neuroinflammation can have widespread effects on brain function and structure. The principal brain cells, including both neurons and glial cells, are sensitive to immune hormones, such as cytokines, and inflammation. Cytokines induced in the brain have been linked to impaired learning and memory and symptoms of depression (Bourgognon 2020, Chaves-Filho 2019). Thus, neuroinflammation contributes mechanistically to mood disorders and cognitive impairment. Indeed, neurodegenerative diseases including Alzheimer's disease, Parkinson's disease, and amyotrophic lateral sclerosis (ALS) are characterized by neuroinflammation. Neuroinflammation seems to be a critical factor in the progression of these diseases and may contribute to their etiology as well (Tiwari 2021).

Neuroinflammation is particularly dangerous because the brain contains abundant PUFAs. About 40% of the lipid content of neuronal membranes are PUFAs, which are susceptible to oxidation/peroxidation (Gentile 2020). Oxidation/peroxidation of neuronal membranes and myelin damages the neurons and other cells, further driving neuroinflammation.

Many "superfoods" have anti-inflammatory actions. The best-characterized of these are: (1) curcumin, which provides the yellow pigment in turmeric, (2) resveratrol, which is found with red pigments in grapes, etc., (3) anthocyanins, which provide the purple/blue pigments in blueberries and black beans, and (4) quercetin, which is also associated with red pigments. These substances act similar to NSAIDs in that they inhibit prostaglandins and down-regulate NFkB, among other anti-inflammatory actions (Li 2016, Maiti 2018, Malaguarnera 2019, Wang 2018, Henriques 2020). The benefits of plant-based diets that provide a wide variety fruits and vegetables are thought to derive at least in part from the anti-inflammatory actions of so-called superfoods.

The High Activity Level of the Brain Requires Extra Energy and Puts it at Risk for Oxidative Stress: Protection by Micronutrients

Because the brain is active all the time, including when we are sleeping, it has a high requirement for energy substrates such as glucose or ketones. As we age, the ability of our brains to take up glucose from the blood declines (Szablewski 2021). This is particularly marked among people with diabetes and brain insulin resistance (Szablewski 2021, Rhea 2019). Poor glucose uptake into the brain is also characteristic of people with Alzheimer's disease, and this likely contributes to cognitive impairment. In addition, the brain's high metabolic activity puts brain cells at risk for oxidative or nitrosative stress. The production of reactive oxygen and nitrogen species that occurs as a necessary feature of metabolism can overwhelm the ability of endogenous antioxidants when brain activity is high. The "extra" reactive species can thus cause oxidative or nitrosative damage to brain cells, compromising the function of the affected cells and inducing or exacerbating neuroinflammation. Oxidative/nitrosative stress contributes in one way or another to nearly all brain disorders (Morris 2016, Onaoolapo 2019). These risks of high activity and oxidative stress can be mitigated, however, by adequate intake of micronutrients: minerals and vitamins that are especially important to support the brain.

B Complex Vitamins are Necessary for Energy Production and can Protect Against Oxidative Stress

The B complex vitamins are eight structurally unrelated molecules that work together to enable cells to generate energy from macronutrients such as glucose. They are also crucial for a variety of other functions that are necessary for brain function, including regulating gene expression and protecting against oxidative stress (Kennedy 2016). Deficiencies of B vitamins are typically associated with symptoms of brain dysfunction, including impairments of learning and memory, dementia, mood disorders, and fatigue (reviewed in Kennedy 2016). Deficiencies of B vitamins are associated also with elevated levels of homocysteine, a potentially toxic amino acid. Excess homocysteine is in turn associated with cognitive impairment, dementia, and cardiovascular disease. Thus, B vitamins are particularly important for the brain.

B vitamins are preferably obtained from the diet. The main sources for B vitamins are leafy vegetables, mushrooms, fruits, nuts, whole/intact grain, dairy, fish, poultry, and red meat. Risk factors for deficiencies stem from inadequate diets (e.g., vegan/vegetarian, Western diet habits, alcoholism), poor absorption from the gut (e.g., due to aging, proton pump inhibitor use, bariatric surgery, autoimmune disease), or increased demand for energy (e.g., in alcoholism, obesity) (Kennedy 2016, Miller 2018). These risk factors are widespread, given the near ubiquity of the Western diet, which does not provide enough fruits, vegetables and whole grains, the increasing popularity of vegan and vegetarian diets that do not include animal products, and drug or surgical treatments and autoimmune conditions such as pernicious anemia that reduce or prevent absorption of B vitamins into the body.

B complex vitamin deficiencies can have serious consequences. For example, lack of thiamine or cobalamin consequent to alcoholism or bariatric surgery can cause permanent brain damage. Given these risks, supplementation is an obvious solution. However, evidence-based recommendations for optimal amounts of B vitamins are are still lacking. This is partly due to limitations of studies. Most studies only assess one B vitamin at a time, when in fact many vitamins work in concert with one another. Thus, the findings from such studies are not readily interpretable. In addition, the amount of B complex vitamins needed likely varies among individuals, for instance based on things such as age, diet, and level of ongoing inflammation or oxidative stress (Kennedy 2016).

Antioxidant Systems in the Brain: Role of Dietary Vitamins C and E, Selenium, and Zinc

The endogenous antioxidant systems that protect the brain from oxidative stress contain minerals obtained from the diet. Glutathione requires the trace mineral selenium, and superoxide dismutase (SOD) requires zinc (Socha 2021, Gomez-Gomez 2019). These antioxidant systems collaborate with antioxidant vitamins C and E to protect PUFAs in membranes, including neuronal membranes (Cansev 2017).

Selenium and zinc are called *trace minerals* because although they are critical for the structure and function of many enzymes, most notably those of antioxidant systems, we don't need large amounts of them. Because selenium and zinc are found in proteins, foods like meat, dairy, poultry, tofu, and seafoods are high in both minerals. However, the richest source of selenium is the Brazil nut. Selenium also occurs in whole-grain breads and pasta, brown rice, and oatmeal. The richest source of zinc is oysters, but is also found in nuts and seeds, beans and other legumes, and mushrooms. Although selenium and zinc are key for antioxidant systems expressed throughout the body, low levels of zinc and selenium have been associated with cognitive impairment and dementia, indicating that the brain is dependent upon these minerals (Socha 2021). Because these minerals are commonly found in a diet of varied foods that contain proteins, whole grains, and nuts, selenium and zinc deficiencies are typically seen only in malnutrition associated with poverty, eating disorders, reliance on Western diet, and aging.

Aging presents particular challenges to the brain, due to "wear and tear" and eventually *inflammaging*. Aging also increases risk for malabsorption of nutrients from the gut. Many elderly people experience a reduction in appetite, which can contribute to risk for malnutrition and insufficient intake of antioxidants, further increasing risks of oxidative/nitrosative stress in the brain. The loss of antioxidant capability with aging may be contributing to *cognitive frailty,* a susceptibility to cognitive impairment and dementia (Gomez-Gomez 2019). Indeed, total antioxidant capability correlates with cognitive function, underlining the potential importance of adequate intake of antioxidant vitamins and minerals, and supplementation if necessary.

Calcium, Magnesium, Sodium and Potassium Regulate Neuronal Activity

Although calcium is famous for its role in the health of bones and teeth, the nervous, endocrine, and immune systems all require calcium to function. Among other things, calcium is critical for neurotransmitter and hormone release. Calcium is so important that it is mobilized from teeth and bone if one's diet is deficient, to protect calcium levels in the brain.

The best sources of dietary calcium are dairy foods, including yogurt, cheese, and milk. Some green vegetables, such as kale, broccoli, Chinese cabbage, and spinach also contain calcium. Tofu is a source for calcium. Diets may also need to include vitamin D as well, because vitamin D helps cells to absorb calcium. Although our bodies are able to synthesize vitamin D if exposed to sunlight, as we age this ability may diminish, and it may be necessary to take supplements. Other things to consider relate to bioavailability of calcium, because some foods, such as spinach, contain phytic and oxalic acids that bind calcium and reduce its uptake into our bodies.

Magnesium is an often underappreciated mineral that is involved in a wide variety of bodily functions, including protein synthesis, regulation of gut and nervous system activity, and blood sugar. Magnesium is necessary for the synthesis of glutathione, the body's endogenous antioxidant. In the nervous system, magnesium regulates neuronal excitability and glutamate receptors that are involved in learning, memory, and pain. Magnesium deficiency is associated with seizures, whereas increased dietary intake is associated with lower risk of stroke (Kirkland 2018). Good sources of magnesium include nuts (especially almonds), spinach, black beans, and whole wheat. Avocado, potatoes with skins, brown rice, and bananas are also good sources.

Sodium and potassium work together to regulate nervous system excitability among other things. Sodium and potassium levels need to be in a balance, but the Western diet tends to provide too much sodium, and not enough potassium. Sodium is used as a preservative in many prepared foods, and we seem to have an innate preference for it. However, sodium plays a role in the regulation of blood pressure, and high-sodium diets have been linked to increased risk of hypertension and stroke (Nowak 2018). Recent evidence suggests that the ratio of sodium to potassium is more important, such that high intakes of potassium may balance high sodium intake (Nowak 2018). Dietary sources of potassium include banana and avocado.

The Brain Needs Building Blocks for Proteins, Neurotransmitters/Signaling Molecules, and Membranes

In addition to producing our thoughts and perceptions, the brain is constantly re-wiring itself, thereby providing the biological basis of neuroplasticity, including learning and memory. This requires the production of proteins which ultimately derive from amino acids sourced from the diet. The production of most neurotransmitters and *neuromodulators* such as the biogenic amines (e.g., dopamine, norepinephrine, serotonin, glutamate, GABA), and neuropeptides (such as oxytocin, endorphins), are also reliant on dietary protein. Production of the neurotransmitter acetylcholine depends on choline from the diet as well. Good sources of amino acids in the diet include mushrooms, poultry, beef, fish, tofu, beans, eggs, and dairy.

The essential fatty acids, omega-3 and omega-6 PUFAs, are "essential" because they must be obtained from the diet. These essential fatty acids provide a significant proportion of the lipids that form cell membranes in the brain. Because PUFAs are vulnerable to oxidative damage, we need an adequate supply of new substrates to maintain brain cell health. The essential fatty acids also provide the precursors for lipid-based neurotransmitters and neuromodulators, such as endocannabinoids. Endocannabinoids are synthesized from omega-6 fatty acids. Good sources of these fatty acids are vegetables, especially green leafy vegetables. The emphasis should be on green, because the fatty acids are contained in the chloroplasts that make vegetables green. Seafood, such as cold-water fish and algae, also provides essential fatty acids. Importantly, fish oil supplements have not been found to be as protective as the whole foods from which they are derived.

Which is Best: Single Item Supplements and "Superfoods" or Diet Patterns?

The findings from observational studies such as REGARDS and others that correlate incidence of neurological conditions with diet strongly support the importance of fruits and vegetables, as well as whole/intact grains for brain health (Jennings 2020, Morris 2018). The likely mechanisms that account for this finding involve antioxidant and anti-inflammatory actions demonstrated by pre-clinical studies, using laboratory animals and *in vitro* techniques. Such studies have supported the idea that intake of vitamins (e.g., B, C, D), anti-inflammatory substances (e.g., curcumin), and antioxidants (e.g., vitamin C, E, plant polyphenols, fish oils) can protect against cognitive impairment. The findings have led to increasing popularity of products containing plant-based substances that purport to protect or "boost" brain function. Do these products really work?

Studies designed to answer this question have typically recruited people at risk for cognitive impairment, who are then given specified amounts of a single agent and are later assessed to determine any protective effects. Such studies include control groups that receive a placebo and are matched to the experimental groups with respect to demographics (e.g., race/ethnicity, socioeconomic status, gender). Thus, the studies are designed to detect reliable differences between people based solely on whether they received the supplement. The findings from these types of studies, however, typically show small, variable, or no effects (Forbes 2015, Jennings 2020). Why don't these studies show the benefits suggested by pre-clinical studies?

The reasons why single-ingredient supplements or extracts are largely ineffective for improving cognitive function may be that antioxidants must work in systems to avoid the "redox conundrum". Supplement preparations do not contain other food ingredients that may improve absorption or modify the activity of the supplemented substance. The supplement either may not reach parts of the brain in amounts that are required for effect, or they may have limited effects because of relative shortages of the rest of the substances in the antioxidant system. In general, the biggest effects are seen in clinical trial populations, in which participants are included due to evidence of a pre-existing deficiency. Most aspects of brain function are tightly regulated based on needs or activity, and any excess precursors, for instance, are excreted. Supplements may simply be discarded by the body as unnecessary. For some substances, supplementation may be risky. Some metals and fat-soluble vitamins may accumulate in tissues, even leading to toxicity. It is difficult to ascertain the precise requirements for vitamins and minerals for each individual, which could impair the ability of a study that uses standard dosing to reveal positive effects. Nonetheless, the much more reliable effects seen with specific dietary patterns, such as the Mediterranean diet, argue for a whole food approach to brain health and cognitive support.

Diet Patterns Designed for Brain Health: MIND and Ketogenic

Based on the recognition that overall diet patterns exert more impact on cognitive function than intake of specific "superfoods," standardized diet patterns have become attractive for providing guidelines about brain-healthy diets. Two of these have been utilized in clinical trials. During these trials, adopting specific diets has produced beneficial effects on cognitive performance.

The MIND (Mediterranean-DASH Intervention for Neurodegenerative Delay) Diet

The Mediterranean dietary pattern is associated with slower cognitive decline and lower risk of dementia (Cherian 2019, Jennings 2020). The Mediterranean diet was found to be associated with reduced brain atrophy (Agarwal 2020). The diet's key features are plant-based foods such as fruits, berries, vegetables, leafy greens, whole grains, olive oil, legumes, and nuts, as well as fish. These foods are rich in essential nutrients and contain bioactive substances that have anti-inflammatory and antioxidant properties. The diet may exert a neuroprotective effect by reducing oxidative stress and inflammation. Importantly, these Mediterranean diet patterns also limit the consumption of red meat, fatty foods, processed foods, and sweets. (Agarwal 2020). To aid in systematic study of Mediterranean diet pattern effects, and to provide specific recommendations for how to adopt a brain-healthy diet, the MIND diet recommends the following:

> DO eat: 3 or more servings of whole grain/day, 6 or more servings of green leafy vegetables per week plus daily servings of other vegetables, 2 or more servings of berries per week, one or more servings of fish per week, 2 or more servings of poultry per week, 3 or more servings of beans per week, and 5 or more servings of nuts per week. Olive oil is the recommended oil, and one alcoholic beverage is allowed per day.

> LIMIT: Red meat and red meat products (e.g., bacon, sausage, hot dogs, lunch meat, etc.) to less than 4 servings per week, fast food and fried food to less than one serving per week, butter or margarine to less than 1 tsp per day, cheese to less than once a week, and pastries and sweets to less than 5 servings per week (from Cherian 2019).

Studies of the MIND diet have shown that it can indeed protect against cognitive impairment associated with aging (van den Brink 2019). One possible limitation, however, is that it was designed prior to studies showing the importance of gut health. Future studies may help to optimize the diet further. For example, it is possible that the blanket limitations on cheese may be excessively strict. It is possible that some high-quality probiotic dairy, such as yogurt and some soft cheeses, might be beneficial or not harmful. In addition, the diet allows 5 servings of sweets per week, which might be harmful.

Although the Mediterranean diet is the best-known traditional diet pattern that is associated with health benefits, other regional diets, such as the Nordic and Okinawa diets, are also associated with better cognitive function (Gomez-Gomez 2019). These diets are based on traditional local foods, such as fish or sweet potatoes, that are low in refined carbohydrates and processed foods. Traditional local diets encourage cooking local foods, and can support social, cultural, and emotional aspects of eating.

The Ketogenic Diet

Although the ketogenic diet is currently best known as a diet to aid in weight loss, it was originally formulated as a treatment for epilepsy (Ulamek-Koziol 2019). The key feature of the diet is that it is very low-carbohydrate. In the absence of carbohydrate, the liver must generate fuel for metabolism by converting fat into ketones, which cells of the brain can use as a substitute for glucose. The major advantage for the brain is that metabolizing ketones generates fewer reactive oxygen and nitrogen species. Utilizing ketones for energy may be less likely to cause oxidative/nitrosative stress.

The standard keto diet is configured such that 70% of calories are derived from fat, 20% from protein, and 10% or less from carbohydrate. The keto diet eliminates foods including sugary sweets, sugar-containing condiments, and starchy tubers, such as potatoes, that are associated poor health outcomes. It also restricts consumption of all fruits, grains, and legumes. Allowed foods include dairy, eggs, fish, poultry, red meat, and red meat products.

The best documented benefits for the ketogenic diet have been found for children with treatment-resistant epilepsy (Ulamek-Koziol 2019). Epilepsy is characterized by uncontrolled electrical activity in the brain or seizures that cause oxidative stress and damage to the brain. The damage to the brain can facilitate further seizure activity. Seizure control is particularly important for children, as the seizures can impair cognitive development.

The recognition of the role of oxidative stress in many different neurological disorders is spurring interest in ketogenic diet interventions for dementia, migraine, schizophrenia, traumatic brain injury, and others (Neth 2020, Gross 2019, Sarnyai 2019, Arora 2020). This is a developing story, but there is some evidence that a ketogenic diet may improve glucose uptake to the brain (Neth 2020). Glucose uptake decreases during aging and becomes marked in dementia, especially Alzheimer's disease. One preliminary study showed an improvement in peripheral metabolic markers and some Alzheimer's disease-specific markers after 6 weeks (Neth 2020). Thus, the ketogenic diet seems promising for a variety of challenging brain disorders.

The classic ketogenic diet, however, is hard to follow. This is in part because following the ketogenic diet can lead to persistent gastrointestinal symptoms, such as diarrhea. The classic ketogenic diet does not allow many vegetables, and allows no grains or legumes. These restrictions have negative implications for gut microbe populations. There are also concerns about the long-term safety of a diet high in fat, particularly saturated fat. Consequent to these concerns, modifications to the ketogenic diet have been developed, notably the "Med-Keto diet." The Med-Keto diet includes vegetables and whole grains. In this way, the Med-Keto diet preserves the benefits of restricting high-energy refined carbohydrates but preserves the fiber and other nutritional benefits of whole/intact grains.

"Healthy Gut, Healthy Brain"

Thanks to the close anatomical and functional connections of the brain with the gut, the condition of the gut plays a critical role in maintaining and modulating brain function. The brain's tremendous need for energy requires a healthy gut barrier to absorb nutrients. The sensitivity of the brain to inflammation means that immune programming by the gut can have either beneficial or deleterious effects on the brain. Further, a diverse population of microbes in the gut helps maintain the gut barrier, and helps to program immune cells. Some microbes produce substances, such as neurotransmitters (e.g., serotonin, GABA), that can influence the nervous system. Other substances produced by microbes can directly downregulate inflammation in the brain (Dempsey 2019, Estrada 2019). On the other hand, disruption of gut microbe populations can impair gut barrier function and impair their ability to protect the brain.

Chemical agents used in food production, such as herbicides and insecticides, as well as pollutants in the air and water, can act as neurotoxins. Some of these chemicals are implicated in the etiology of neurological disorders, including Parkinson's disease and autism spectrum disorders (Dempsey 2019). Many of these chemicals disrupt gut microbe populations. For instance, the herbicide glyphosate, known by the trade name Roundup®, encourages the growth of pathogenic gut microbes while being toxic to beneficial commensals (Dempsey 2019). Glyphosate induces inflammation in the gut, and is associated with evidence of increased permeability or gut leakiness (Qiu 2020). Many insecticides are directly neurotoxic (Dempsey 2019). Insecticides such as malathion have been also observed to disrupt gut microbe populations in farmworkers. Residues of toxins on food can be expected to exert outsize effects on gut microbes, as the microbes are directly exposed to them during digestion. Some microbes can convert toxins into less dangerous chemicals, and thereby protect the brain. Currently, the interactions among gut microbes, chemical agents, and pollutants are a developing story. Findings to date underline the importance of maintaining a healthy, diverse gut microbial population; consuming a diet that is low in pesticide or herbicide residues can help achieve this objective. Eating local, homegrown, or organic foods can also minimize pesticide and herbicide consumption.

A key pathophysiological feature of brain disorders, from depression to neurodegenerative disorders, is neuroinflammation. Short-chain fatty acids (SCFAs) produced by gut microbes, such as butyrate and acetate, are absorbed into the body and can reach the brain. SCFAs act upon aryl hydrocarbon receptors, which are expressed on the surface of immune cells, including microglia of the brain. SCFA activation of these receptors down-regulates inflammation. SCFAs also inhibit neuroinflammation by influencing epigenetic mechanisms of inflammatory gene regulation (Dempsey 2019). These protective actions of SCFAs may contribute to the health benefits of a high-fiber diet, as the microbes that produce SCFAs are supported by dietary fiber. On the other hand, the low-fiber, high-energy Western diet is associated with pro-inflammatory bacterial species such as *Escherichia coli* (Estrada 2019). In this way, microbes provide mechanistic links between diet and brain health.

> **Key Points**
>
> - Many lines of evidence including from pre-clinical, epidemiological, observational, and clinical trial studies, demonstrate that dietary patterns emphasizing fruits, vegetables, whole grains, nuts, seeds, good-quality dairy, seafood, poultry, and limited red meat from mammals are consistently associated with better cognitive function during aging than diets that emphasize high-energy, low-nutrition, processed foods.
> - Green leafy vegetables seem particularly important for the brain, possibly because they contain omega-3 and omega-6 essential fatty acids. Omega-3 is also found in seafood, including algae.
> - All diets that improve or protect cognitive function limit consumption of sugar and refined carbohydrates.
> - Vitamins B, C, and E, along with the trace minerals selenium and zinc, have been shown to contribute to the brain's antioxidant systems. These antioxidant systems help protect against neuroinflammation.

- Vitamin and mineral deficiencies can occur in many circumstances: with advancing age, after bariatric surgery, during proton pump inhibitor usage (e.g., for gastric reflux disease or heartburn), or when eating a typical Western diet.
- Supplements of vitamin and minerals are effective for preventing deficiencies but do not "boost" brain function. However, vitamin and mineral requirements may increase over the lifespan.

References

Agarwal P, Morris MC, Barnes LL. Racial Differences in Dietary Relations to Cognitive Decline and Alzheimer's Disease Risk: Do We Know Enough? Frontiers in Human Neuroscience, 14:359, 2020.

Attuquayefio T, Stevenson RJ, Oaten MJ, Francis HM. A four-day Western-style dietary intervention causes reductions in hippocampal-dependent learning and memory and interoceptive sensitivity. PLoS ONE, 12(2): 0172645, 2017.

Arora N, Mehta TR. Role of the ketogenic diet in acute neurological diseases. Clinical Neurology and Neurosurgery, 192:105727, 2020.

Barr E, Barak B. Microglia roles in synaptic plasticity and myelination in homeostatic conditions and neurodevelopmental disorders. Glia, 67:2125-2141, 2019.

Bourgognon J-M, Cavanagh J, The role of cytokines in modulating learning and memory and brain plasticity. Brain and Neuroscience Advances, 4:1-13, 2020.

Cansev M, Turkyilmaz M, Sijben JWC, Sevinc C, Broersen LM, van Wijk N. Synaptic Membrane Synthesis in Rats Depends on Dietary Sufficiency of Vitamin C, Vitamin E, and Selenium: Relevance for Alzheimer's Disease. Journal of Alzheimer's Disease, 59:301-311, 2017.

Chaves-Filho AM, Macedo DS, de Lucena DF, Maes M. Shared microglial mechanisms underpinning depression and chronic fatigue syndrome and their comorbidities. Behavioral Brain Research, 372:111975, 2019.

Cherian L, Y. Wang Y, Fakuda K, Leurgans S, Aggarwal N, Morris M. Mediterranean-Dash Intervention for Neurodegenerative Delay (MIND) Diet Slows Cognitive Decline After Stroke. Journal of the Prevention of Alzheimer's Disease, 6:267-273, 2019.

Dempsey JL, Little M, Cui JY. Gut microbiome: an intermediary to neurotoxicity. Neurotoxicology, 75:41-69, 2019.

Estrada JA, Contreras I. Nutritional Modulation of Immune and Central Nervous System Homeostasis: The Role of Diet in Development of Neuroinflammation and Neurological Disease. Nutrients, 11:1076, 2019.

Forbes SC, Holroyd-Leduc JM, Poulin MJ, Hogan DB. Effect of Nutrients, Dietary Supplements and Vitamins on Cognition: A Systematic Review and Meta-Analysis of Randomized Controlled Trials. Canadian Geriatrics Journal, 18:231-245, 2015.

Gentile F, Doneddu PE, Riva N, Eduardo Nobile-Orazio E, Quattrini A. Diet, Microbiota and Brain Health: Unraveling the Network Intersecting Metabolism and Neurodegeneration. International Journal of Molecular Sciences, 21, 7471, 2020.

Gomez-Gomez ME, Zapico SC. Frailty, Cognitive Decline, Neurodegenerative Diseases and Nutrition Interventions. International Journal of Molecular Sciences. 20:2842, 2019.

Gross EC, Klement RJ, Schoenen J, D'Agostino DP, Fischer D. Potential Protective Mechanisms of Ketone Bodies in Migraine Prevention. Nutrients, 11:811, 2019.

Henriques, JF, Serra D, Dinis TCP, Almeida LM. The anti-neuroinflammatory role of anthocyanins and their metabolites for the prevention and treatment of brain disorders. International Journal of Molecular Sciences, 21:8653, 2020.

Jennings A, Cunnane SC, Minihane AM. Can nutrition support healthy cognitive aging and reduce dementia risk? BMJ, 369:m2269, 2020.

Kázmierczak-Baránska J, Boguszewska K, Karwowski BT. Nutrition Can Help DNA Repair in the Case of Aging. Nutrients, 12:3364, 2020.

Kennedy DO. B Vitamins and the Brain: Mechanisms, Dose and Efficacy-A Review. Nutrients, 8:68, 2016.

Kirkland AE, Sarlo GL, Holton KF. The role of magnesium in neurological disorders. Nutrients, 10:730, 2018.

Li Y, Yao J, Han C, Jiaxin Yang J, Tabassum Chaudhry M, Wang S, Liu H Yin Y. Quercetin, Inflammation and Immunity. Nutrients, 8:167, 2016.

Maiti P, Dunbar GL. Use of curcumin, a natural polyphenol for targeting molecular pathways in treating age-related neurodegenerative diseases. International Journal of Molecular Sciences, 19:1637, 2018.

Malaguarnera L. Influence of reseveratrol on the immune system. Nutrients, 11, 946, 2019.

Medawar E, Huhn S, Villringer A, Witte AV. The effects of plant-based diets on the body and the brain: a systematic review. Translational Psychiatry, 9:226, 2019.

Miller JW. Proton Pump Inhibitors, H2-Receptor Antagonists, Metformin, and Vitamin B-12 Deficiency: Clinical Implications. Advances in Nutrition, 9:511S-518S, 2018.

Morris G, Walder K, Puri BK, Berk M, Maes M. The Deleterious Effects of Oxidative and Nitrosative Stress on Palmitoylation, Membrane Lipid Rafts and Lipid-Based Cellular Signalling: New Drug Targets in Neuroimmune Disorders. Molecular Neurobiology, 53:4638-4658, 2016.

Morris MC, Wang Y, Barnes LL, Bennett DA, Dawson-Hughes B, Booth SL. Nutrients and bioactives in green leafy vegetables and cognitive decline. Neurology, 90:e214-e222, 2018.

Napoletano F, Schifano F, Corkery JM, Guirguis A, Arillotta D, Zangani C, Vento A. The Psychonauts' World of Cognitive Enhancers. Frontiers in Psychiatry, 11:546796, 2020.

Neth BJ, Mintz A, Whitlow C, Jung Y, Sai KS, Register TC, et al. Modified ketogenic diet is associated with improved cerebrospinal fluid biomarker profile, cerebral perfusion, and cerebral ketone body uptake in older adults at risk for Alzheimer's disease: a pilot study. Neurobiology of Aging, 86:54-63, 2020.

Nowak KL, Fried L, Jovanovich A, Ix J, Yaffe K, You Z, Chonchol M. Dietary Sodium/Potassium Intake Does Not Affect Cognitive Function or Brain Imaging Indices. American Journal of Nephrology, 47:57-65, 2018.

Onaolapo AY, Adebimpe Yemisi Obelawo AY, Onaolapo OJ. Brain Ageing, Cognition and Diet: A Review of the Emerging Roles of Food-Based Nootropics in Mitigating Age-Related Memory Decline. Current Aging Science, 12:2-14, 2019.

Pearson KE, Wadley VG, Mc Clure LA, Shikany JM, Unverzagt FW, Judd SE. Dietary patterns are associated with cognitive function in the REasons for Geographic And Racial Differences in Stroke (REGARDS) cohort. Journal of Nutritional Science, 5:C38, 2016.

Qiu S, Fu H, Zhou R, Yang Z, Bai G, Shi B. Toxic effects of glyphosate on intestinal morphology, antioxidant capacity and barrier function in weaned piglets. Ecotoxicology and Environmental Safety, 187:109846, 2020.

Rajaram S, Jones J, Lee GJ. Plant-based dietary patterns, plant foods and age-related cognitive decline. Advances in Nutrition, 10:S422-S436, 2019.

Rhea EM, Banks WA. Role of the blood-brain barrier in central nervous system insulin resistance. Frintiers in Neuroscience,15:521, 2019.

Sarnyai Z, Kraeuter, A-K, Palmer CM. Ketogenic diet for schizophrenia: clinical implication. Current Opinion in Psychiatry, 32:394-401, 2019.

Socha K, Klimiuk K, Naliwajko SK, Soroczynska J, Puscion-Jakubik A, et al. Dietary Habits, Selenium, Copper, Zinc and Total Antioxidant Status in Serum in Relation to Cognitive Functions of Patients with Alzheimer's Disease. Nutrients,13:287, 2021.

Szablewski L. Brain glucose transporters: Role in pathogenesis and potential targets for the treatment of Alzheimer's Disease. International Journal of Molecular Sciences, 22:8142, 2021.

Tiwari RK, Moin A, Rizvi WMD, Shahid AMA, Bajpai P. Modulating neuroinflammation in neurodegeneration-related dementia: can microglial toll-like receptors pull the plug? Metabolic Brain Disease, 36:829-847, 2021.

Ulamek-Koziol M, Czuczwar SJ, Januszewski S, Pluta R. Ketogenic diet and epilepsy. Nutrients,11:2510, 2019.

van den Brink A, Brouwer-Brolsma EM, Berendsen AAM, van de Rest O. The Mediterranean, Dietary Approaches to Stop Hypertension (DASH), and Mediterranean-DASH Intervention for Neurodegenerative Delay (MIND) Diets Are Associated with Less Cognitive Decline and a Lower Risk of Alzheimer's Disease—A Review. Advances in Nutrition, 10:1040-1065, 2019.

Wang J, Song Y, Chen Z, Leng SX. Connection between Systemic Inflammation and Neuroinflammation Underlies Neuroprotective Mechanism of Several Phytochemicals in Neurodegenerative Diseases. Oxidative Medicine and Cellular Longevity, 2018:1972714, 2018.

- THE MULTIVARIATE APPROACH TO LOW-STRESS HEALTHY EATING

- WHAT ABOUT WINE?

- SOME TRICKS FOR INSTITUTING A MULTIVARIATE DIET

- ORGANIZING FEATURES OF THE MULTIVARIATE APPROACH

- RECIPES

- SALADS: GETTING THE CRUNCH AND FLAVOR IN

- SOUPS AND STEWS: A CHANCE TO BE CREATIVE

- FLATBREADS

- CASSEROLES: AN AGE-OLD WAY TO COMBINE MANY INGREDIENTS INTO AN EASY TO PREPARE DISH

- BREAKFAST AND DESSERT: SWITCHING THEM AROUND

Food provides sustenance for mind and body, from the molecular to the spiritual levels. At one level, food provides nutrients enabling the cells of our bodies to function. But at another level, diet choices reflect our self-image and how much we value ourselves. What we eat is also symbolic of who we are in our culture and society. Food can express caring and nurturing. Eating with other people can establish or reinforce social bonds. Thus, what we eat affects every aspect of our lives. To make food choices that support feeling well physically, mentally, and spiritually we must give thought to the many layers of meaning in food.

Below are key concepts that can help optimize our health and diet:

Giving thought to the nutritional value of food: We literally "are what we eat" at the molecular level. To be healthy and feel well, we need to consume a diet that provides adequate vitamins and minerals, proteins, essential fatty acids, and complex carbohydrates. Many of these are lacking in typical Western diet foods.

Giving thought for how foods affect inflammation: Inflammation induces the sickness syndrome of low mood, fatigue, "cognitive fuzziness," pain, and sleep problems that often lie at the heart of not feeling well. The foods we eat can either induce or exacerbate inflammation or help regulate it. Indeed, the effects of foods on inflammation are the principal factors that determines whether they are "healthy."

Giving thought for how food influences the condition of our bodies: Food affects how we feel via the mind-body pathway of *interoception*, which signals the condition of our bodies. Interoceptive pathways let us know when we have eaten enough food, and when we have damage or inflammation. Together these can help regulate appetite but can also give rise to pain.

Giving thought to how foods affect our gut and its microbes: The gut is the first place in our bodies that interacts with food. It is responsible for absorbing nutrients while keeping pathogens out. Foods that we eat can either help or compromise this barrier function. Microbes resident in the gut influence both the immune and nervous systems and regulate both the gut barrier and inflammation (Wastyk 2021). Diet is the most important influence on the kinds of microbial populations in our gut.

Giving thought to how our diets contribute to our moods and energy levels: Recent studies have verified that eating better DOES make us feel better (Chatterton 2018, Jacka 2017, Li 2017). This means wellness requires making an effort to choose to eat the fresh vegetables and whole/intact grains that can help regulate inflammation. Even if it feels hard, it will be worth it.

Giving thought to the emotional meanings of food reward: The rewarding value of certain foods can lead us to turn to them when feeling stressed or disappointed. Because certain foods can be associated with celebrations and positive social experiences, we learn to associate positive emotions with them. One way to address this is to avoid pairing sugary foods with celebrations and happy times by substituting healthier options, such as colorful salads.

Giving thought to the ways in which diet can perpetuate sociocultural disparities: Relatively inexpensive Western diet foods are often the only foods easily available in low-income "food deserts." This puts residents in those areas at risk for malnutrition, depression, obesity, and type 2 diabetes. These conditions also put people at risk for cognitive impairment as they age and elevate risk of dementia. The chronic stress associated with poor diet can also favor decision-making that prioritizes short-term benefits over long-term effects. The resulting impulsive behavior can create additional challenges for wellness.

Giving thought to how food choices affect the way food is produced: Choosing foods from local or smaller, high-quality, organic producers helps keep them in business. Picking such products sends a message about what consumers expect and are willing to pay for.

Giving thought to vulnerability of food quality to environmental pollution: Toxins are ubiquitous in our modern environment, and hence in our foods. Growing your own food or buying organic produce and grains can reduce exposure to toxins, like glyphosate and malathion, that are associated with food production.

Whereas addressing these issues is critical to taking back our health, this is easier said than done. Moving away from over-reliance on easily accessible, immediately rewarding Western diet foods can be particularly challenging for those who are busy or experiencing stress. Western diet foods are especially pernicious because although they can satisfy some emotional drivers of appetite in the short term, they contribute to inflammation and nutritional deficiency that worsen symptoms in the long term. This can lead to a self-sustaining loop whereby stress and habits contribute to inflammation, which feeds back to worsen symptoms of mood, pain, and sleep problems. This cycle is difficult to escape.

The Multivariate Approach to Low-Stress Healthy Eating

"Healthy eating is a way of life, so it is important to establish routines that are simple, realistically, and ultimately livable." – Horace (born 65 BCE; Roman poet during reign of Augustus, translated from Latin)

This two-thousand-year-old quote encapsulates a critical but age-old issue: healthy routines must be routinely do-able. A healthy mind and body require a diverse diet that provides the necessary proteins, essential fats, vitamins, and minerals, as well as fiber-rich and fermented foods that support a healthy and diverse microbial population. Such a diet must also be convenient, rewarding, and flexible enough to accommodate cultural aspects of food that support personal and ethnic identity. One way to achieve this is to adopt a "multivariate diet" approach.

A multivariate diet approach includes "base" dishes such as salads, soups, casseroles, and flatbreads. These incorporate many different ingredients and can be mixed and matched to an available set of ingredients based on, for example, seasonal availability of fresh vegetables and fruit, cultural preferences, or cost.

The approach combines features of diet types (Mediterranean, vegetarian, vegan) that studies have shown to improve inflammation, mood, and pain symptoms (Dragan 2020, Jacka 2017). Thus, the multivariate diet approach relies on whole/intact grains, incorporates green leafy vegetables, and reduces reliance on large servings of meat. Foods containing fiber, such as beans, grains, whole fruits and vegetables, and fermented foods such as plain Greek yogurt, help support diverse microbe populations. Fermented foods can especially provide the Old Friends that support healthful microbe populations (Wastyk 2021).

Controlling appetite requires regulating emotions and increasing awareness of body signals such as satiety. Eating food slowly can help with this awareness. The multivariate diet approach supports appetite-regulating strategies such as mindful eating and intuitive eating by including many different ingredients with contrasting tastes and textures, along with herbs and spices, all of which increase the complexity of the taste experience. Added complexity helps to slow down eating and enable awareness of satiety-related cues from the gut. In this way, multivariate dishes can satisfy both "head factors" and "gut factors." Additionally, cooking itself is a health behavior that can enhance feelings of well-being and social connectedness (Farmer and Cotter, 2021).

What About Wine?

Although alcohol consumption is associated with numerous health risks and alcohol consumption can cause chronic disease, several lines of evidence suggest that drinking a moderate amount of red wine is associated with better health. Moderate means no more than 1 to 2 glasses per day. Maximum consumption before alcohol use is considered risky is based on sex, weight and other risk factors, and clinical guidelines generally recommend a maximum of one glass per day for all women and many men. The Mediterranean diet, linked widely to positive health outcomes, typically includes red wine. Correlational studies have linked a diet rich in green vegetables, and low to moderate amounts of alcohol, to higher scores on cognitive tests among older adults (Morris 2018, Pearson 2016). These diet effects could not be accounted for by other variables such as socio-economic status. Why would red wine be good for health?

There are many different varieties of red wine, but they all seem to contain antioxidant and anti-inflammatory polyphenols, notably resveratrol, quercetin, anthocyanins, and many others (Dimitrovska 2013, Landrault 2001, Myrtsi 2021, Rothwell 2013). Red wine is fermented with the skins of the grape and the whole fruits are thrown into vats. This technique extracts dozens of compounds, which based on their structure should have antioxidant properties. These other compounds have not been studied, but the health benefits of red wine may follow from the interactions, or synergy, of the many different compounds present. The fermentation process may also be important. Microbes can metabolize antioxidants, which may in turn make these products may be more bioactive or bioavailable (Li and Sun, 2019). Most red wines, and some white wines, undergo a second fermentation with lactic acid bacteria, which can also increase the potential bioactivity of the antioxidants in wine (Virdis 2021). Therefore, there is a scientific basis for recommending a glass of red wine with dinner. However, the wine should be "dry" and not sweet due to residual sugar.

What about white wine? White wine has a much lower level of antioxidant and anti-inflammatory agents, because these substances are mostly found in the skins and seed of grapes (Rothwell 2013). Whereas red wine is made by fermenting the whole grapes including skins and seeds, white wine is only fermented juice. Thus, although white grapes contain the same antioxidant potential as red grapes, most wines made from them have much less antioxidant content. However, if you strongly prefer white wine to red, look for *orange wine*. Orange wine is made using a traditional wine-making style whereby the white grapes are left "on the skins" for a while. This is similar to the technique of making rosé wine from red grapes. Orange wine has a more robust flavor than white wine and is reported to contain antioxidant capabilities in the range of the lighter-bodied red wines (Landrault 2001).

What if you can't drink wine, or don't want to? Not to worry. The multivariate diet approach contains lots of fresh fruits, vegetables, and nuts, all of which contain antioxidants and anti-inflammatory agents. For instance, blueberries, cranberries, black rice, tomatoes, dark chocolate, and red onions are among the foods that contain quercetin, anthocyanins, and resveratrol (Rothwell 2013).

Some tricks for instituting a multivariate diet:

Eliminating extra sugar: Sugar is everywhere and many of us have grown up eating sugary foods and beverages. But it has become quite clear that added refined sugars contribute to adverse health conditions including diabetes, cardiometabolic syndrome, non-alcoholic fatty liver disease, and Alzheimer's disease.

Reducing the amount of sugar in the diet can be a challenge. The potentially addictive qualities of sugary foods, as well as the near ubiquity of added sugars in processed foods, make them difficult to avoid. Indeed, the addition of sugars to processed foods is likely an important contributor to the association of processed-food diets with adverse health outcomes. Another problem with habitually eating sugary foods is that taste receptors for sweet can become desensitized with high exposure to the taste (Kinnamon and

Finger, 2013). This means that frequent consumption of sweet foods and beverages can make sugary foods seem less sweet over time, encouraging the addition of even more sugar. Fortunately, reducing sugar exposure can restore sensitivity of the receptors. Basically, the less sugar you eat, the less you need to experience the sensation of sweetness.

There are ways to replicate the pleasurable aspects of sweet tastes. The first step is to avoid processed foods as much as possible. Baking at home means that you know exactly what is in your food, and you can experiment with ways to make food just how you like it. One trick to reduce sugar in baked goods is to substitute baking spices such as cinnamon, ginger, cardamon, nutmeg or clove (Peters 2014, Peters 2018). Another trick is to add whole fruit or citrus zest. Although ripe fruit contains sugars, whole fruits contain fiber and possibly other substances that can help slow the uptake of sugars into the body, reducing the risk of hyperglycemia.

Diversifying protein sources: Dietary protein is important for many cellular functions, especially in the brain. Unfortunately, the main sources of protein in the Western diet come from processed meats, especially beef and pork, that are linked to increased risk of conditions such as colorectal cancer and cardiovascular disease (Wolk 2017). In contrast, the Mediterranean and multivariate diet approaches rely on smaller amounts of animal protein, such as chicken, fish, seafood, or unprocessed beef and pork, that are incorporated into dishes containing other ingredients such as greens, grains, beans, or pasta. Multivariate plant-based diets avoid these animal proteins altogether. Meat-based protein can be substituted with plant-based protein sources, including high-protein grains such as quinoa or gluten-based meat substitutes such as seitan; beans, lentils, and bean-based products such as tofu and tempeh; nuts and nut-based dairy and cheeses; or mushrooms. Fermented animal milk such as plain yogurt and kefir can also substitute for meat protein, and likewise fermented plant-milk yogurt and kefir can support plant-based diets. Plant-based protein sources have an added benefit of providing fiber that can help support healthy diverse microbial population. Notably, vegetarian and vegan diets are associated with reduced risks of cardiometabolic disease and with better cognitive function than the Western diet (Pearson 2016).

Adapting "traditional" cooking: Many traditional diets, such as the Southern diet, have been criticized because they rely on unhealthy cooking techniques such as excessive frying, starchy ingredients, too many saturated animal or *trans* fats, and lack of variety of ingredients. Nonetheless, traditional diets support emotional meanings of food and may not be entirely "unhealthy" (Teicholz 2019). Traditional diets can be modified in ways that retain some key ingredients and flavors but provide more nutrition. For instance, the Southern diet traditionally relied on greens, such as collard and mustard greens, beans, sweet potatoes, yams, and corn. These are all nutritious ingredients. Rather than frying them in bacon grease they can be roasted or sautéed in vegetable oils. Authenticity can be maintained by including traditional spices. For example, cumin, curry, and cardamon help provide South Asian flavors, and *kan kan kan*, a spice mix of peanut powder, chili powder, allspice, and Maggi bouillon cubes mashed together, can provide West African flavors. These can be used to enhance stews or soups.

Getting kids to eat a healthy diet: Children can be "picky" eaters, suspicious of foods that are new or have an unusual texture or aren't sweet. Children should be encouraged to try many different foods, because poor eating in childhood can have lifetime consequences, including diabetes and obesity and the long-term consequences of those conditions. One way to get kids interested in fruits and vegetables is to get them involved in gardening (DaCosta 2017). As Ron Finley says (Finley 2013), "If kids grow tomatoes, they eat tomatoes." In fact, "hands-on" gardening and cooking programs designed to improve eating behavior in children are substantially more effective than nutritional instruction (DaCosta 2017). For instance, an elementary school intervention in which families were given healthy multicultural recipes led both children and parents to cook, appreciate, and eat more diverse foods (Chen 2014). The flexibility of the multivariate diet approach means that kids can be creative or experiment with different ingredients and spices.

The freezer is your friend: A common barrier to cooking "from scratch" is being too busy, especially mid-working week (Lavelle 2016). This may be particularly challenging in wintertime when it is harder to find fresh vegetables. We have found that in the summertime, growing food or going to farmer's markets often results in more produce than we can eat. So, we freeze the extra in meal-size portions in Tupperware-type containers in the summer, which can easily be used when needed. Pro tip: put a date on it on the container, and purge older food after a year or so.

Leftovers are a blessing: One of the most effective strategies our family has used is to prepare enough food to generate leftovers. It is nice to come home after a long day of work and have a pot of chili or soup that just needs to be reheated. Moreover, soups and stews often taste even better the next day. It is less work to double the amount of ingredients to put in a casserole than to make two separate meals. Leftovers can be quickly heated in a microwave or oven.

Anyone can cook! Many people fear of cooking "from scratch," especially if they did not learn how to cook as children (Lavelle 2016). People who think they can't cook often think so because they tend to overcook food, or they don't use many herbs or spices in the dishes they make. They may also feel overwhelmed by recipes than contain long lists of ingredients that might be hard to obtain, or ones that require complicated cooking techniques. The multivariate approach, however, relies on simple cooking techniques that use minimal heating times to avoid oxidation of ingredients, and a flexible array of possible ingredients that can be "just thrown together." Recipes have an easy basic structure that can encourage experimentation.

Organizing features of the multivariate approach

There are some common features which form the bases for attractive and tasty dishes that can be thrown together quickly or can be served as part of a sophisticated meal. Here are four important features:

Color: Humans are visual creatures, and much of what we consider appetizing is based on visual appeal. So, for instance, gray foods are not usually considered attractive. But foods with color tend to catch our eye. Red and yellow peppers, tomatoes, and blueberries, for instance, add a visual pop to a dish. White cheese can provide color contrast. This is particularly important for salads because they are often cold, and therefore don't give off strong aromas; enticing smells also drive motivation for food. Importantly, color in fruits and vegetables is associated with anti-inflammatory and antioxidant capabilities.

Texture: Dishes are most rewarding to eat when the ingredients provide a complex chewing experience. So, a salad with just one kind of lettuce will be less interesting than one that has multiple varieties, or where some of the lettuce is chopped. Add crunchy things like walnuts, pine nuts, pistachios, sunflower or pumpkin seeds, or chewy things such as dried fruit. Dried or fresh fruit, especially cranberries or tart cherries, also give a splash of color and can give a salad a nice fruity tang. Similarly, for casseroles, nuts can add crunch, and olives, capers, or pickled vegetables can add a briny tang. Gourmet soup recipes often call for "processing" and straining soups before serving, but leaving skins (such as tomato or peppers) in the soup increases the nutrition and contributes a more interesting texture.

An acid: That nice little tang is provided by foods that contain acids, such as acetic acid (found in vinegar) or ascorbic acid (vitamin C, found in citrus). Foods with tang include citrus (e.g., lemons and limes), red peppers, tart fruit, and sharp cheese. Balsamic or rice vinegar works well to complement the flavors of vegetables and tangy fruit.

A protein: To make a dish feel satisfying and be nutritious, it needs some protein in it. There are many high-protein ingredients that work well with a multivariate approach, including cheeses, lentils or beans, tofu or tempeh, nuts, fish, chicken, mushrooms, and shredded pork, beef, or seitan.

Liberal use of herbs and spices: Changing diets usually means getting used to new flavors or textures. Western diet foods are characterized by sweet or salty tastes, with smooth, oily, high-fat textures. Low-sugar, low-salt, or low-fat foods can be perceived as less appetizing (Peters 2014, Peters 2018, Haldar 2018). This is one likely barrier to changing eating behavior. However, such low-salt and low-fat foods can be made more attractive by adding spices. Curry mixes, turmeric, garlic, oregano, basil, ground chile, and baking spices such as cinnamon, ginger, nutmeg, cardamom, or clove, can improve hedonic perceptions of low-sugar desserts (Peters 2018). In addition, foods containing herbs and spices seem to contribute to satiety. People who consumed the same foods, with and without herbs and spices, reported that they felt fuller, more satisfied, and less motivated to eat more food after they had eaten the food seasoned with spices (Halder 2018). In this way, spices can make food both more appetizing and more satisfying.

Basically, the multivariate diet approach involves combining a variety of different ingredients to create healthy dishes that are emotionally satisfying to eat.

The following are recipes that you don't need a lot of time or cooking experience to make. We know they are easy and quick to prepare because they are family recipes we relied upon during busy times in our lives.

1. Salads: Getting the Crunch and Flavor In

Studies show that green vegetables and salads correlate with better cognitive function in older people (Morris 2018). This may well be true for younger people as well.

What we think of as "salad" is just a mix of different ingredients, usually served cold. They often involve green leafy vegetables, especially different kinds of lettuce, spinach, or kale. These green leafy vegetables can serve as a bed for ingredients such as nuts, beans, baked tofu, meat, fish, or cheese. Eaten with a nice piece of whole grain bread, a salad can form the basis for a meal that can be quick, easy, and consistent with any of the diets associated with healthy aging.

Salads need not rely on leafy greens, however. Whole grains such as bulgur wheat, wild rice, and quinoa, also make delicious and nutritious salads. These grains can be mixed with herbs, dried fruits, nuts, chicken, mushrooms, and any many other ingredients. Salads can even be made mostly with beans, meat, or fish (e.g., tuna salad). Mashed garbanzo beans, chicken, salmon, and tuna can serve as the base of such salads, and can be served on lettuce to include greens. In this way, ingredients associated with Mediterranean diet can be combined together in way that reinforces appropriate serving sizes (4 ounces or less of meat).

Some examples of salads:

Default Mode Salad

This is the salad we make every day. When making this salad becomes habitual, it only takes about 10 minutes to put together.

    Mesclun or mixed greens mix

    1/3 bell pepper (red, yellow, or green), sliced and cut into bite-sized pieces

    6-8 cherry tomatoes, halved

    6 small fresh mozzarella balls (sliced in thirds), or 1/3 cup feta or goat cheese crumbles

    Pine nuts, or other nuts such as walnuts or almonds (one handful, optional)

    Olive oil

    Balsamic vinegar

Combine ingredients, and drizzle with olive oil and balsamic vinegar.

Basic Greek

This is an elaboration of the default mode salad that goes well for picnics or with Mediterranean main dishes.

    Mixed greens or "mesclun mix"

    Red or green onion

    Cherry or Roma tomatoes

    Cucumber (sliced or diced)

    Feta or goat cheese

    Kalamata (or other Mediterranean) olives

    Balsamic vinegar and olive oil, for dressing

Combine ingredients, and drizzle with olive oil and balsamic vinegar.

Baked Salmon or Seafood Salad

This is basically a default mode salad with salmon and lemony herbs. It can be made with other fish or shrimp and can serve as a main dish in warm weather.

> Sockeye salmon or other firm fish filets (e.g., tuna, mahi mahi), or shrimp (shelled and de-veined)
>
> Olive oil
>
> Garlic powder
>
> Balsamic vinegar
>
> Lemon juice
>
> Red or green onion (diced)
>
> Cherry tomatoes (sliced in half)
>
> Lemon thyme, lemon balm, or lemon verbena
>
> Basil leaves
>
> Mixed salad greens or "mesclun mix"

Rinse fish, pat dry, rub with olive oil and sprinkle with garlic powder and sea salt (optional). Roast at 350 F for about 20 minutes. Let cool, and then flake into a bowl while monitoring for remaining bones. Drizzle with about a tablespoon of balsamic vinegar and lemon juice. For shrimp, rinse and pat dry. Add them to a bowl with about a tablespoon of olive oil, 1 tsp garlic powder, 1 TBS oregano, and squirt of sriracha or other hot pepper sauce. Stir and marinade for 30 minutes, then sauté in a pan until the shrimp are pink and opaque.

Combine greens with the tomatoes, onions, and herbs. Top with roasted salmon and/or other fish and shrimp.

Amy's Curried Chicken Salad

Curry spices go perfectly with chicken. This salad is perfect for picnics, Parties, or potlucks.

For the dressing, mix together:

> Crème fraiche (1/4 cup) or mayonnaise (but not as tasty)
>
> Greek yogurt (plain unsweetened, 1/4 cup)
>
> Lemon juice (1 tsp)
>
> Honey (1/2 tsp)
>
> Curry powder (any kind/your favorite, 1 tsp, or to taste)
>
> Sumac (1/4 tsp or to taste, optional)
>
> Garlic (1 clove, minced)
>
> Black pepper (freshly ground, to taste)

For the salad, mix together:

Chicken (cooked, chopped into bite size pieces, 2.5 cups) and/or

shiitake mushrooms (roasted) or tofu

Green onions (sliced or minced, about 3 stalks) or red onion (1 small, diced)

Celery (two stalks chopped or sliced, optional)

Almonds (sliced, ½ cup)

Raisins (black or yellow, ½ cup)

Combine the ingredients and serve over a bed of leafy greens.

*Note: for extra deliciousness, if cooking the chicken, tofu, or mushrooms yourself, they can be marinated in olive oil and curry powder for ½ hour in refrigerator before cooking.

Chickpea Salad

This very flexible recipe provides a high-protein, plant-based, tuna salad-like option. It is great in sandwiches, paired with a green salad, as an appetizer served on endive leaves or crackers, or wrapped in cabbage or lettuce leaves.

1 can chickpeas, with the water (i.e., aquafaba), drained off.

Celery (~2 stalks, chopped)

Carrots (~1-2 carrots, chopped)

Dill pickle (~½ pickle, chopped)

Red onion (~1/8 cup, chopped)

~1-2 TBS vegan mayonnaise (optional, but it does taste nice)

~ 1 TBS German mustard

Lemon juice (~1 TBS)

Chopped garlic (~2 cloves)

Dill, parsley and/or other herbs

Salt and pepper

Smash the chickpeas with the back of a fork or a potato masher until they are flaky in texture, like canned tuna. Stir in chopped vegetables and dressing ingredients until everything is combined evenly. Adjust quantities to taste.

Other vegetables can be added or substituted per your taste and preferences. Other suggestions include bell peppers, green onions, cucumber, cherry tomatoes, capers, or finely chopped kale (pre-massage the kale lightly with olive oil and salt for 30 seconds to avoid bitterness).

You can also change the flavor profile by changing up the spices in the dressing and/or your choices of chopped vegetables. For example, you could substitute cumin, coriander, turmeric, and paprika for the dill for more Middle Eastern flavors.

Caprese Salad

These serving suggestions include two ways to make this salad: traditional and multivariate.

Traditional Caprese Salad (4 servings)

> Fresh mozzarella balls, 2 large (approximately 3 inches diameter)
>
> Heirloom ripe tomatoes, medium size
>
> Fresh basil leaves
>
> Extra virgin olive oil
>
> Balsamic vinegar
>
> Freshly ground black pepper

Cut the mozzarella balls and tomatoes into 1/3 inch slices (approximately). Trim stems from fresh basil leaves. Place the mozzarella slices on a serving plate or individual dishes. Layer tomato slices followed by basil leaves onto the cheese, and drizzle with olive oil and balsamic vinegar. Grind fresh black pepper on each, according to taste.

Multivariate Caprese Salad

> Fresh mozzarella balls, large or small
>
> Cherry, grape, Roma, or heirloom tomatoes
>
> Fresh basil leaves
>
> Fresh oregano leaves (optional)
>
> Mesclun mix, Romaine, or favorite green leafy vegetables
>
> Extra virgin olive oil
>
> Balsamic vinegar
>
> Freshly ground pepper

Cut the mozzarella and tomatoes into bite size pieces, Cherry tomatoes can be halved. Tear basil and oregano, if used, into large bite-sized pieces.

Cover the bottom of a side salad bowl with greens. Layer the cheese, tomatoes, and herbs over the greens and drizzle with olive oil and balsamic vinegar. Grind some fresh black pepper over the salad.

Whole Grain Salad

Whole/intact grains are surprisingly filling, and they go well with just about any seasoning style (Mediterranean, South or East Asian, South American, etc.). This recipe is more Mediterranean, and I like it best with bulgur or wild rice.

Quinoa, bulgur, barley, wild rice or black rice, or other intact grain

Cooked chicken, beef, salmon, tofu and/or roasted mushrooms

Bell peppers (fresh or roasted)

Fresh greens, such as arugula, spinach, parsley, or dandelion

Basil, oregano, lemon thyme, lemon verbena, rosemary, or other favorite herbs

Kalamata or other olives

Zucchini cubes, sautéed briefly in white wine and olive oil

Lemon juice, fresh 1 TBS

Marinated artichokes, chopped into bite-sized pieces

Feta or goat cheese, crumbled

Garlic, fresh minced, or powdered

Cook the grains (usually 1 cup grain to 2 cups water or broth) in a medium saucepan. Remove from heat and let sit for 10 minutes with the lid off the pan.

Toss in all the other ingredients. Serve in a bowl, or over a bed of greens.

Roasted Mushroom Salad

This is an elegant salad that is both easy and suitable for entertaining.

Mushrooms (shiitake, oyster, or hen of the woods)

Olive oil (for roasting)

Poultry seasoning

Garlic powder

Nutmeg

Cayenne pepper

Mixed greens or "mesclun mix"

Pine nuts

Hard cheese (parmesan, Romano, Spanish), very thinly sliced

Red or other bell pepper (fresh, sliced into bite-size pieces)

Extra virgin olive oil (for dressing)

Balsamic vinegar

Fresh black peppercorns

Slice or tear mushrooms into bite-sized pieces and toss them in olive oil, herbs, and spices. Roast at 325-350 F until the released liquid is nearly gone and parts of the mushrooms are getting crispy (about 30 minutes).

In a wide salad bowl, spread greens evenly across the bottom and layer with red pepper, pine nuts, cheese, and mushrooms. Drizzle with olive oil and balsamic vinegar and grind black pepper over it (if desired).

Ani and Steve's "Mezeh Bowls"

"Our friend Corey who has a TERRIBLE diet and is in no way vegetarian came over, not really interested in the food because it 'probably wouldn't fill him up.'. After a few drinks he was hungry so he put together one of our "rabbit food" mezeh bowls and was absolutely shocked at how good it was, surprised that it didn't even need meat to satisfy his hunger."

1 cup quinoa (rinsed and cooled, with drizzled with lemon, seasoned to add taste)

Mesclun mix

Fresh spinach

Walnuts, chopped

Garlic minced, sliced, or roasted!

1 red pepper

1 cucumber

½ bunch green onions chopped

1 pack roasted mushrooms or 1 whole roasted eggplant, or both!

½ cup artichoke hearts

½ cup Kalamata olives

Tzatziki or hummus as "dressing"

Feta cheese sprinkled on top

Tzatziki

Greek yogurt

Cucumber (about a 2-inch chunk)

Garlic (1 clove, peeled)

Grate cucumber into a medium-sized bowl. It will be juicy! Then grate in the garlic clove. Stir in the yogurt and taste. Add more cucumber and garlic if desired.

Make a base of lettuce, add quinoa, add veggies plus pickled stuff, sprinkle walnuts and cheese on top. Add globs of hummus or tzatziki to mix in as you eat. Great as a bowl or wrapped in a flatbread such as pita or naan.

2. Soups and Stews: A Chance to be Creative

Soups and stews are especially well-suited for the multivariate approach because you can throw everything you need for a healthy nutritious meal into one pot: grains, greens, a protein, colorful vegetables, and herbs and spices. They generate fewer dishes to wash and provide more than one meal. Importantly, soups and stews provide opportunities to be creative and combine seasonal or culturally meaningful ingredients.

Mom's Minestrone

This is our family's traditional vegetable soup.

> V-8 juice
>
> Broth, chicken or vegetable (2 cups)
>
> 3 cans of beans (dark kidney, light kidney, cannelloni), drained
>
> 1 large can diced tomatoes
>
> 1 medium carrot, or so (diced)
>
> 1 package frozen spinach (thawed), or equivalent in fresh spinach, collards, or other greens
>
> Napa or other cabbage
>
> 1 medium white or yellow onion, chopped
>
> Other vegetables, such as mushrooms, that you have lying around and need to use
>
> 2 TBS oregano
>
> 2 TBS garlic powder
>
> 1 TBS marjoram
>
> ¼ tsp cayenne
>
> 1 TBS anise seeds
>
> One cup hearty dry red wine (optional)
>
> 1 cup dried pasta, such as seashells
>
> Fresh parsley, chopped (optional)
>
> Italian cheese (Parmesan or Romano), grated

In a large pot, combine all the ingredients except the pasta, and bring to a boil. Then reduce heat to low. Shortly before planning to serve, cook the pasta as directed on its package, and drain. To serve, put one large spoonful of cooked pasta into a large bowl and ladle soup over it. Garnish with fresh parsley and Parmesan or Romano cheese.

<h1 style="text-align:center">Pam's Black Bean Chili</h1>

This is a thick and spicy chili, made with anthocyanin-rich black beans.

> Olive oil
>
> 1 cup finely chopped onion
>
> 1 clove or more garlic, minced
>
> 1/2 cup finely chopped carrot
>
> I large finely chopped red bell pepper

Sauté 5 minutes.

Add the following:

> 1 TBS chili powder
>
> 1 tsp cumin
>
> 1 14.5- oz can diced tomatoes
>
> 2 15-oz cans black beans (Pam purées half of the beans to make chili thicker)
>
> 1/4 cup canned chopped green chiles
>
> 3/4 cup water
>
> 3/4 cup orange juice
>
> 1/4 tsp salt

Simmer 20 minutes.

Before serving, stir in 2 TBS chopped cilantro.

Garnish with cheddar cheese, sour cream, or Greek yogurt.

Add some La Torre brand chipotle peppers to taste. These are hot and flavorful.

If doubling for a crowd, don't double chili powder.

<h2 style="text-align:center">Mushroom Chowder</h2>

This is a hearty, mushroom-y soup that goes well with some fresh garlic bread and Default Mode Salad.

> Lots of mushrooms! Portobella, shiitake, oyster, sliced into large pieces
>
> 4 small/medium golden (or other colorful) potatoes
>
> 16 oz white wine
>
> ½ to 1 cup water
>
> ¼ cup olive oil

1 pint half-and-half (or if vegan, puree ½ cup cashews, ideally after pre-soaking the nuts in water. Blend the pureed nuts with ¾ cup unsweetened plant milk, and use as cream)

3 green onions, sliced

½ head of garlic, minced

Garlic powder, cayenne, poultry seasoning, and marjoram, to taste

Wash and cut potatoes into ~half-inch cubes.

Place the potatoes in a medium size pot, and cover with the wine, and water. Bring to a boil and then let simmer until the potatoes become tender (~45-60 minutes)

When the potatoes begin to soften, add the mushrooms and oil, and half the minced garlic, along with spices. Stir so that the mushrooms become moistened.

When the mushrooms have shrunk down, released their liquid, and become soft, add the half-and-half. Stir, taste, and add more spices if desired.

Add sliced green onions, and let the chowder warm up, but not to a boil.

Serve and enjoy!

Hearty Cupboard Mushroom Chili

This chili goes together quickly and is nice for chilly weather. It is also perfect for using up "dibby dabs" of vegetables (such as eggplant or squash), meat, or sauces. Just throw them in!

Black, pinto, kidney, or other beans (3 15-oz cans)

1 jar green salsa (such as Hatch Valley®) (12-16 oz)

1 jar red salsa (12-16) oz

I can diced tomatoes (15 oz)

Corn kernels, fresh, frozen, or canned (about 15 oz)

Mushrooms (2-4 portabello caps or similar amount of shiitake) and/or cooked chicken, beef, turkey, tofu, or other available protein

Garlic powder (1 TBS)

Oregano (1 TBS)

Chile powder (ancho, chipotle, or "chili powder") to taste.

Green or red onions (sliced) to garnish

Cheese (extra-sharp cheddar or pepper Jack, grated) to garnish

Avocado (fresh, sliced into chunks) to garnish

Greek yogurt, to garnish

Slice mushrooms into large bite-sized pieces (remembering that they shrink). In a large pot combine contents of cans and jars and bring to a boil. Add mushrooms and seasonings and simmer until mushrooms are tender. This takes longer for portobello (15-30 minutes) than shiitake (5 minutes). Other ingredients (cooked vegetables and meat) can be added now if desired, to heat. Serve in large bowls, sprinkle green onion, grated cheese, and avocado over the chili and a dollop (spoonful) of yogurt. It's ready to eat!

Multivariate Fish Soup

This soup is based on a theme similar to the classic Italian (cioppino) and French (bouillabaisse) versions of fish soup. Fish and shellfish are combined in a tomato and broth base with tomatoes and onions and other vegetables. It is designed to work with whatever the daily catch is, so it is naturally multivariate. This version uses V-8 juice as part of the soup base, making it just a little heartier in texture than the traditional version, but more nutrient-dense.

V-8 juice (46 oz bottle)

Fish stock or clam juice, or vegetable broth (8 oz)

White wine, 2 cups

Tomatoes, 1 28-oz can

Onion

Fennel bulb, sliced into pieces

Garlic (about 4 cloves, minced)

Garlic powder (1 TBS)

Oregano (1 TBS)

Basil (1 TBS)

Marjoram (1 TBS)

Coriander (1 tsp at least)

Cayenne (1/4 tsp)

Smoked paprika (1 tsp)

Turmeric (1 tsp at least)

Fish filets (1 ½ lbs) such as cod, mahi mahi, grouper

Shrimp (1 lb) raw, shelled and deveined

Shellfish such as mussels and clams (smaller ones are more tender/not tough; about 20 each)

Fresh parsley, chopped for garnish if desired.

Lemon wedges for squeezing

In a large pot, combine the V-8, clam juice, wine, tomatoes, onion, fennel, and fresh garlic with the dried spices and bring to a boil. Turn off heat and let broth rest.

Prepare fish filets by removing any remaining bones, tough connective tissue, or bloody parts. Cut into one-inch pieces. Reheat the broth and add fish. Turn off heat when the fish pieces look cooked.

Twenty to thirty minutes before desired serving time, bring broth to a boil, and add the shrimp and shellfish. The shellfish are done when their shells open. The shrimp will be cooked by then. Discard any unopened shells. Serve in large bowls, garnished with parsley, a generous squeeze of fresh lemon, and some fresh crusty bread.

3: Flatbreads

Flatbreads may be the most ancient of cooked foods (Wikipedia 2022). Charred crumbs of multigrain flatbread have been found in the Eastern Mediterranean area, dating back 14,000 years. This is around 4,000 years before there is evidence of agriculture in the region! The most basic flatbreads are breads made of grain or bean flour mixed with water and cooked in ovens, grilled over fires, or pan-fried. Most flatbreads also contain oils, or dairy, eggs, vegetables, or spices. Flatbread varieties are extremely diverse and are found in most if not all cultures, on all inhabited continents. They include pizza, tortilla, pita, naan, scallion pancakes (cong you bing), bannock, blini, and so many more.

Flatbreads are fantastic because there is so much you can do with them. They can be eaten flat with toppings, such as pizza, or rolled up and filled with vegetables, meats, or cheese, such as burritos. They can be served with, or part of, main dishes such as curries. Here are some examples of things you can do with flatbreads:

Sally's Whole Wheat Pizza Dough

We make pizza with our 30-year-old sourdough starter. This regular yeast recipe is based on the fantastic food blog Sally's Baking Addiction (#sallysbakingaddiction, https://sallysbakingaddiction.com/homemade-whole-wheat-pizza-crust-recipe/) that uses yeast. It makes two 12-inch pizzas.

> Yeast (1 TBS), Sally recommends instant yeast such as Red Star® Platinum, but active dry yeast works too, although rise time is longer)
>
> 1 and ½ cups warm water (105-115 degrees F)
>
> 1 TBS olive oil
>
> 1 TBS honey
>
> 1 teaspoon salt
>
> 1 ¼ cups whole wheat flour (real whole wheat flour, not "white" whole wheat flour)
>
> Olive oil for brushing crust

Mix the yeast and warm water and let it sit for 5 minutes or until it becomes dissolved and foamy. This is called "proofing" the yeast, and if it does not dissolve and get foamy it is dead and you need to start again with new yeast. In a large bowl, mix the successfully proofed yeast with the olive oil, honey, and salt. Add the 3 cups of flour, ½ cup (or so) at time. Towards the end you may need to use your hands to mix it.

Knead dough for 5 minutes or so. If it is too sticky you can add up to 1/3 cup more whole wheat flour. It should be smooth and elastic. Sally recommends poking the dough with a finger to tell when it is ready to rise. If it slowly bounces back, it is ready. Shape the dough into a ball and place it in a large bowl that has been coated lightly with olive oil. Roll the dough ball around until it is coated all over. Cover with plastic wrap or a tea towel and let it rise in a warm place. I use an oven preheated to 110 degrees and then turned off. I put the dough in the oven and sign on the outside: DOUGH INSIDE. This helps prevent mishaps.

When the dough has doubled in size (1-2 hours), punch it down to deflate the air and knead it briefly (you may need a little flour on your hands). Divide the dough into two equal balls and put them into separate oiled bowls. Let them "rest" covered with plastic wrap or tea towel for 20 minutes. Preheat the oven to 475 F.

Grease or spray two baking pans with non-stick spray or olive oil. Sprinkle with cornmeal flour. Put each dough ball on a pan and flatten it out into a 12-inch round using your hands. Lift up or pinch the edges to create a lip around the outside of each pizza. Brush the top with olive oil (or pesto) to prevent the dough getting soggy. Top with favorite toppings and bake for 15 minutes or until crust is lightly browned. Slice the pizza and serve hot.

Our default mode pizza: After 20 years this is still our favorite pizza to make at home. I use sourdough starter instead of yeast, with mostly organic white flour and about ½ cup Bakers Bran with olive oil. No salt or honey in the dough, but we do add garlic powder and dried oregano. When spread out in rounds on pizza pans, the pizzas are topped with pesto sauce, minced fresh garlic, mushrooms, Kalamata olives, feta cheese (crumbles or ½ inch cubes) chopped red pepper, sliced green onions, and "pizza cheese" (a mix of mozzarella and other Italian cheeses). We bake it at 350 F for about 25 minutes. This yields a crust that is more like bread than typical pizza dough, which is cooked at higher temperatures for shorter times, as described above. I keep meaning to try baking the pizza the hot and quick way, but we keep still liking it the slower way.

"Homemade Flatbread" (adapted from Sunset Magazine)

I make these with about a cup of sourdough starter instead of yeast. You can top them with anything. They are good for picnics or potlucks. Bring along hummus or tzatziki or any favorite dip and these flatbreads are great. They are also perfect to serve with Middle Eastern or South and Central Asian stews.

> 2 teaspoons yeast
>
> ¾ cup warm water
>
> ¼ cup whole wheat flour
>
> 2 ¼ cups all-purpose (white) flour
>
> ½ cup full-fat plain, unsweetened yogurt
>
> 2 TBS olive oil

For finishing: olive oil; flaky salt, sesame, poppy or other favorite seeds, ground nuts such as pistachios or almonds, etc.

In a large bowl, mix water and yeast (to proof it, see above), or use a cup of sourdough starter if you have some. Add the whole wheat flour and ¼ cup of the all-purpose flour and let rest for 15 minutes. It should start bubbling. Add yogurt and stir. Add in remaining 2 cups of flour, then knead the dough for 2 minutes or so. Let it rest for 10 minutes, then knead it again and put it in an oiled bowl, covered with a tea towel, and let rise on the counter for 2 hours.

After two hours, punch down the dough and divide it into 4-6 balls. Dust them with flour and let them rise again for about an hour. Then, using either your hands or a rolling pin, stretch or roll the dough until it is about 1/4 inch thick.

For pan or griddle cooking: heat pan or griddle to medium-high, add a "nub" of butter and cook flatbreads on both sides until golden brown.

To grill: place the flatbreads directly onto an oiled grill (or even on the floor of a pizza oven). Flip the flatbreads halfway through cooking.

Brush the flatbreads with olive oil while they are still warm and top with salt, seeds, or nuts.

Ani and Steve's Breakfast Burritos

Brown rice spiced with garlic and Mexican seasonings

Chipotle-spiced mushrooms or eggplant, OR BOTH

Spinach or kale

Fajita veggies (sautéed onion, pepper)

Salsa

A can of chopped green chiles

1 pack of tofu, or chicken, cut into small squares, marinated in extra virgin olive oil, garlic, Mexican spices

Optional: Add scrambled eggs for breakfast style

Combine ingredients and use as taco or burrito fillings, or wrap filling a flat bread.

Seafood Tacos

Sockeye salmon filets (grilled or roasted), or other fish or shrimp

Greens or cabbage (sliced or grated)

Greek yogurt with sriracha sauce (to taste)

Avocado, chopped and tossed in 1-2 TBS lime juice

Pico de gallo:

¼ cup diced red onion

½ cup diced tomato,

¼ cup chopped cilantro

Above ingredients tossed with about 2 TBS lime juice

Whole wheat tortillas

Grill or roast fish filets and flake into large pieces while checking for bones. For shrimp, shell them, then boil, or grill. They are easier to eat in a taco if cut into thirds.

Prepare the greens. Prepare a small bowl cup of Greek yogurt mixed with 3-4 drops of siracha sauce, or more if you like it really spicy, and set out small bowls of pico de gallo, and avocado. Heat a grill to medium, and grill tortillas until lightly browned (5-10 minutes).

Layer yogurt, greens, pico de gallo, salmon, and avocado onto a tortilla, fold it up, and enjoy!

Will's Multivariate Burritos

This recipe uses a basic burrito (rolled-up flatbread) base but combines Mexican and South Asian ingredients and spices.

Onions

Tomatoes

Bell peppers

Beans (unsalted), such as pinto beans or black beans

Garlic powder or garlic

Spinach leaves

Matcha powder

Red chili powder

Turmeric

Yellow curry, and/or combinations with various Indian-blend spices, e.g., tandoori spices

Avocado

Greek yogurt

Whole wheat tortillas

Sauté the onion, garlic, and pepper until they start to soften. Add in the matcha powder, chili powder, turmeric, and yellow curry and sauté for 30 seconds. Add the tomatoes and spinach, stirring until the spinach wilts. Add beans and stir together until the mixture is warm.

Warm a tortilla. Spread the tortilla with mashed avocado and Greek yogurt. Place a scoop of the bean mixture in the center. Fold in the ends of the tortilla and roll into a burrito.

Multivariate Santa Fe-Style Enchiladas

Santa Fe-style enchiladas are not rolled up, but instead are layered. This recipe layers the tortillas in a casserole dish, which allows for more ingredients between the layers. It is baked, reducing the amount of fat that would be used if they were fried, as is traditional.

Tortillas (whole wheat or corn, about 12 medium-sized)

Shredded chicken or beef, and/or mushrooms, shrimp or tofu, seitan, lentils, or whole beans

One can vegetarian refried beans (15 oz)

One cup sliced green onions

1 can (4 oz) sliced black olives

12 oz of Pepper Jack cheese, grated (or cheddar or regular Jack cheese, if preferred. For a vegan option, see * below)

Hatch Valley green salsa (12 oz jar)

Red enchilada sauce

6 oz extra-sharp cheddar cheese (or you can use more Pepper Jack or plant-based nacho sauce if preferred)

Greek yogurt (or plain, unsweetened plant-based yogurt)

1 avocado, sliced (optional for garnishing)

Other ingredients as desired or available: chopped cilantro, chopped garlic, roasted eggplant, fresh tomatoes, bell peppers, corn, or zucchini

Layer tortillas along the bottom of a large casserole dish. For a square dish you can tear the tortillas in half to make them cover. Layer half the beans over them, and spoon half the green salsa (if making two layers; more than two can be pretty tall). Evenly sprinkle half the olives, green onions, protein (meat, mushrooms, shrimp, tofu, etc.), and Pepper Jack cheese over the layer. Add another layer of tortillas and then repeat with the rest of the ingredients. Layer more tortillas, and cover with red enchilada sauce and Cheddar or extra Pepper jJack cheese. Bake at 350 F for 30-40 minutes.

*To make a plant-based, nacho cheese-like sauce that can be substituted for the cheese above and/or used in casseroles or as a dip, blend the following together in blender or food processor. Note that this sauce is thick and starchy. Don't leave the blender running unattended or you may overheat it!

2 cups boiled peeled potatoes

1 cup boiled carrots

½ cup soaked and pureed cashews (optional)

1 cup unsweetened plant milk or alternatively, ½ cup water plus 1/3 cup olive oil

½ cup nutritional yeast

2 TBS lemon juice

Salt to taste (e.g., 1-2 tsp)

1 tsp chopped garlic

¼ cup chopped onion

Chili, black pepper, chicken-flavored seasoning, or other spices to taste

Bhindi Masala (Okra Curry) (2-4 servings) with Naan

This recipe was inspired by a dish served at The Spice Room in Sydney, Australia. Okra is nutritious and easy to grow, but many people dislike the "sliminess" inside. This curry eliminates the sliminess. It is delicious served with naan or over spiced whole grain rice.

1lb fresh okra

3 TBS extra virgin olive oil

1 large onion, diced (any variety will work)

1 tsp ginger powder or fresh grated ginger

Minced garlic to taste (1 clove to 1 head, depending on your preference)

1-2 large tomatoes diced (or 4 small tomatoes or 1 can diced tomatoes)

½ tsp turmeric

1 tsp ground coriander

~½ tsp red chili powder (to taste depending on spice preference)

Indian curry spice mix (make out of each individual spice or buy pre-made Indian masala spice mix: look for, cumin, fenugreek or kasoori methi, jeera)

½ cup Greek yogurt

1 tsp garam masala (or regular curry powder)

A few sprigs of cilantro leaves

Wash, dry, and cut okra to desired size (recommend ½ inch pieces). Fry in shallow oil, on medium to high heat for about 7 minutes, until the sliminess goes away, and the sides of the okra get lightly browned. Remove from pan and keep aside, leaving any leftover oil in pan.

To make masala sauce, sauté chopped onion and garlic in remaining oil, until just translucent. Add chopped tomatoes and continue to sauté until they are mushy and saucy. Add turmeric, chili powder, and some of your spice mix, sauté 1 minute. Add ½-1 cup of water, stirring in to loosen gravy. Add more spice mix to taste. Simmer 5-7 minutes. The gravy should get darker, thicker, and richer with flavor. Add cooked okra, lower heat, and lightly simmer until sauce is thickened and coating the okra. Remove from heat and add Greek yogurt, stirring in quickly to avoid curdling. Taste often, adding more spices to taste if needed, or more Greek yogurt if too spicy. Serve with naan or over rice.

4. Casseroles: An age-old way to combine many ingredients into an easy to prepare dish

The word "casserole" originates from the French word for a large baking dish, in which food is both cooked in and from which it is served. Casseroles traditionally contain grains or pasta, chopped vegetables, and often chopped meats, fish, cheese, or eggs. Examples include cassoulet, ragout, moussaka, lasagna, shepherd's pie, and good old American macaroni and cheese. They are attractive because they can include many good ingredients in one dish, making them convenient to prepare and serve. Seasoned with spices, they are delicious and satisfying to eat. The beauty is that you can make them with your favorite ingredients, and they can be adapted to what is on hand in the cupboard or garden.

Favorites include:

Mushroom, Spinach and Barley Casserole

This recipe is a riff on a recipe from *Sunset Magazine*. It can be made with other grains, such as bulgur or quinoa. It makes quite a lot.

> 1 1/2 lbs or more mixed mushrooms, sliced
>
> 1 cup red wine
>
> ½ cup or so olive oil
>
> Dried herbs, such as thyme, marjoram, cayenne
>
> ½ teaspoon ground nutmeg
>
> 1 head garlic, coarsely chopped, divided
>
> 1 cup barley
>
> 2 ½ cups mushroom broth
>
> 1 10-oz jar roasted red peppers
>
> 1 cup pine nuts
>
> 1 cup or so olive tapenade
>
> 1 10-oz package frozen spinach, thawed and drained
>
> 16 oz full fat ricotta cheese
>
> 8-12 oz shredded parmesan cheese (bag)
>
> Puff pastry to cover the top

Toss sliced mushrooms with the herbs and nutmeg, olive oil and red wine, and roast until most of the liquid released is gone.

Remove from oven, and stir in half of the chopped garlic, and the olive tapenade.

Cook barley in mushroom broth until the broth is absorbed and barley is tender. Add chopped roasted red peppers, pine nuts, and the rest of the garlic. Stir!

In a large casserole dish, layer the mushrooms evenly across the bottom.

Add half of the spinach, and sprinkle cheese over it.

Layer the barley/pepper mix on top.

Add the rest of the spinach.

Layer ricotta evenly, and sprinkle with the rest of the cheese.

Lay thawed puff pastry on top.

Bake at 350 F about 40 minutes. It is ready when the pastry puffs up and is a golden brown,

Plant-based notes: While there are good commercial plant-based ricotta and Parmesan cheeses on the market, they can be expensive and, in some cases, include a lot of processed ingredients. You can make quick homemade vegan substitutes for the cheeses:

For plant-based ricotta, mash together the following:

1 package extra-firm tofu

1 tsp chopped garlic

2 TBS nutritional yeast

1-2 TBS lemon juice

1-2 TBS tahini (optional)

1-2 TBS miso (optional)

Olive oil to taste (optional)

2 TBS finely diced shallots or onion (optional)

Dash of nutmeg

Salt and black pepper to taste

Oregano, basil and/or parsley

The optional ingredients provide depth of flavor and can be used or not as available and to taste preference.

For plant-based Parmesan, pulse the following in a food processor until it is the consistency of grated Parmesan cheese:

½ cup Brazil nuts (preferred), cashews, pine nuts, or other nuts. Sunflower or hemp seeds can also work!

¼ cup nutritional yeast

Diced garlic and salt to taste

Refrigerator Lasagna (also known as "Farmer's Market Lasagna")

This is a favorite multivariate dish for times when you have perishable ingredients, or "dibby dabs" of ingredients that need to be used. These are suggested ingredients, but the key features are the no-boil lasagna noodles and a sauce. The noodles cook in the sauce.

> No-boil lasagna noodles
>
> Good quality pasta sauce (24-oz jar)
>
> Portobello mushroom caps (3 or so)
>
> Eggplant
>
> Zucchini
>
> Kalamata olives
>
> Feta or ricotta cheese
>
> Mozzarella or "pizza cheese" mix (8 oz)

Any other ingredients, such as red onion, artichokes, squash, red bell peppers, etc.

If using mushrooms or eggplant, it is best to roast them briefly first. Otherwise, the lasagna starts out too tall for the casserole dish. Cut the vegetables into bite-sized chunks and toss with olive oil and garlic powder, and chunks of garlic cloves, if desired. Roast at 325 or 350 F for 15 minutes or so, until the mushrooms shrink.

In a casserole dish, layer ¼ of the pasta sauce into the bottom and cover with a single layer of uncooked lasagna noodles. Layer another ¼ of the pasta sauce and ½ each of the other ingredients, except the pizza cheese (use only ¼). Layer more lasagna noodles on top, repeat the layering (including pasta sauce), using the rest of the ingredients (except for pasta sauce and pizza cheese). Cover with another layer of lasagna noodles, the rest of the pasta sauce, and cheese. You can also accent this top layer with slices of fresh mozzarella and dollops of pesto sauce. Bake uncovered at 350 F for 30-40 minutes. When done, the lasagna should be bubbling and the cheese on the top will be melted and getting brown.

To make a tasty plant-based version without using commercial shredded vegan cheese, I recommend substituting homemade plant-based alfredo sauce for the cheese layer. You can make a quick plant-based alfredo sauce by blending 1 box of silken tofu with olive oil, lemon juice, chopped garlic, salt, nutmeg, and black pepper to taste. It provides a high-protein sauce that pairs well with most vegetables, tomato sauces and/or pesto sauces in both lasagna as well as with other pastas and casseroles.

Multivariate Mac & Cheese

This "gourmet-style" mac & cheese has been a favorite dish in our family since our daughters were little. It goes together quickly and provides highly desired leftovers. The base dish involves pasta, cheese, and canned mushroom soup instead of a roux or other white sauce. Canned soup as a base is convenient, and this dish goes together in 30 minutes. Canned mushroom soup also has fewer calories than the butter-based white sauces typically used in "gourmet" style mac & cheese. Any kind of pasta can be used, but we prefer bowties/farfalle with cheddar cheese, and whole wheat or tricolor rotini with the Italian cheese mix.

Two cups grated cheddar, or "Italian blend" cheese, including mozzarella

12 oz dried pasta (whole wheat or tricolor if available)

2 cans cream of mushroom soup (10 oz each)

Dried herbs: oregano, garlic, marjoram, cayenne (or other favorite herbs, 1 tsp-1 TBS, except for cayenne)

Dijon-style mustard (1-2 TBS)

Onions (we like green, but red, yellow, or white work)

Mushrooms (shiitake are delicious but others work; roasted portobellos are best)

Sliced olives (Kalamatas work well with Italian cheese, and black olives work well with cheddar)

Capers (pickled, about ¼ to ½ cup)

Marinated artichokes (1 ½ cups chopped)

Boil water for pasta. Meanwhile prepare onions and mushrooms, and grate cheese (if necessary). Cook pasta according to directions, drain, and return to pot. Add the mushroom soup, recommended water if the soup is condensed, and herbs. Stir well and add the rest of the ingredients. It is easiest to add the cheese last. Spray a baking dish (e.g., casserole dish) with cooking spray and pour the mac & cheese into it. Sprinkle with more cheese (if desired) and bake at 325-350 F for 30 minutes or so.

Chiles Rellenos Casserole

Chiles rellenos is a traditional Mexican dish in which large mild chiles, such as poblano, are stuffed with cheese, dipped in egg, and deep-fried. To avoid the frying, I have developed this recipe to approximate my favorite version, from La Estrellita restaurant in Seattle. It is one of our family favorites now. La Estrellita served it in individual baking dishes, with two stuffed chiles smothered in sauce and topped with a crispy egg and cheese mix. I make my version with all of the chiles together in a rectangular casserole dish to make it easier to do for a family.

Whole poblano chiles (fresh or canned, seeded) 10-12 (enough to fill the dish)

Salsa (red or green, good quality, 16 oz)

Green onions (about 1 cup sliced)

Black olives (sliced, 4 oz)

Cheddar cheese (grated)

Pepper Jack or Jack cheese (cut into sticks or pieces that fit inside the chiles)

Chili powder (I prefer ancho, but others work well too)

Eggs (6-8, separated)

Flour (about a quarter of a cup)

Spray a rectangular casserole dish with cooking spray and arrange chiles evenly along the bottom. Remove any seeds or stem remnants, and stuff the insides of the peppers with Jack cheese. Cover with salsa, olives, and green onions. Separate the eggs such that the whites end up in a medium to large bowl. The yolks can be dropped into a small bowl. Stir the yolks to blend them. Add chile powder to the whites and beat them with a hand or table mixer until stiff. Sift in the flour gradually during this process. When the eggs whites are stiff, fold in the blended yolks and one third of the cheddar cheese. Spoon the mixture over the stuffed chiles gently, and sprinkle with the rest of the cheddar cheese. Bake uncovered in a pre-heated 350 F oven. The egg mixture will poof up like a soufflé, so be sure there are no oven racks above. When the egg has poofed up and is moderately browned, it is done (usually 30-45 minutes).

Paella

Paella is a naturally multivariate, rice-based dish originally from Valencia, Spain. It is the inspiration for other rice-based casseroles or one-pot dishes such as jambalaya, arroz con pollo, and even the "Spanish rice" my mother used to make. It gets its name from the wide shallow pan, or paella, in which it is traditionally cooked. Regional variety is based on what kind of ingredients are available, so some are entirely meat-based, others are fish and seafood-based, and still others are plant-based. There are many, many recipes for paella. Because I am allergic to red meat, I prefer to make seafood or mushroom paella. The base for this dish is short-grain rice (such as arborio), a protein (fish, meat, seafood, snails, tofu, or mushrooms), saffron, and garlic. Other ingredients often used are tomatoes, onions, beans, and fresh peas.

Rice (short-grained, such as arborio, 2 cups)

Broth (chicken or vegetable, 2-2 ½ cups)

White wine (1-1 ½ cups)

Fish (1/2 lb, cut into 1-inch pieces)

Shrimp (1/2 lb, peeled and de-veined, but tails can be left on)

Shellfish (littleneck clams, small mussels, ½ lb)

Onion (1 white or yellow, chopped)

Garlic (3-6 cloves chopped)

Olives (e.g., Kalamata, sliced, 3/4 cup or so)

Tomatoes (fresh or canned, 14 oz, or 1 ½ cup)

Mushrooms (e.g., shiitake, trumpet, or oyster 6-8 oz, sliced)

Olive oil (about 3 TBS)

Saffron threads (1 "pinch")

Turmeric (1 tsp)

Marjoram (2 tsp)

In a large saucepan (or paella!), sauté onion and garlic briefly (~1 minute at medium-high heat). Add fish or protein and cook on all sides. Add broth and wine carefully. Bring to boil, then add rice and spices, being sure that the rice is evenly distributed in the pan. Add the shrimp and shellfish. Cook over medium-high heat. Don't stir the rice, but if things start to look dried out, add more broth or wine. If it starts to burn on the bottom, lower the heat. After about 10 minutes, add the tomatoes, olives, and mushrooms. The rice is done when it is tender and still moist. The shells of the shellfish should be open. If rice is stuck to the bottom of the pan, that is considered a sign of a true paella (according to Mark Bittman, https://markbittman.com).

Breakfast and Dessert: Switching Them Around

Because metabolic hormones, including insulin and cortisol, are higher in the morning after waking than they are at night, it is better to consume more calories earlier in the day. To stay healthy and feel well, it is better to eat breakfast than dessert. But many people don't eat breakfast, even though not eating breakfast is associated with elevated risks of diabetes and obesity. Why not?

Some people feel too busy in the morning to make breakfast. Others feel like it is too hard to get the usual breakfast foods (eggs, bacon, pancakes, etc.) down in the morning. These recipes can be made in advance and go down easily in the morning.

<h3 style="text-align:center">Fruit Crisp with Greek Yogurt</h3>

"Crisp" is usually considered to be an oat-based sweet dessert dish, but this version is really just granola and fruit with yogurt. It can be made in the evening. Because it is a casserole, it lasts for several days. This makes it convenient for busy mornings, and it can easily be taken to work in a container. It does not contain added sugar, beyond the honey in the granola. Instead, it relies on generous amounts of spices to bring out the flavor of the fruit.

> Granola (low sugar) purchased or from the recipe below
>
> Raisins (golden or black) or currants
>
> Nuts (coarsely chopped) if desired, especially if there aren't many in the commercial granola
>
> Seeds (especially flax seeds), if there aren't many in the commercial granola
>
> 4 TBS butter or coconut oil, melted
>
> Fresh fruit (apples, peaches, berries, or other favorite or seasonal fruit)
>
> Cinnamon, ginger, nutmeg, anise, clove, cardamom, Chinese 5 Spice powder, at least 1 tsp of each, but to taste (clove is stronger, generally less is needed)
>
> Greek yogurt

Mix the granola, raisins, nuts and seeds, and melted butter.

Chop the fruit into bit-size pieces and mix with the spices.

Butter or spray a casserole dish and fill with the fruit, spreading it evenly. Top with the granola mixture and bake for 20-30 minutes at 350 F.

Serve with a big dollop of Greek yogurt. Store covered in the refrigerator.

Mom's Tasty & Easy Granola

2 cups rolled oats

2 cups of mixed nuts and seeds (such as almonds, walnuts, sunflower seeds, flax seeds, pumpkin seeds)

1 cup or more dried fruit, such as currants, white raisins, or dried cranberries

3 big tablespoons of good honey

3 tablespoons coconut oil

½ teaspoon good quality vanilla extract

Star anise (ground), cinnamon, cardamom, ginger, and/or other spices; to taste. I use about a teaspoon of each, maybe slightly less of the star anise because it is strong.

Preheat oven to 300 F.

Put oats in a wide bowl and add spices. Stir the oats and spices together well.

Chop nuts coarsely to provide about 1 cup. Put in a 2-cup measuring cup. Add seeds to fill the measuring cup. Add contents to oats.

Add the dried fruit to the oats & nuts.

Add honey, coconut oil, and vanilla.

Mix with your clean hands. Be sure that if the coconut oil was solid when added to the mixture, it melts from the heat of your hands, and is thoroughly mixed in and not clumped.

Line a cookie sheet with parchment paper and spread the granola evenly along it.

Bake 15-20 minutes, until it is lightly toasted. Be VERY CAREFUL not to overcook it or it will taste like burnt popcorn.

Store in plastic containers up to 2 weeks or so.

(Adapted from a recipe by Elizabeth Rider)

Tiramisu with Fruit

This is an easy way to make a fairly authentic-tasting tiramisu, without having to mess with egg yolks and double boilers. Tiramisu is traditionally eaten in its originating country Italy as an afternoon "pick-me-up." We find that as breakfast it is a delicious and sustaining way to start the day. It also seems to make a splash when brought to school potlucks or dinner parties. The dish is usually made with "ladyfinger" cookies, but we find that vanilla wafers are not as sickly sweet, and they suck up more espresso without falling apart than ladyfingers. Any kind of fruit can be used, but we find more robust and less juicy fruit, such as blueberries or strawberries, are best if the tiramisu is not expected to be eaten in one day.

Heavy whipping cream (1 pint)

Mascarpone (Italian cream cheese; 16 oz, room temperature)

Greek yogurt (1 cup)

Vanilla extract, 2 TBS

Marsala (Italian sherry), 2 TBS

Espresso (4-6 oz)

Dark chocolate

Seasonal fruit (blueberries, strawberries, peaches etc.)

Vanilla wafers (good quality, 1 12-oz box)

Prepare ingredients:

Grate dark chocolate. For best results use a stand-up grater and cover counters. Dark chocolate seems to be charged and flies around after you grate it.

Wash and slice fruit (if necessary).

Make or acquire espresso.

Pour whipping cream into large bowl and add vanilla and marsala. Whip until it is thick with standing peaks. Fold in Greek yogurt and mascarpone.

Layer ingredients:

Soak vanilla wafers in espresso and line the bottom of a trifle bowl or deep casserole dish. To avoid sogginess, don't soak the wafers for the bottom layer completely. Spoon and spread 1/3 of the whipped cream mixture over the wafers, then layer ½ of the fruit. Cover the fruit with 1/3 of the grated dark chocolate. Make another layer of vanilla wafers, 1/3 cream mixture, rest of fruit, and 1/3 chocolate. For the final layer, layer espresso-soaked wafers and cover with the rest of the cream mixture, and cover with chocolate. Cover and refrigerate at least two hours before serving. Enjoy!

References

Chatterton ML, Mihalopoulos C, O'Neil A, Itsiopoulos C, Opie R, Castle D, Dash S, Brazionis L, Michael Berk M, Jacka F. Economic evaluation of a dietary intervention for adults with major depression (the"SMILES" trial). BMC Public Health, 18:599, 2018.

Chen Q, Goto K, Wolff C, Bianco-Simeral S, Gruneisen K, Gray K. Cooking up diversity. Impact of a multicomponent, multicultural, experiential intervention on food and cooking behaviors among elementary-school students from low-income ethnically diverse families. Appetite, 80:114-122, 2014.

DaCosta P, Moller P, Frost MB, Olsen A. Changing children's eating behaviour- A review of experimental research. Appetite, 113:327-357, 2017.

Dimitrovska M, Tomavska E, Bocevska M. Characterisation of Vranec, Cabernet Sauvignon and Merlot wines based on their chromatic and anthocyanin profiles. Journal of the Serbian Chemical Society, 78:1309-1322, 2013.

Dragan S, Serban M-C, Damian G, Buleu F, Valcovici M, Christodorescu R. Dietary patterns and interventions to alleviate chronic pain. Nutrients, 12:2510, 2020.

Farmer N, Cotter EW. Well-being and cooking behavior: using the positive emotion, engagement, relationships, meaning, and accomplishment (PERMA) model as a theoretical framework. Frontiers in Psychology, 12, article 560578, 2021.

Finley R. A guerilla gardener in South LA. TED Talk, www.ted.com/talks/ron_finley_a_guerrilla_gardener_in_south_central_la?language=en 2013.

Haldar S, Lim J, Chi AC, Ponnalagu S, Henry CJ. Effects of two doses of curry prepared with mixed spices on postprandial ghrelin and subjective appetite responses—a randomized controlled crossover trial. Foods, 7:47, 2018.

Jacka FN, O'Neil A, Itsiopoulos C, Opie R, Cotton S, Mohebbi M, et al. A randomised, controlled trial of dietary improvement for adults with major depression (the 'SMILES' trial). BMC Medicine, 15:181 2017.

Landrault N, Poucheret P, Gasc F, Cros G, Teissendre P-L. Antioxidant capacities and phenolics levels of French wines from different varieties and vintages. Journal of Agriculture and Food Chemistry, 49:3341-3348, 2001.

Lavelle F, McGowan L, Spence M, Caraher M, Raats MM, Hollywood L, McDowell D, McCloat A, Mooney E, Dean M. Barriers and facilitators to cooking from 'scratch' using basic or raw ingredients: A qualitative interview study. Appetite, 107:383-391, 2016.

Li l, Sun B. Grape and wine polymeric polyphenols: Their importance in enology. Critical Reviews in Food Science and Nutrition, 59:563-579, 2019.

Li Y, Lv M-R, Wei Y-J, Sun L, Zhang J-X, Zhang H-G, Li B. Dietary patterns and depression risk: A meta-analysis. Psychiatry Research, 253:373-382, 2017.

Kinnamon SC, Finger TE. A taste for ATP: neurotransmission in taste buds. Frontiers in Cellular Neuroscience, 7:264, 2013.

Moore K, Hughes CF, Ward M, Hoey L, McNulty H. Diet, nutrition, and the ageing brain: current evidence and new directions. Proceedings of the Nutrition Society, 77:152-163, 2018.

Morris MC. Nutrition and the risk of dementia: overview and methodological issues. Annals of the New York Academy of Sciences, 1367:31-37, 2016.

Morris, MC, Wang, Y, Barnes, LL, Bennet DA, Dawson-Hughs, B, Booth, SL. Nutrients and bioactives in green leafy vegetables and cognitive decline. Neurology, 90:e214-e222. 2018.

Mujcic R, Oswald AJ. Evolution of well-being and happiness after increases in consumption of fruit and vegetables. American Journal of Public Health, 106:1504-1510, 2016.

Myrtsi ED, Koulocheri SD, Iliopoulos V, Haroutounian SA. High-throughput quantification of 32 bioactive antioxidant phenolic compounds in grapes, wines and vinification byproducts by LC–MS/MS. Antioxidants, 10:1174, 2021.

Nagpal R, Neth BJ, Wang S, Craft S, Yadav H. Modified Mediterranean-ketogenic diet modulates gut microbiome and short-chain fatty acids in association with Alzheimer's disease markers in subjects with mild cognitive impairment. EBioMedicine., 47:529-542, 2019.

Pearson KE, Wadley VG, McClure LA, Shikany JM, Unverzagt FW, Judd SE. Dietary patterns are associated with cognitive function in the REasons for Geographic And Racial Differences in Stroke (REGARDS) cohort. Journal of Nutritional Science, 5:e38, 2016.

Peters JC, Marker R, Pan Z, Breen JA, Hill JO. The influence of adding spices to reduced sugar foods on overall liking. Journal of Food Science, 83:Nr 3, 2018.

Peters JC, Polsky S, Stark R, Pan Z, Hill JO. The influence of herbs and spices on overall liking of reduced fat food. Appetite, 79:183-188, 2014.

Rothwell JA, Perez-JimenezJ, Neveu V, Medina-Ramon A, M'Hiri N, Garcia Lobato P, Manach C, Knox K, Eisner R, Wishart D, Scalbert A. Phenol-Explorer 3.0: A major update of the Phenol-Explorer database to incorporate data on the effects of food processing on polyphenol content. Database, 10.1093/database/bat070, 2013.

Teicholz N. Diets are not one-size-fits-all. So why do we treat dietary guidelines that way? The Washington Post, May 2, 2019.

Virdis C, Sumby K, Bartowsky E, Jiranek V. Lactic acid bacteria in wine: technological advances and evaluation of their functional role. Frontiers in Microbiology, 11:612118, 2021.

Wastyk HC, Fragiadakis GK, Perelman D, Dahan D, Merrill BD, Yu FB, Topf M, Gonzalez CG, Van Treuren W, Han S, Robinson JL, Elias JE, Sonnenburg ED, Gardner CD, Sonnenburg JL. Gut-microbiota-targeted diets modulate human immune status. Cell, 184:4137–4153, 2021.

Wikipedia contributors, "Flatbread," *Wikipedia, The Free Encyclopedia,* https://en.wikipedia.org/w/index.php?title=Flatbread&oldid=1073772315 (accessed April 23, 2022).

Wolk A. Potential health hazards of eating red meat. Journal of Internal Medicine, 281:106-122, 2017.

Acetylcholine: A neurotransmitter used by the autonomic nervous system and in the brain. Acetylcholine has anti-inflammatory effects on immune cells such as macrophages, and this is likely a major way that mind-body modalities that activate the vagus nerve lower levels of inflammatory mediators in the body.

Adipokines: Hormone-like factors released from fat tissue that influence metabolism and inflammation. Some adipokines are also cytokines.

Advanced Glycation End-Products (AGEs): Proteins that have been changed structurally by the additions of sugars. AGEs can form in the blood during hyperglycemia or they can form in food during cooking. AGEs can induce inflammation and are linked to the complications of diabetes.

Advanced Lipid Oxidation End-Products (ALEs): These form after lipids are oxidized. Lipids may become oxidized in the blood or in tissues such as blood vessels or cell membranes. They serve as damage signals and induce inflammation.

Allodynia: When normally not-painful stimuli, such as food or light touch, feel painful.

Allostatic load: The "price the body pays" to meet challenges and maintain homeostasis. Higher loads are associated with more wear and tear on the body, and higher risk for disease.

Alpha-7 nicotinic cholinergic receptor: A receptor for acetylcholine found on pro-inflammatory immune cells. Release of acetylcholine from the vagus nerve acts on this receptor to inhibit activation of NFkB and reduce inflammation producing release of cytokines from these immune cells.

Antioxidant: A chemical that can prevent other chemicals from being damaged by oxidation. Antioxidants may be found in the body or in food.

Arousal Systems: Brain networks that activate and co-ordinate brain functions, such as motivation, mood, and cognition. Arousal systems use neurotransmitters such as serotonin, dopamine, histamine, and norepinephrine. Arousal systems are influenced by drugs including antidepressants and psychostimulants (e.g., amphetamine, cocaine).

Autonomic Nervous System: The part of the nervous system that is involved in coordinating physiological functions such as respiratory, cardiovascular, gastrointestinal, and immune systems.

Bacteroides: A type of gram-negative, anaerobic, rod-shaped bacteria that are commonly found in the human intestine. Bacteroides assists with breaking down food and producing needed nutrients and energy. If Bacteroides escape the gut they can cause infections and abscesses.

Bifidobacteria: A type of gram-positive anaerobic bacteria that live in the gastrointestinal tract of mammals. These are major components of the human gut microbiome and are often used as probiotics.

Bioavailability: The rate and quantity of substances absorbed into the body by the gut. If a substance has poor bioavailability, even eating large amounts of it may not provide benefits, because it does not get taken up into the circulation.

Biogenic amines: These are compounds made by life forms that contain one or more amine groups (i.e., NH_3, a nitrogen with three hydrogens attached). Examples of biogenic amines are serotonin, dopamine, histamine, melatonin, and putrescine.

Brain-Derived Neurotrophic Factor (BDNF): A molecule released in the nervous system in response to neural activity that triggers the establishment of new connections or synapses between neurons. BDNF is a key factor supporting *neuroplasticity*.

Brain Insulin Resistance: Brain insulin resistance occurs in the context of hyperglycemia and high levels of insulin (hyperinsulinemia). This causes fewer receptors for insulin to be made in the brain, reducing insulin's actions there.

Catastrophizing: An attitude or habit of approaching challenges by focusing on how difficult they are, rather than how to manage them.

Central Sensitization: Sometimes also called "wind-up," central sensitization involves changes in brain responses to pain that occur when pain persists, such that pain signals are more easily transmitted and are increased in magnitude.

Calcitonin gene-related peptide (CGRP): A peptide hormone involved in vasodilation and transmission of nociceptive, or pain-related signals. CGRP can suppress appetite and contributes to gastric acid secretion. CGRP can also inhibit inflammatory actions of immune cells.

Clostridia bacteria: A type of rod-shaped bacteria that are usually gram positive. They may live in soil, water, and the intestinal tract, but grow only in the absence of oxygen. Some clostridia bacteria can cause disease in humans, including Clostridium botulinum (cause of botulism), Clostridium tetani (cause of tetanus), C. perfringens (cause of food born illness from raw meat and gangrene). Other clostridia bacteria are beneficial, because they produce the short chain fatty acid butyrate. Butyrate serves as the main energy source for the gut cells that absorb nutrients. Butyrate can also reduce inflammation.

Commensal Microbes: Bacteria, viruses, and fungi that normally live in the gut. They do not cause disease, and many have beneficial actions, such as producing vitamins and fuel for gut cells.

Corticotropin-releasing hormone (also known as corticotrophin-releasing factor) (CRH or CRF): CRH or CRF is a peptide hormone involved in stress response. CRH stimulates release of adrenocorticotropin hormone (ACTH) in the pituitary. ACTH triggers release of cortisol.

Cortisol: A hormone produced by the adrenal gland that co-ordinates metabolism, the immune system, and the body's responses to challenges. When challenges are not met, cortisol and the systems it influences become dysregulated, leading to inflammation, metabolic diseases, and brain dysfunction.

Cytokines: Hormone-like chemicals produced by immune cells, as well as a few other cells. Cytokines regulate inflammation and other immune responses. Some cytokines signal the presence of inflammation to the brain.

Damage-Associated Molecular Patterns (DAMPs): These molecular signals are produced by cells when they are damaged by, for instance, injury or inflammation. DAMPs signal other cells to respond to the damage.

Default Mode Network: A constellation of brain regions mostly located along the midline of the brain that is most active when we are "being" rather than "doing." It helps construct our sense of our emotional and physical self and interacts with the Executive Control and Salience Networks to respond to challenges and regulate emotions. An important influence on this network is interoception.

Dendritic cells: These are cells of the immune system that process and present antigens to T cells of the immune system. Dendritic cells wait in tissues that are in contact with the external environment, such as skin, digestive tract, lungs, and nose. When activated they migrate to lymph nodes where they interact with T cells to initiate an immune response. Thus, dendritic cells serve as "sentinels" for the immune system.

Diabetes Distress: The negative emotional impact from worries and frustrations of managing diabetes.

Dorsal vagal complex: A collection of three brain nuclei in the caudal, dorsomedial medulla oblongata: the nucleus of the solitary tract, the area postrema, and the dorsal motor nucleus of the vagus. The dorsal vagal complex is the major integration center for the autonomic nervous system. It receives sensory information from the vagus nerve, including signals related to inflammation and gut hormones that influence food intake. The motor neurons in this complex regulate heart and gut function and help control inflammation.

Dysbiosis: This is an imbalance in microbes such that some species overgrow. It is associated with low microbial diversity, usually because of antibiotic use and/or a poor diet. Dysbiosis leads to increased inflammation and is commonly seen with a wide variety of chronic conditions, including metabolic syndrome and neurological disorders.

Endogenous Antioxidants: These are substances produced in the body that scavenge free-radicals and help prevent against oxidative stress. Examples are the glutathione and superoxide dismutase systems, uric acid, and melatonin.

Enteric glial cells: These are glial cells that are associated with the cell bodies and axons of enteric neurons, which are neurons that innervate the digestive tract. These cells support communication between neurons and can modulate gut-brain communication and inflammation.

Epigenetic Modifications: These are permanent or semi-permanent changes in the way that genes are expressed. They occur due to environmental influences, and thus are major mechanisms for "nurture" effects on "nature."

Epithelial cells: These are cells that form layers that line both the outer surface of the body and hollow organs and glands. They may be arranged in single or multiple layers depending on their location. Many produce mucus or other secretions and some may have cilia, which are tiny hairs. Some serve as the chemoreceptive "taste cells of the gut", which produce hormones that help regulate digestion and eating behavior.

Executive Control Network: A collection of brain regions, mostly in frontal and parietal lobes, that make decisions about behavior. For example, executive control networks help decide whether we should eat a specific food.

Firmicutes: A type of bacteria with a thick cell wall. Most bacteria in this phylum are gram-positive, and many produce endospores which can survive in extreme conditions.

Growth factors: Any of a variety of signaling molecules that can encourage cell proliferation, differentiation or maturation, development, or wound healing. Cytokines and hormones such as epidermal growth factor, insulin, and some interleukins and neurotropins, are examples of growth factors.

Helminths: These are worm-like parasites, including flukes, tapeworms, and roundworms.

Hyperalgesia: When normally painful stimuli, such as hot chili peppers or intestinal distension, feel even more painful.

Inflammation: The body's first line of defense against pathogens and first response to tissue injury. It involves the release of damaging chemicals from immune cells that can kill pathogens, but it must be tightly regulated to prevent damage to our own tissues.

Inflammaging: The development of chronic, low-grade inflammation that is associated with aging and is thought to contribute to aging-related diseases.

Insula: A cortical brain region that serves as a major neural center for processing interoceptive signals that may originate from the gut, heart, skin, and other peripheral systems. The insula is involved in signaling hunger, disgust, pain and other sensations.

Insulin: A hormone made by beta cells in the pancreas that triggers cells to take up glucose and amino acids from the blood. It has other actions that regulate metabolism, including fat storage and appetite.

Insulin Resistance: Insulin resistance occurs when cells lose sensitivity to insulin. This can result in glucose not being taken up into cells to use for their energy needs, leading to persistent high levels of glucose in the blood, a condition called hyperglycemia.

Interleukin-10 (IL-10): An anti-inflammatory cytokine that is released by immune cells while they are in the regulatory or anti-inflammatory state. One effect of IL-10 Is to prevent induction of pro-inflammatory responses that would otherwise be triggered by the presence of lipopolysaccharide and other bacterial products.

Interoception: The sense of the condition of our bodies. This sense includes pain, hunger, satiety, and inflammation.

Intuitive Eating: An approach to eating that rejects the idea of "diets" and instead relies on non-judgmental attention to signals from the body to help decide how much to eat.

Lipopolysaccharide: These are molecules that are made up of lipids and carbohydrates. Lipopolysaccharides are major components of the cell wall of gram-negative bacteria, and are used by immune cells as signals of the presence of potentially dangerous bacteria (i.e., as Pathogen-Associated Molecular Patterns (PAMPs). Lipopolysaccharide can "program" immune cells to be pro-inflammatory. It is sometimes called "endotoxin".

(Commensal) Microbe-associated molecular patterns (MAMPs): These are parts of microbes that immune cells can detect. MAMPs may influence immune cell function and inflammation.

M2 anti-inflammatory phenotype: Macrophages can change their state and predominant functions to take on different phenotypes. The M2 anti-inflammatory phenotype is a macrophage state where the macrophage encourages the resolution of inflammation (e.g., by releasing anti-inflammatory cytokines), and the clean-up and repair after inflammatory responses, for example cleaning up dead cells (i.e., phagocytosis of apoptotic cells) and repairing collagen.

Macrophages: A type of white blood cell that can engulf and kill microorganisms, remove dead cells, and stimulate and regulate response of other immune system cells. They can also produce growth factors that help keep other cells healthy.

Microbial Diversity: This describes how many different kinds of microbes are living in a tissue such as the gut. Generally, the more diverse the microbe population is, the healthier we are.

Mindful Eating: An approach to eating that involves paying close attention to the sensory characteristics of food and body signals, such as hunger and satiety, as well as to the emotions that occur around eating and food. Like intuitive eating, it emphasizes acceptance.

Negative Feedback: This is a key feature of regulatory systems. When a response is made to address a challenge, successful results of the response serve to turn it off. An example might be the response to hypoglycemia. When the liver detects low blood sugar, it releases glucose from its stores into the blood. When the levels of glucose go up, the liver detects this *negative feedback* signal and stops releasing glucose into the blood.

Neurogenic Inflammation: This is inflammation caused by pro-inflammatory mediators released by peripheral nerves. It can cause swelling, redness, and pain. It also contributes to migraine headache.

NFkB: NFkB is a genetic transcription factor that activates inflammation.

Neuroinflammation: Neuroinflammation is a term for when inflammation occurs within the brain, spinal cord, or peripheral nerve.

Non-alcoholic fatty liver (NAFL) is a general term for a number of liver conditions in which the main characteristic is excessive accumulation of fat in the liver in persons who drink little to no alcohol. This can cause liver inflammation and dysfunction.

Non-alcoholic hepatic steatosis (NASH) is an aggressive form of non-alcoholic fatty liver, where the liver is significantly inflamed. This may lead to progressive liver scarring, called cirrhosis, and can cause liver failure.

Nrf2: A genetic transcription factor that activates anti-inflammatory processes and the endogenous antioxidant response.

Old Friend Bacteria: They include *Bifidobacteria*, *Clostridium* clusters IV and XIVa, *Lactobacillus*, and others. Some produce butyrate and they play a pivotal function in gut barrier health. This is because butyrate serves as the principal source of energy of the gut epithelial cells. Some of them also produce the inhibitory neurotransmitter GABA, which can influence the neurons in the gut. GABA can also influence immune cells to reduce inflammation. They are called Old Friends because they are found in fermented foods and beverages that humans have consumed for thousands of years.

Opiate-Induced Hyperalgesia: The condition that develops when opiates are used long-term. Chronic suppression of pain transmission by opiates leads to compensatory amplification of pain transmission, leading to more pain.

Oxidative Stress: This is when there are too many reactive oxygen species for the antioxidants present to neutralize. This can happen due to inflammation or hypoglycemia. The result can be damage to cells, especially in the mitochondria. This leads to dysfunction and even death of the cells.

Pathobionts: Commensal microbes that are normally non-pathogenic but can cause or contribute to disease in some conditions, such as overgrowth.

Pattern Recognition Receptors: These are found on immune and other cells that detect molecular patterns that are associated with infection or tissue damage. Activation of these receptors triggers bodily responses, such as inflammation.

Pathogen-Associated Molecular Patterns (PAMPs): These are parts of microbes or other potential pathogens, such as cells walls or genetic material, that can't easily change or mutate. They serve as signals of potential danger and are detected by pattern recognition receptors.

Peroxynitrate: A reactive nitrogen species that is produced during metabolism and inflammation. It serves as a signaling messenger within the cell and regulates DNA repair and gene expression. But during oxidative stress, peroxynitrate contributes to insulin and glucocorticoid resistance.

Peyer's patches: Areas of lymphoid tissue in the small of the small intestine. These are involved in the development of immunity to antigens present in the gut.

Plasticity: The ability of the brain to change its functions, and even structure, to adapt to changes in the environment or other kinds of challenges. This is the basis of learning and cognitive and behavioral flexibility.

Pre-biotic: Dietary components or supplements that nourish specific microbes. Most food is pre-biotic in some way.

Probiotic: Live micro-organisms that confer beneficial effects to the host.

Prostaglandins: Lipid molecules derived from arachidonic acid that are used as signaling molecules to regulate a variety of physiological functions, such as clot formation, vasodilation, fever, uterus contraction, and gastric mucus secretion. Prostaglandins are one of the first signals generated after infection or damage to tissues. They are the target of the Non-Steroidal Anti-Inflammatory Drugs (NSAIDs) such aspirin or ibuprofen.

Proton Pump Inhibitors (PPIs): These are medications that reduce the amount of acid secreted in the stomach. PPIs are frequently prescribed for Gastroesophageal Reflux Disease (GERD) to reduce acid reflux.

Poly-unsaturated fatty acids (PUFAs): These are fatty acids that contain more than one carbon to carbon double bond. Omega-3 and Omega-6 fatty acids are commonly known examples of PUFAs.

Reactive Oxygen/Nitrogen Species (ROS/NOS): These are small molecules that can steal hydrogens or electrons. They can bind onto other molecules and thus damage them. In normal physiology, they are important because they can transfer energy. They are also key weapons for defense against pathogens.

Receptor for Advanced Glycation End Products (RAGE): A transmembrane receptor which was named for its ability to bind advanced glycation end products, which are proteins or lipids that have been modified through reaction with sugars. Activation of RAGE results in activation of pro-inflammatory genes. It is involved in the inflammatory pathophysiology of diabetes and Alzheimer's Disease.

Salience Network: A network of brain regions that work together to determine the importance of perceived situations or stimuli.

Sickness Syndrome: This is a constellation of symptoms that are induced by inflammation and are mediated by the brain. The symptoms include fatigue, low mood/depression, anhedonia, cognitive impairment, sleep dysfunction, and social isolation. These symptoms are most prominent during acute illness, but also occur with the stress of chronic illness. They can be ameliorated by anti-inflammatory interventions.

Social Self: One's perception of social esteem, status, and acceptance by others.

Substance P: This is a peptide used as a signaling molecule by sensory nerves and in brain circuits that are involved in interoception and emotion regulation. It is released from sensory nerves in response to extremely noxious stimuli that are likely to cause tissue damage, such as high heat and extreme pressure. Substance P can trigger inflammation and signal pain.

Superoxide dismutase (SOD): SOD is an enzyme that breaks down superoxide radicals, which are produced as a biproducts of metabolism and can cause cell damage if not regulated. SOD converts superoxide radicals into ordinary oxygen and hydrogen peroxide. SOD is a powerful endogenous anti-oxidant.

Sympathetic chain (sympathetic motor ganglia): This is a connected set of ganglia (clusters of neurons) that run beside the spinal column and coordinate physiological responses to challenges.

Sympathetic Nervous System: The branch of the autonomic nervous that coordinates responses to challenges and physiological perturbations. These responses include increasing blood pressure, heart rate, and blood sugar.

T cells: A type of white blood cells that circulate in peripheral tissues or the blood. They differentiate into helper, regulatory, cytotoxic or memory T cells. When activated, helper T cells secrete cytokines, regulatory T cells control immune reactions, and cytotoxic T cells kill infected or cancerous cells.

T-helper 17 (Th17) cells: These are white blood cells characterized by production of the cytokine interleukin-17, which strongly promotes inflammation.

Treg: A specialized type of white blood cells that acts to suppress the immune response. Tregs can inhibit T cell proliferation and cytokine production.

Trimethylamide-N-oxide (TMAO): TMAO is a microbial product derived from nutrients (e.g., carnitine, lysine, and choline) in red meat, eggs, fish, and dairy. TMAO can induce oxidative stress and impair neuroplasticity and may contribute to heart disease and neurodegeneration

Vagus Nerve: The principal nerve of the parasympathetic system. It innervates a wide variety of internal organs including the throat, gut, lungs, heart, liver, pancreas, some reproductive tissues, and parts of the outer ear. It is a key pathway for interoception.

Visceral Hypersensitivity: This is when pain-related sensory nerves that innervate the gut and other internal tissues become more sensitive and react to non-painful stimuli as if they are damaging. This can occur as a consequence of chronic inflammation, and it can persist even after the inflammation has healed.

Xenobiotics: Chemicals such as colorings, sweeteners, toxins, pesticides, pollution, and other things that would not normally be part of a diet and may contribute to inflammation.